BioMed Bots Assurance

This book presents a comprehensive analysis of the historical progression, present condition, and prospective trajectory of biomedical robotics through the lens of engineering. The analysis investigates the transformative impact on healthcare delivery, with a focus on precision, adaptability, and integration of artificial intelligence.

BioMed Bots Assurance: Securing Robotics, Healthcare, and IT Convergence commences by providing readers with an extensive exposition of the swiftly progressing field of biomedical robotics, thereby establishing a solid foundation for a meticulous scrutiny of its transformative capacity within contemporary healthcare. This book explores multiple challenges that happen during the integration of robotics into healthcare facilities, with extra focus on implementation protocols of robust IT security. It bestows in-depth knowledge of responsible and ethical use of biomedical robotics in health care through its care analyses on privacy concerns and ethics issues. The authors include several case studies that show the realization of successful biomedical robotic systems in real-world environments, address the regulatory landscape, and offer guidance on maintaining healthcare standards.

The book is crafted for a wide-ranging audience, including undergraduate and postgraduate students, professionals, researchers, and practitioners in the fields of biomedical engineering, robotics, healthcare technology, and information technology (IT) security. It serves as an extensive resource covering fundamental concepts, advanced research, and practical applications within the realm of biomedical robotics.

BioMed Bots Assurance

Securing Robotics, Healthcare, and IT Convergence

Edited by
Rajalakshmi Murugesan, Shanthi Jeyabal,
Bhisham Sharma, and Subrata Chowdhury

CRC Press
Taylor & Francis Group
Boca Raton London New York

CRC Press is an imprint of the
Taylor & Francis Group, an **informa** business

Designed cover image: Rajalakshmi Murugesan

First edition published 2026
by CRC Press
2385 NW Executive Center Drive, Suite 320, Boca Raton FL 33431

and by CRC Press
4 Park Square, Milton Park, Abingdon, Oxon, OX14 4RN

CRC Press is an imprint of Taylor & Francis Group, LLC

ISBN: 9781032910949 (hbk)
ISBN: 9781032910956 (pbk)
ISBN: 9781003561309 (ebk)

DOI: 10.1201/9781003561309

Typeset in Times
by Newgen Publishing UK

Contents

About the Editors

Rajalakshmi Murugesan is an accomplished academic and researcher with 12 years of experience in Control and Instrumentation Engineering. She is currently serving as an Assistant Professor in the Department of Mechatronics Engineering at Thiagarajar College of Engineering, Madurai, India. She holds a PhD from Anna University, Chennai and specializes in areas including mathematical modeling, artificial intelligence, machine learning, biomedical engineering, and unmanned aerial vehicles (UAVs). Dr. Murugesan has an extensive publication record and has contributed to multiple book chapters. Notably, she was awarded the Best Young Researcher Award in Mechatronics by Novel Research Academy, Pondicherry. Further showcasing her academic excellence, she was completed her prestigious Young Scientist Fellowship (YSFS) at IIT Palakkad for the academic year 2023–2024, where she advanced her research endeavors. An active member of professional bodies such as ISTE, ISHRAE and BEIESP, Dr. Murugesan continues to inspire innovation and foster excellence in engineering education and research.

J. Shanthi obtained her PhD from Anna University, Chennai, India. She is currently working in fault detection in through-silicon via of 3D IC, FinFET modeling, and biosensor applications. Her research interests also include VLSI physical design of 2D and 3D ICs, through-silicon vias, machine learning algorithms, optimization algorithms, processor architectures, and device modeling.

Subrata Chowdhury is currently working as an Associate Professor in the Department of Computer Science and Engineering at Sri Venkateswara College of Engineering & Technology (Autonomous), Chittoor, Andhra Pradesh, India. He completed his Bachelor of Computer Applications from I.K. Gujral Punjab Technical University in 2008, followed by a Master of Computer Applications from VIT Vellore in 2015. He earned his PhD in Computer Science from VISTAS, Chennai, in 2021. Dr. Chowdhury has authored and edited over 15 books on various topics and emerging technologies. He has published more than 100 research articles in SCI-indexed journals, Scopus-indexed conferences, and book chapters, as well as presented papers at numerous national and international conferences. He also holds several patents, some of which have been granted. With an H-index of 20, he is actively involved in the global research community. He is a member of the United Nations Laboratory for Sustainability, where he has contributed by authoring seven books, editing around 20 books, and contributing to over 30 book chapters. Dr. Chowdhury has served as a session chair in numerous IEEE, Springer, and ACM conferences, and has delivered keynote talks, faculty development programs (FDPs), workshops, and seminars at various academic and research institutions. Dr. Chowdhury is a professional member of various academic and technical societies, including IEEE, IET, ISTE, IAENG, and ACM. He also serves on the editorial boards of reputed journals from Springer, Elsevier, IEEE Transactions, and ACM.

Bhisham Sharma received his Ph.D. in Computer Science & Engineering from PEC University of Technology (formerly Punjab Engineering College), Chandigarh, India, and is currently working at the Centre of Research Impact and Outcome (CRIO), Chitkara University, Punjab. With 15 years of teaching and research experience at reputed universities across India, he serves as an Associate Editor for Engineering Applications of Artificial Intelligence (Elsevier), Computers & Electrical Engineering (Elsevier), International Journal of Communication Systems (Wiley), Human-centric Computing and Information Sciences (HCIS), and PLOS ONE; a Technical Editor for Computer Communications (Elsevier); and as an Editorial Board Member for Scientific Reports (Springer Nature) and Discover Applied Sciences (Springer). He is also a Guest Editor for several Q1 journals, including Computers & Electrical Engineering (Elsevier), Sensors (MDPI), Security and Communication Networks (Hindawi), Current Medical Imaging (Bentham Science), and Environmental Science and Pollution Research (Springer). Dr. Sharma has reviewed over 500 manuscripts for prestigious journals published by IEEE, Wiley, Springer, Elsevier, Taylor & Francis, MDPI, and others. His research interests span wireless communication, wireless sensor networks, wireless mesh networks, next generation networking, network security, Internet of Things, UAV, medical image processing, artificial intelligence, deep learning, machine learning, and edge/fog computing, with more than 140 research publications in reputed SCI and Scopus-indexed journals, international conferences, and book chapters. He also holds several patents, some of which have been granted.

Contributors

A Ganesh Ram, Department of Instrumentation Engineering, MIT Campus, Anna University, Chennai, Tamilnadu, India

A J Sunija, Department of Chemistry, Thiagarajar College of Engineering, Madurai, Tamilnadu, India

Abinaya S, Thiagarajar College of Engineering, Madurai, Tamil Nadu, India

Aliaa Salim, Department of Computer Science, Southern University and A&M College, Baton Rouge, Louisiana, United States

Arora Swati Chitkara, University Institute of Engineering and Technology (CUIET), Chitkara University, Punjab, India

Bhattacharjee Rituraj, Department of Instrumentation and Control Engineering, Manipal Institute of Technology, Manipal, Karnataka, India

C Meenakshi, Department of Computer Applications, VISTAS, Chennai, Tamilnadu, India

C V Nisha Angeline, Thiagarajar College of Engineering, Madurai, Tamil Nadu, India

Choudhary Keshav, Department of CSE (AIML), Haldia Institute of Technology, Haldia, WB, India

G Mohanbabu, Department of ECE, J.N.N. Institute of Engineering, Chennai, Tamilnadu, India

G Y Rajaa Vikhram, Dept. of EIE, SRM Institute of Science and Technology, Kattankulathur, Kattankulathur, Tamil Nadu, India

Garg Kamal Deep, Department of Computer Science and Engineering Chitkara University, Rajpura, Punjab, India

Ghosh Joyita, Department of CSE (AIML), Haldia Institute of Technology, Haldia, WB, India

Gunasekaran Prabhakar, Thiagarajar College of Engineering, Madurai, Tamilnadu, India

Gupta Subir, Department of CSE (AIML), Haldia Institute of Technology, Haldia, WB, India

Ismail Rashad, Department of Mathematics, Faculty of Science and Arts, King Khalid University, Abha, Asser Province, Saudi Arabia

J Justin Paul, Dept.of BME, KIT – Kalaignarkarunanidhi Institute of Technology, Coimbatore, Tamil Nadu, India

J Shanthi, Thiagarajar College of Engineering, Madurai, Tamilnadu, India

Jeyaraj Josephine Pon Gloria, Department of ECE, Vel Tech Rangarajan Dr. Sagunthala R&D Institute of Science and Technology, Chennai, Tamilnadu, India

K Suganya, School of Arts Sciences, Humanities and Education, SASTRA Deemed University, Thanjavur, Tamil Nadu, India

K Moniga, Department of ECE, SSM Institute of Engineering and Technology, Dindigul, Tamilnadu, India

Kalra Karan, Department Of Computer Science and Engineering Chitkara University, Rajpura, Punjab, India

Karnan Hemalatha, School of Chemical and Biotechnology, SASTRA Deemed University, Thanjavur, Tamil Nadu, India

Kishore Kumar D S, Dept.of BME, KIT – Kalaignarkarunanidhi Institute of Technology, Coimbatore, Tamilnadu, India

Krishnappa Krutthika Hirebasur, Southern University and A&M College, Baton Rouge, Louisiana, United States

Kumari Kanishka, Department Of Computer Science and Engineering Chitkara University, Rajpura, Punjab, India

Kumari Shalini, Chitkara University Institute of Engineering and Technology, Chitkara University, Rajpura, Punjab, India

Lokesh Ramachandrappa, Senior Application developer, Goldline Technologies, Baton Rouge, Louisiana United States

M Premkumar, Department of Artificial Intelligence and Data Science, SSM Institute of Engineering and Technology, Dindigul, Tamilnadu, India

M Surya, School of Advanced Sciences, VIT Chennai., Chennai, Tamilnadu, India

M Vijai Varshshan, Thiagarajar College of Engineering, Madurai, Tamil Nadu, India

M Vijayakarthick, Department of Instrumentation Engineering, MIT Campus, Anna University, Chennai, Tamilnadu, India

Mukherjee Subhradip, ECE Department, MVJ College of Engineering, Bengaluru, Karnataka, India

Muthuramalingam S, Thiagarajar College of Engineering, Madurai, Tamil Nadu, India

N Vinoth, Department of Instrumentation Engineering, MIT Campus, Anna University, Chennai, Tamilnadu, India

P Revathy, Kongu Engineering College, Perundurai, Tamilnadu, India

Pathak Dheeraj, Department of CSE (AIML), Haldia Institute of Technology, Haldia, WB, India

Prabha Chander, Chitkara University Institute of Engineering and Technology, Chitkara University, Rajpura, Punjab, India

R Sangeetha, Department of ECE, SRM Madurai College for Engineering and Technology, Sivagangai, Tamil Nadu, India

R Madhura, Dayananda Sagar College of Engineering, Bengaluru, Karnataka, India

R Manasa, Dayananda Sagar College of Engineering, Bengaluru, Karnataka, India

R S Varsha, Dept. of EIE, SRM Institute of Science and Technology, Kattankulathur, Kattankulathu, Tamil Nadu, India

Raj Yash, Department of CSE (AIML), Haldia Institute of Technology, Haldia, WB, India

Rajalakshmi Murugesan, Department of Mechatronics, Thiagarajar College of Engineering, Madurai, Tamilnadu, India

Ratana Warren, Department of Computer Science, Southern University and A&M College, Baton Rouge, Louisiana, United States

Roy Dipankar, Department of CSE (AIML), Haldia Institute of Technology, Haldia, WB, India

S Anupallavi, Department of Artificial intelligence and Machine learning, Acharya Institute of Technology, Bangalore, Karnataka, India

S Balachandran, School of Arts Sciences, Humanities and Education, SASTRA Deemed University, Thanjavur, Tamil Nadu, India

S Hariharan, School of Chemical and Biotechnology, SASTRA Deemed University, Thanjavur, Tamil Nadu, India

S Harini, Thiagarajar College of Engineering, Madurai, Tamil Nadu, India

S Meenakshi, Thiagarajar College of Engineering, Madurai, Tamilnadu, India

S Meyyappan, Department of Instrumentation Engineering, MIT Campus, Anna University, Chennai, Tamilnadu, India

S. R. Ashokkumar, Faculty of Engineering and Technology, M S Ramaiah University of Applied Sciences, Bangalore, Karnataka, India

Selvaraj Ravindrakumar, Dept.of BME, KIT – Kalaignarkarunanidhi Institute of Technology, Coimbatore, Tamilnadu, India

Soni Antra, Department Of Computer Science and Engineering Chitkara University, Rajpura, Punjab, India

T Sebasheela, Dept.of BME, KIT – Kalaignarkarunanidhi Institute of Technology, Coimbatore, Tamilnadu, India

T Theivanai, Dept.of BME, KIT – Kalaignarkarunanidhi Institute of Technology, Coimbatore, Tamilnadu, India

V Sarveshwaran, Thiagarajar College of Engineering, Madurai, Tamil Nadu, India

Wadhawan Kashish, Department Of Computer Science and Engineering Chitkara University, Rajpura, Punjab, India

1 The Future of Driving

Exploring Human Machine Collaboration in Modern Vehicles

Kamal Deep Garg, Kanishka Kumari, and Kashish Wadhawan

1.1 INTRODUCTION

The rapid advancement of autonomous vehicles (AVs) technology is transforming the future of transportation, evaluating how humans interact with machines on the road. As artificial intelligence, machine learning, and sensor technologies continue to evolve, AVs are becoming more capable of handling complex driving scenarios with minimal human intermediation. However, the success of autonomous driving depends not only on technological advancements but also on effective human-machine collaboration. Ensuring seamless interaction between drivers, pedestrians, and AV systems is crucial for improving safety, enhancing trust, and addressing challenges related to mixed traffic environments and pedestrian interactions. Studies indicate that pedestrian behaviour around AVs is influenced by prior experiences with human drivers, making it necessary to develop AV-pedestrian interaction models that mirror human driving behaviour [1].

Human-machine collaboration in AVs involves multiple aspects, including in-vehicle agents (IVAs), external human-machine interfaces (EHMIs), advanced driver assistance systems (ADAS), and decision-making algorithms that determine how AVs respond to real-world conditions. While automation reduces human errors and enhances efficiency, it also raises concerns about safety, pedestrian interaction, ethical dilemmas, and the socio-economic impact of AV adoption. The transition from human-driven to fully autonomous vehicles presents challenges that require careful consideration of technological reliability, user trust, and regulatory frameworks.

This paper explores four key areas of human-machine collaboration in AVs. First, it examines how IVAs and EHMIs make communication between drivers, passengers, and AV systems possible, ensuring a smooth transition between manual and automated driving. Second, it discusses safety concerns, including the role of ADAS (Advanced Driver Assistance Systems) in accident prevention and the challenges of pedestrian interaction in mixed-traffic environments. Third, it evaluates the social, ethical, and economic implications of AVs, focusing on job displacement, mobility equity, and ethical dilemmas in AV decision-making. Finally, it highlights current challenges and future research directions, addressing sensor reliability, cybersecurity risks, human-machine interaction, and infrastructure readiness.

DOI: 10.1201/9781003561309-1

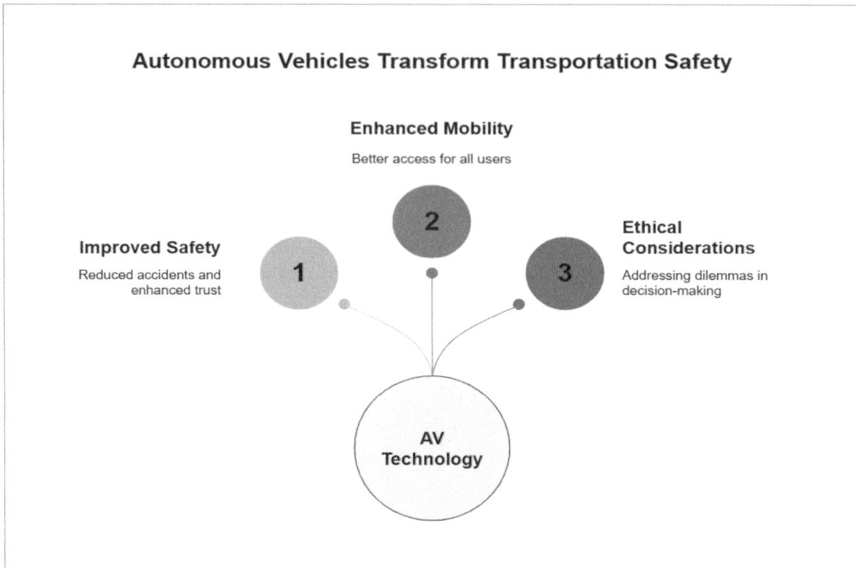

FIGURE 1.1 Role of AV technology in transforming transportation safety.

As AVs become increasingly integrated into urban environments, addressing these challenges is important to ensure their safe, efficient, and socially responsible implementation. Figure 1.1 illustrates the incorporation of AV technology that greatly improves transportation safety by reducing accidents, increasing mobility, and taking beliefs into account while decision-making. By enhancing human-machine collaboration, AVs can revolutionize transportation, reducing accidents, improving mobility access, and shaping the future of smart cities. AVs are rapidly advancing, promising safer and more efficient transportation systems. However, their widespread adoption depends on overcoming several key challenges, including technological reliability, ethical concerns, and regulatory frameworks that ensure safe integration into existing road networks [2].

1.1.1 Research Contribution

This research work outlines the following challenges and prospects of human-machine collaboration. The following are the work's goals:

a) To examine the potential pros and cons of the use of both human and artificial intelligence in automobile systems of the present day.
b) To ascertain the current state of the proposed autonomous driving technology and potential impacts on transportation in the future.
c) To understand possible obstacles and restrictions on human-machine cooperation nowadays in automobiles and offer remedies.

The novelties of this chapter are machine learning algorithms applied to IoT-based systems for enhancing the accuracy and convenience of driving current cars. Figure 1.1 shows the role of AV technology in transforming transportation safety.

1.2 LITERATURE REVIEW

This section explores prior studies and methodologies that have contributed to the development of AVs, highlighting key findings and research gaps.

A study in 2020 [3] focuses on cross-cultural autonomous vehicle-pedestrian interactions, revealing behavioural variations between Sri Lanka and Germany. The research creates experimental frameworks for EHMI design, focusing on non-verbal cues and adaptive AV interfaces. It proposes global usability standards and machine learning for pedestrian intent detection for future AV systems. A 2021 collaboration [4] examines and assesses EHMI technology for self-driving cars. The team performed experimental validations, evaluated technical factors, and looked at pedestrian-vehicle interactions. To improve AV safety and usability, the study produced recommendations for the efficient deployment of EHMIs, addressing communication issues and conforming to industry standards.

Researchers [5] explored the effectiveness of a multimodal EHMI for driverless vehicles using virtual reality. They designed experiments, analysed pedestrian-vehicle interactions, and assessed user responses. Their research provided insights into optimizing EHMI design for safer and more intuitive communication between autonomous vehicles and pedestrians. Another group of authors [6] reviewed the effects of AVs on several topics, such as public health, safety, economy, land use, and public behaviour. They investigated the interrelated impacts of AVs on infrastructure and society by synthesizing results from other studies, identifying research gaps, and offering a comprehensive analysis. Further research [7] focused on enhancing human-machine collaboration in automated driving through an intelligent two-phase haptic interface. They developed a control system, conducted simulations and real-world tests, and analysed driver responses. Their research aimed to improve transition handling, safety, and adaptability in automated driving environments. Experts also examined user interfaces for automated vehicles, focusing on human-machine interaction, usability, and driver engagement. They explored interface design, communication strategies, and user experience challenges. Their research provided insights into improving trust, transparency, and interaction efficiency, contributing to the development of intuitive and user-friendly interfaces for future automated driving systems. Developers [8] also developed a design space for in-vehicle interaction that is focused on human sensors and actuators by conducting a thorough assessment of 327 articles. Their work provided key insights for upcoming adaptive car interfaces, which identified input-output modalities, multimodal interactions, and user approval.

A group of scholars [9] analysed the integration of artificial intelligence and the Internet of Things (IoT) in autonomous vehicles, addressing safety standards, object detection, cybersecurity, and V2X (Vehicle-to-Everything communication) privacy challenges. They also explored applications of autonomous trucks, buses, cars, shuttles, helicopters, rovers, and underground vehicles across various sectors and countries, providing insights into intelligent transportation systems. Another team collectively examined the integration of 5G technology with AVs. They discussed current advancements in AV automation levels, enabling technologies, and the specific requirements of 5G networks [10]. The team analysed emerging techniques for integrating 5G with AVs, assessed the impact of 5G and beyond 5G technologies on AV performance, and identified potential security concerns. They also reviewed recent standardization activities and projects related to 5G-enabled AV technologies, providing insights into existing challenges and future research directions to advance AV development in the 5G era.

Table 1.1 presents the previously conducted studies in the context of exploring human-machine collaboration in modern vehicles. Despite the recent progress in these techniques, difficulties such as sparse datasets, drawn-out decision-making procedures, privacy and security issues, and the ongoing requirement for heuristic development and optimization remain important topics for more study.

TABLE 1.1
Comparative analysis of human-machine interaction models in AVs

Reference/ Year	Model	Advantages	Limitations	Futuristic Approach
[3] (2020)	Cross-cultural AV-pedestrian interaction study.	Highlights cultural differences in AV-pedestrian interactions.	Limited geographic scope (only Sri Lanka and Germany considered); does not address real-world implementation challenges.	Broaden research to include more cultural settings and refine EHMI designs.
[4] (2021)	EHMI for Autonomous Vehicles	Improved pedestrian-vehicle interaction, enhanced communication through external HMI	Limited real-world deployment, lack of standardized design principles	Develop standardized EHMI protocols and conduct large-scale real-world testing
[5] (2021)	Multimodal EHMI in Virtual Reality	Realistic VR-based testing, better understanding of pedestrian behaviour	Limited to virtual simulations, challenges in real-world implementation	Extend VR studies to real-world applications, integrate AI-based behaviour prediction

TABLE 1.1 (Continued)
Comparative analysis of human-machine interaction models in AVs

Reference/ Year	Model	Advantages	Limitations	Futuristic Approach
[6] (2021)	Autonomous Vehicle Impact Analysis	Comprehensive societal impact study, insights into land use, economy, and safety	Theoretical analysis without empirical validation	Conduct empirical studies to validate the theoretical findings
[7] (2022)	User Interfaces for Automated Vehicles	Focus on driver engagement, usability, and trust in AVs	Limited empirical testing in real-world settings	Implement real-world testing for better validation
[8] (2022)	Design Space for Human Sensor and Actuator-Focused In-Vehicle Interaction	Identifies multimodal input-output modalities for enhanced AV interaction	Limited real-world testing; some novel modalities (e.g., olfactory, cerebral) lack practical implementation	Investing Implement real-world testing of novel interaction modalities and explore adaptive interfaces for future AVs
[9] (2022)	AI and IoT in AVs	Enhanced automation, improved safety and efficiency	Security and privacy concerns, data management challenges	Develop robust cybersecurity frameworks, optimize AI for real-time decision-making
[10] (2024)	5G Integration in Autonomous Vehicles	Low latency, high-speed communication, improved safety	Early-stage integration, security risks	Enhance security measures, develop hybrid 5G-B5G integration models

Addressing these challenges will be essential for the continued advancement and real-world deployment of these technologies.

1.3 HUMAN-MACHINE COLLABORATION IN AUTONOMOUS VEHICLES

The collaboration between humans and machines in AVs is crucial for ensuring safety, trust, and seamless interaction between drivers and vehicle systems. As

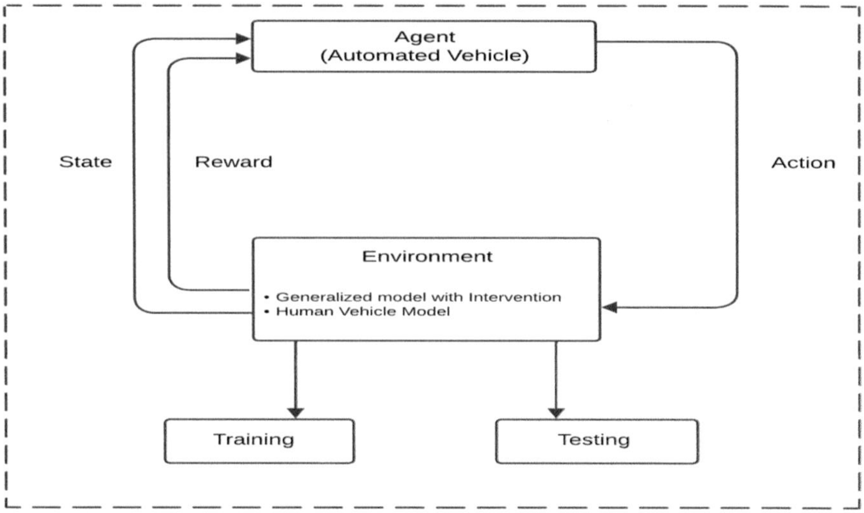

FIGURE 1.2 Reinforcement learning control framework for AVs.

automation levels progress, human intervention reduces, but the need for effective human-vehicle interaction (HVI) remains essential. IVAs and EHMIs are emerging technologies that bridge the gap between human drivers, passengers, pedestrians, and AVs. Additionally, transitioning between manual and automated driving modes poses significant challenges in terms of user adaptability and system reliability.

Tracking body components and the kinematics of the body, like head posture, body alignment, position of hands, feet, and trunk, presence of infants, and so on, is essential for interaction, safety, and assessing driver or passenger behaviour. From an ergonomic perspective, checking driver posture is also crucial when driving. Research has indicated that bad posture is a factor in long-distance drivers' discomfort. As such, in addition to the sections on activity, mood, and distraction detection that were previously covered, posture recognition is examined independently [11]. The reinforcement learning control framework for automated vehicles is shown in Figure 1.2. The model, which is a combination of a human vehicle model and a generalized one wherein the instruments are involved, stresses the supervisory role of the agent (AV) in its interaction with the environment. The agent learns the right way to do this as it receives a state and a reward from the environment. Hence, the trained agent will be tested to validate its capability. The cycle of reinforcement learning consists of the agent's learning as a result of its interactions with the nearby environment which becomes the basis of its improvement in the framework, which is exemplified in this situation.

1.3.1 Role of In-Vehicle Agents and External Human-Machine Interfaces

Integrating smart interfaces and AI-driven systems in vehicles is reshaping how drivers and AVs interact. IVAs and EHMIs are two key technologies facilitating this transition. IVAs are AI-powered virtual assistants integrated into the vehicle's system to enhance user experience and safety. Well-designed IVA interfaces can significantly improve the driving experience by reducing cognitive overload and making real-time information easier to process. By providing intuitive interactions, these systems allow drivers to quickly understand alerts and make informed decisions without distractions [7]. These agents provide real-time driving assistance by monitoring traffic, road conditions, and vehicle diagnostics. They also detect driver fatigue, distraction, or stress and respond accordingly to ensure a safer driving experience.

Additionally, IVAs personalize interactions by adjusting driving preferences, infotainment, and navigation based on user behaviour, making them an essential intermediary between human drivers and the autonomous system. This enables a smooth transition between manual and automated control while maintaining driver awareness. Human-vehicle interaction systems must be designed to actively engage drivers to prevent over-reliance on automation [12].

While IVAs manage in-car interactions, EHMIs facilitate communication between AVs and pedestrians or human-driven vehicles. Emerging intelligent in-vehicle interaction technologies are improving driver experience, making AV interfaces more adaptable to different users and driving scenarios [13]. These interfaces improve road safety by providing clear signals that indicate the vehicle's intentions. Visual indicators include LED displays, light signals, or projections communicate actions like stopping, yielding, or accelerating. Auditory cues include sounds or voice alerts, informing pedestrians and cyclists about the AV's next move. Standardized gestures are also being explored to establish universal communication methods between AVs and road users.

By implementing these external communication methods, EHMIs contribute to building public trust and ensuring safer interactions in mixed-traffic environments. However, standardization remains a challenge, as different manufacturers may implement varying designs, leading to inconsistencies in pedestrian understanding and response.

Figure 1.2 shows the reinforcement learning control framework for AVs. As AV technology advances, studies highlight that human-AI interaction mechanisms should be designed with adaptability in mind, ensuring inclusivity for a diverse range of users, including those with varying levels of technological familiarity. Effective IVAs and EHMIs must incorporate clear, intuitive communication strategies that align with human cognitive patterns, allowing both drivers and pedestrians to quickly assess vehicle intentions, react accordingly, and develop long-term trust in autonomous systems [14]. From driver experience and communication tactics to safety concerns and standardization issues, human-AI interaction in autonomous vehicles offers both potential and challenges depicted in Figure 1.3.

1.3.2 Transition Between Manual and Automated Driving

A seamless transition between manual and automated driving is one of the most significant challenges in AV development. While full automation at level 5 eliminates human intervention, semi-autonomous vehicles at levels 1 to 3 still require drivers

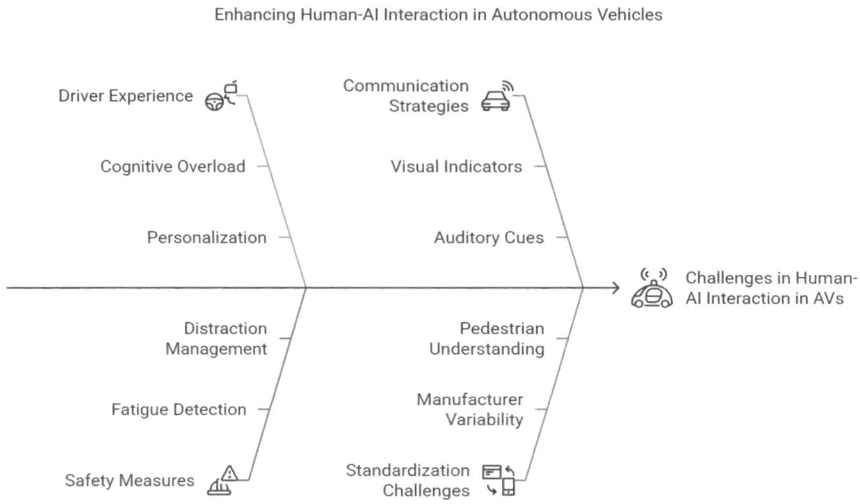

FIGURE 1.3 Enhancing human-AI interaction in AVs.

to remain engaged and ready to take control when necessary. Effective collaboration between humans and machines is essential to prevent delays in response times and ensure safe vehicle operation.

For semi-autonomous vehicles, drivers must remain prepared to take control when AV systems struggle, such as in unpredictable traffic conditions, sudden pedestrian crossings, or aggressive driving behaviour from human-operated vehicles. Environmental challenges such as heavy rain, fog, and snow can also affect sensor performance, requiring manual intervention. Additionally, construction zones and detours often require human decision-making, as AV systems may not always recognize temporary road changes accurately. Ensuring that drivers remain attentive during these scenarios is a major concern, as over-reliance on automation can lead to slower reaction times. Studies suggest that a well-structured transition process from manual to autonomous driving is crucial in maintaining driver awareness. Gradual exposure to automation, combined with periodic system prompts to keep drivers engaged, has been shown to reduce response delays and improve safety when human intervention is required [15]. To mitigate this, IVAs and HMI feedback mechanisms, such as visual alerts, auditory warnings, and haptic feedback, are crucial in maintaining driver awareness and engagement. Human-machine interfaces must incorporate multimodal interaction methods, including voice and gesture controls, to prevent driver disengagement in semi-autonomous vehicles [16].

User acceptance of AV technology depends largely on trust, system transparency, and adaptability. A major factor influencing trust is the predictability of AV behaviour. Research highlights that effective human-vehicle cooperation relies on clear communication between AVs and drivers, particularly during control transitions [17]. Drivers and pedestrians must feel confident that the vehicle will act in a safe and expected manner.

Clear communication is necessary to inform drivers when and why intervention is required. Gradual exposure to automation through driver training programs can also help users develop familiarity with AV systems, reducing hesitation in real-world scenarios. A well-designed human-machine interface should focus on intuitive interaction methods that keep the driver informed and engaged without causing cognitive overload. Ensuring a seamless transition between manual and automated driving requires a dynamic feedback system that keeps drivers actively engaged, even when AVs are in control. Research highlights that multimodal alert mechanisms—combining visual cues, auditory signals, and haptic feedback—help drivers maintain situational awareness, reducing reaction time when intervention is needed. By integrating adaptive learning algorithms, AVs can personalize these alerts based on individual driver behaviours, minimizing cognitive overload and improving handover efficiency [18].

To maximize safety and efficiency, human-machine collaboration in autonomous vehicles must focus on developing intelligent IVAs for personalized interaction, enhancing EHMI designs for standardized pedestrian communication, and implementing adaptive transition mechanisms to maintain driver awareness. By addressing these challenges, autonomous vehicles can achieve safer integration into real-world environments, ensuring a balance between human intuition and machine intelligence.

1.4 SAFETY AND PEDESTRIAN INTERACTION IN AUTONOMOUS VEHICLES

AVs have become more integrated into modern transportation systems, ensuring safety and effective interaction with pedestrians, which remains a critical concern. While AVs are designed to minimize human errors, challenges persist in making them adaptable to unpredictable road scenarios. ADAS and EHMIs play a crucial role in accident prevention and pedestrian communication. Additionally, the interaction between AVs and human-driven vehicles in mixed-traffic environments presents challenges that must be addressed to ensure seamless coexistence.

1.4.1 Advanced Driver Assistance Systems and Accident Prevention

ADAS have been developed to enhance road safety by assisting drivers and sometimes taking over critical driving functions. These systems leverage AI-powered decision-making, sensor fusion, and real-time data analysis to reduce accident risks. Features such as Adaptive Cruise Control (ACC), Automatic Emergency Braking (AEB), Lane Keeping Assist (LKA), and Blind Spot Detection (BSD) contribute to minimizing human errors and preventing collisions. ADAS act as an intermediary step toward full autonomy by automating certain driving functions while controlling the human driver. Intelligent automation systems are expanding ADAS capabilities, allowing AVs to make more precise adjustments to changing traffic conditions [9].

One of the most significant benefits of ADAS is its ability to react faster than human drivers in emergencies. Automatic Emergency Braking, for example, detects sudden obstacles or potential collisions and applies the brakes if the driver fails to respond

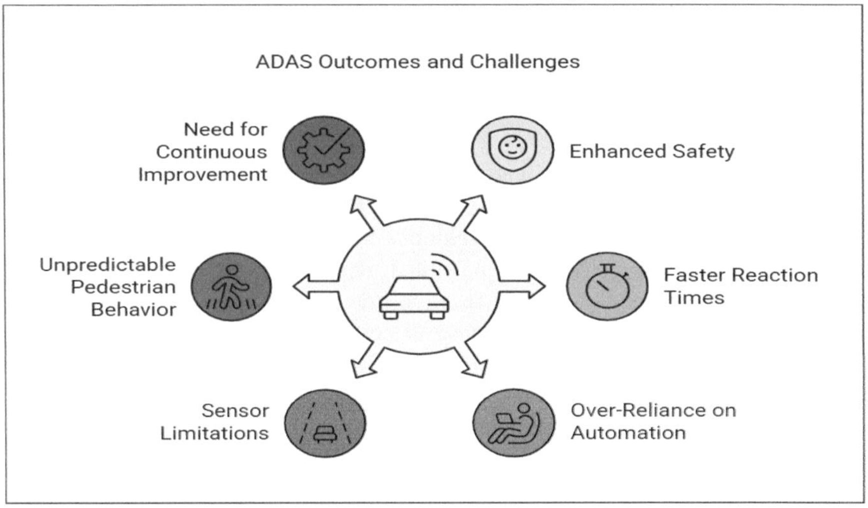

FIGURE 1.4 ADAS outcomes and challenges.

in time. Similarly, Lane Keeping Assist prevents unintentional lane departures, which is especially useful in cases of driver distraction or drowsiness. These technologies significantly reduce the likelihood of accidents caused by human errors such as misjudgement, fatigue, or inattentiveness. However, while ADAS improves safety, it also introduces challenges such as over-reliance on automation. Drivers may become complacent, assuming that the vehicle will handle all scenarios, which can lead to delayed reactions when human intervention is required.

Furthermore, sensor limitations pose another challenge in accident prevention. ADAS rely on cameras, radar, LIDAR, and ultrasonic sensors to detect objects and road conditions. Adverse weather conditions such as heavy rain, fog, or snow can impair sensor functionality, reducing the system's accuracy. Additionally, unpredictable pedestrian behaviour remains a major concern, as ADAS cannot always anticipate sudden movements by pedestrians. To enhance effectiveness, continuous improvements in machine learning algorithms, sensor robustness, and fail-safe mechanisms are necessary to ensure that ADAS functions reliably in diverse road conditions. Recent research highlights that integrating machine learning with roadside units can further improve ADAS functionality by detecting abnormal driving behaviours in real-time. By analysing vehicle movement patterns, these systems can provide early warnings to AVs and human drivers, reducing the likelihood of accidents before they occur [19]. While there are many advantages of ADAS, such as increased safety and quicker reaction times, there are drawbacks as well, like sensor limits and an excessive dependence on automation shown in Figure 1.4.

1.4.2 Challenges in Mixed Traffic Environments

As AVs become more common, they will need to coexist with human-driven vehicles, cyclists, and pedestrians, creating a mixed traffic environment. Unlike

AVs, human drivers exhibit varying levels of skill, judgment, and behavioural unpredictability. This difference in driving styles can lead to misunderstandings and potential safety risks. AVs rely on programmed algorithms to follow traffic rules consistently, but human drivers often make split-second decisions based on intuition and situational awareness. As a result, AVs may struggle to predict and react to aggressive or unconventional driving behaviours exhibited by human-operated vehicles. One of the primary concerns in mixed traffic environments is how AVs communicate their intentions to human drivers and pedestrians. EHMIs are being developed to bridge this communication gap. EHMIs use visual displays, light signals, and auditory cues to inform pedestrians and other road users about the AV's next action. For example, an AV approaching a crosswalk may display a signal indicating that it is yielding to pedestrians, thereby reducing confusion and ensuring safe passage. However, the effectiveness of EHMIs depends on standardization and widespread public awareness.

The way pedestrians interpret AV signalling methods varies significantly across cultures and personal experiences. This inconsistency highlights the importance of standardizing EHMI communication techniques to ensure that all road users can safely and reliably predict AV behaviour [4]. If different manufacturers implement varying communication methods, it may lead to inconsistent interpretations, posing safety risks.

Another challenge in mixed-traffic environments is pedestrian interaction with AVs. Unlike human-driven vehicles, AVs do not rely on direct eye contact or gestures to communicate with pedestrians. Pedestrians are accustomed to non-verbal cues from human drivers such as hand signals or subtle nods, to determine when it is safe to cross. In the absence of these cues AVs must develop alternative ways to indicate their intentions clearly. Research has shown that pedestrians may initially hesitate to interact with AVs due to uncertainty about how the vehicle will behave.

Studies indicate that pedestrians often hesitate when crossing in front of autonomous vehicles due to unclear communication of AV intentions. Establishing standardized external signalling methods, such as visual or auditory cues, can reduce this uncertainty and enhance pedestrian trust in AV systems. Building trust in AV systems will require widespread education, clear and intuitive signalling mechanisms, and real-world testing to refine pedestrian-vehicle interaction models.

Human-driven vehicles may not always follow predictable patterns. Issues such as sudden lane changes, aggressive overtaking, and disregard for traffic signals create challenges for AVs that rely on predefined rules and structured decision-making. To address these issues, AVs must incorporate advanced AI-driven behavioural prediction models that allow them to anticipate and adapt to the actions of human drivers. Furthermore, regulatory frameworks and updated road infrastructure may be necessary to facilitate safer mixed traffic environments by integrating smart traffic signals, dedicated AV lanes, and standardized AV communication protocols.

Ensuring safety in AV deployment requires continuous advancements in ADAS, improved pedestrian communication methods, and adaptive response mechanisms for mixed-traffic environments. As technology evolves, collaboration between policymakers, manufacturers, and researchers will be essential to establish regulations that promote seamless AV integration while prioritizing road user safety.

utilitarian approach, minimizing overall harm regardless of individual consequences, while others advocate for prioritizing passenger safety above all else. The challenge lies in defining an ethical framework that is widely accepted across different cultures and legal systems. Public trust in AVs will depend on the transparency of their decision-making processes and the ability of regulatory bodies to establish clear ethical guidelines. At the same time, over-reliance on AV signalling systems could lead pedestrians to assume all vehicles will yield, increasing the risk of accidents when interacting with human-driven cars. A careful balance is needed to ensure that AVs communicate effectively without fostering unrealistic safety expectations among road users [22].

Another ethical concern is accountability in the event of an accident. In conventional traffic incidents, the responsibility typically falls on the driver. However, in an autonomous vehicle scenario, liability could extend to multiple stakeholders, including the vehicle manufacturer, software developers, and regulatory bodies. Determining who is legally responsible for an AV-related accident remains a complex issue. Manufacturers must ensure that AVs operate within ethical and legal boundaries while also providing mechanisms for human oversight when necessary.

Beyond accident scenarios, AVs also pose privacy and surveillance concerns. These vehicles rely on extensive data collection, including location tracking, biometric recognition, and behavioural monitoring, to optimize performance and ensure safety. While data-driven intelligence enhances vehicle functionality, it also raises questions about data security and user privacy. Unauthorized access to AV data could lead to security breaches, targeted surveillance, or misuse of personal information. Striking a balance between technological innovation and ethical responsibility is essential to ensuring that AV adoption benefits society as a whole without compromising fundamental rights.

As AV technology continues to advance, addressing these social, ethical, and economic challenges will require collaboration between governments, industry leaders, ethicists, and the public. Developing policies that prioritize job security, equitable mobility access, transparent ethical decision-making, and data privacy will be crucial in shaping a future where AVs enhance society while minimizing unintended consequences.

1.6 CHALLENGES AND FUTURE RESEARCH DIRECTIONS

The widespread adoption of AVs presents significant challenges that must be addressed before they can fully integrate into society. While AVs promise increased safety, efficiency, and convenience, unresolved technological and human-factor challenges continue to hinder their large-scale deployment. Sensor reliability, adverse environmental conditions, cybersecurity threats, and vehicle-to-human communication are key areas requiring further development. Additionally, human-machine interaction must be optimized to ensure that drivers, pedestrians, and passengers can trust and effectively engage with autonomous systems. Addressing these challenges through advanced research and innovation is essential for the successful implementation of AV technology.

1.6.1 Technological Limitations and Sensor Reliability

One of the most critical challenges in AV development is ensuring that vehicles can accurately perceive and respond to their environment in all conditions. AVs rely on an array of sensors, including LiDAR, radar, cameras, and ultrasonic sensors, to detect objects, interpret traffic signals, and navigate roads. However, these sensors are still prone to limitations, particularly in adverse weather conditions. Heavy rain, fog, snow, and glare from sunlight can obscure sensor readings, reducing the accuracy of object detection and increasing the likelihood of errors in decision-making. Weather conditions such as fog and heavy snowfall remain major obstacles, requiring AI-driven sensor fusion to enhance AV perception in challenging environments [23]. While human drivers can adjust their perception based on intuition and experience, AVs depend solely on sensor data, making them vulnerable to misinterpretations. Improving sensor robustness through machine learning advancements and multi-sensor fusion techniques remains a crucial area of research. While 5G can enhance AV sensor performance and reduce latency, its real-world impact is limited in regions with poor network coverage, posing navigation challenges [10].

Cybersecurity is another pressing concern in AV technology. Since AVs are heavily dependent on software, connectivity, and real-time data exchange, they are susceptible to hacking and cyberattacks. Malicious actors could exploit security vulnerabilities to take control of an AV, manipulate traffic systems, or steal sensitive user data. Ensuring the security of AV networks requires robust encryption protocols, intrusion detection systems, and fail-safe mechanisms that prevent unauthorized access. Reducing uncertainty in AV decision-making models is crucial, as even small prediction errors can lead to system failures in real-world conditions [24]. Additionally, regulatory standards must be established to enforce cybersecurity measures across all AV manufacturers and operators. Research in blockchain-based security frameworks and AI-driven threat detection could enhance the resilience of AV systems against cyber threats.

Infrastructure readiness also plays a crucial role in AV deployment. Many urban and rural areas lack the necessary infrastructure to support autonomous driving, including high-precision GPS mapping, intelligent traffic signals, and dedicated AV lanes. The effectiveness of AVs depends on seamless communication with the surrounding infrastructure, yet existing road networks were primarily designed for human-driven vehicles. In order to accommodate AVs, governments and city planners must make investments in smart infrastructure solutions. They should make sure that highways have real-time data-sharing capabilities to improve vehicle coordination and safety. Future human-machine collaboration in cars can benefit from concepts like EESR (Energy Efficient Sector-Based Routing), which was first created for UWSNs (Underwater Wireless Sensor Networks). This will help optimise data flow across autonomous systems for safer and more intelligent driving [25].

1.6.2 Human Factor Issues and Improving Human-Machine Interfaces

Despite the advancements in automation, human involvement remains an essential component of AV operations, particularly in semi-autonomous vehicles. One of the biggest challenges is maintaining driver attention and readiness to take control when necessary. Levels 1 to 3 automation still require human supervision, but over-reliance on automation can lead to automation complacency—a state in which drivers become disengaged and slow to react when manual intervention is needed. Studies have shown that human reaction times increase significantly when transitioning from autonomous to manual control, leading to potential safety risks. Developing an intuitive HHMI that keeps drivers engaged without causing cognitive overload is critical to addressing this issue.

Another challenge is the emotional and psychological response of humans interacting with AVs. Many drivers and pedestrians remain sceptical about AV decision-making, leading to hesitation or distrust in their capabilities. EHMIs, such as visual signals, auditory alerts, and digital displays, are being developed to communicate AV intentions. However, pedestrian behaviour is often unpredictable, and AVs must be designed to anticipate sudden movements and respond appropriately. Research in behavioural modelling and AI-driven prediction systems can improve AV responses to real-world human interactions. Figure 1.6 presents key features of ethical and inclusive AV innovation. The figure highlights the interconnected nature of

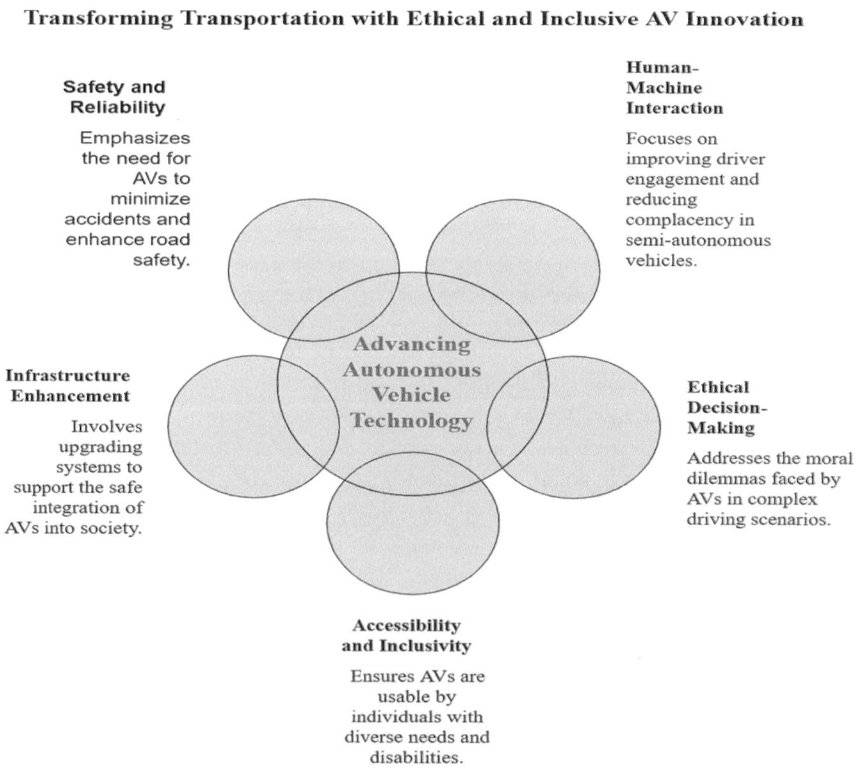

FIGURE 1.6 Framework for advancing AV technology with a focus on ethics and acceptance.

crucial factors like safety, human-machine interface, ethical decision-making, infrastructure improvement, and inclusivity.

Accessibility and inclusivity also need to be prioritized in AV design. While AVs have the potential to improve mobility for individuals with disabilities, current systems may not fully accommodate diverse user needs. Voice-based controls, haptic feedback, and adaptive interfaces must be integrated to enhance usability for individuals with visual, auditory, or physical impairments. Future research should focus on multi-modal interaction systems that provide personalized assistance to different user groups, ensuring that AV technology benefits all members of society. Furthermore, ethical considerations must be addressed regarding the role of AVs in decision-making scenarios. Current AV systems rely on predefined algorithms to make driving decisions, but human morality is complex and context-dependent. Situations involving unavoidable accidents present moral dilemmas—should an AV prioritize passenger safety or minimize overall harm? Standardizing ethical guidelines for AV behaviour remains a challenge, as cultural and legal perspectives on responsibility and risk vary globally. Research in AI ethics and policy-making must work toward establishing internationally accepted frameworks for AV decision-making.

As AV technology continues to evolve, overcoming these challenges will require collaborative efforts between researchers, policymakers, automotive manufacturers, and society. Addressing technological limitations, refining human-machine interactions, and enhancing infrastructure will be key to ensuring that AVs are not only functional but also safe, ethical, and widely accepted. By prioritizing these research directions, AVs can transition from experimental technology to everyday reality transforming transportation for future generations.

Despite significant advancements in smart vehicle technology, accidents caused by human distraction, poor judgment, and errors may continue to persist. AVs are specifically designed to eliminate these human errors by leveraging advanced sensors, AI, and machine learning to make precise, real-time decisions. By removing the unpredictable element of human behaviour, AVs have the potential to significantly reduce crash rates, enhance road safety and minimize fatalities and injuries caused by distracted driving. The widespread adoption of AVs could lead to safer, more efficient roads, with fewer accidents and traffic-related deaths.

1.7 EVALUATION METHODS

This section covers various research methods that have been used to understand the interaction of ADS (Automated Driving System) with pedestrians. To make design and deployment lead to a safer and more efficient shared road environment, such methods should be employed towards understanding pedestrian perspectives of and response to automated vehicles.

1.7.1 Survey-Based Studies

In an evaluation of automatic or automated vehicles, survey-based studies that take the form of in-person interviews or written/online questionnaires are commonly used to address the impact of automated driving technology implementation in the future. It is suggested that a pedestrian behaviour opinion poll should be developed and validated about different driving technologies.

Simulator-Based Studies: A large variety of trainer-based techniques and several virtual environment tools are employed to range over the potential for ADS and pedestrian communication. One new approach studies road user behaviours in specified areas by using the Multiple Participant Simulator (MPS). The MPS allows users to interact simultaneously in the same virtual environment by utilizing two or more independent simulators that are physically connected. By applying the MPS technique in a secured environment, one may evaluate the efficacy of ADS in a variety of traffic scenarios. Synthetic environment, in which multiple traffic participants engage in mutual interactions within a single traffic scenario. Virtual Reality (VR) which is based on simulators uses a similar method to allow the statistical observation of pedestrian behaviour in various aspects. The majority of these gadgets, which are also known as pedestrian simulators, fall into the category of Cave Automatic Virtual Environment (CAVE) settings, which use Head-Mounted Display (HMD) sets and projector screens to create a replication of the environment. One example of this sort of device is VR-based pedestrian simulators, used in various traffic conditions. This simulator produces pictorial feedback for human subjects with the use of an HMD alongside a wearable human motion capture system and dynamic driving simulation. Virtual reality technology is utilized to explore the outward appearance of an autonomous vehicle. For instance, the decision of a pedestrian to proceed to an automated vehicle's crossroads can be changed.

Wizard-Of-Oz-Technique**:** Using a false driverless car in an actual traffic environment, the Wizard-Of-Oz (WoZ) technique examines potential interactions between pedestrians and fully autonomous vehicles. Using a designed automobile seat, a skilled driver can be kept out of sight to simulate an automated system or an invisible controller within the car that can operate the vehicle. The WoZ method is additionally employed to look into:

1. How automobiles convey their intended motions.
2. How pedestrian behaviour is impacted when the driver is not present.

Road-Trial: Another method applied to gather data in ADS-pedestrian interaction is the road trial which is more or less the closest approximation of real life. In this, the instrumented automated pods presently in use on the roads are used to gather the necessary data. With this, cameras are fitted at the exterior of the vehicles to capture the road scene and provide video data feeds. Similar functionalities and travelling at moderate velocities (up to 25 mph in urban environments) over shorter distances in less complex traffic patterns could be said to be similar to level-4 ADS; other examples of applying automated pods as public transportation are Google's driverless pods, Easy Mile EZ10 shuttles, and automated pods themselves. Road trials are undoubtedly better than any other methods and might provide a set of naturalistic data on user requirements and behaviours regarding interaction with ADSs. However, since the current automated pods operate slowly, their functionality is restricted; thus, they do not represent automated technologies entirely. Alternatively, WoZ exercises the actions of users in various types of traffic with the help of a prototype ADS. Another advantage of the WoZ method is gathering data regarding the mode of behaviour towards pedestrians in a real environment. The other simulator studies are suitable to test not only the user's behaviour but also the functioning of ADS.

1.7.2 Enhancing Driver Safety and Situational Awareness in In-Vehicle Information Systems

Even during automated driving periods, drivers must develop and sustain an appropriate level of Self-Assurance (SA) so they can take over control of the car when instructed. As a result, even if they might be participating in other NDRTs, it is imperative to maintain their control loop while communicating context-related information and vehicle status [13]. When designing human-vehicle interfaces, the entire Interaction-Attention Continuum should be taken into consideration, as drivers should be able to seamlessly shift their attention from things unrelated to driving to supervision and ultimately assuming control.

1. Focused interaction: Interaction that is focused is the most prevalent kind. It is challenging to work on another task at the same time as it needs concentrated attention. For example, manually drive, and enter the address in the GPS.
2. Peripheral interaction: The goal of peripheral interaction is to "present information from computing systems to users in a subtle manner, such that it can be perceived in their periphery of attention." It also consists of peripheral data displays, ambient screens and awareness programs. For example, talk to the other passengers and use the steering wheel to adjust the music wheel controls, a hands-free kit, etc.
3. Implicit interaction: "Rely on automatic sensing of people's activity or presence as input for computer-initiated activities" is the definition of implicit interaction. The Internet of Things, omnipresent sensors, and ambient intelligence serve as instances of it. For example, auto lights – auto windshield wipers.

To maintain the SA when the user is using a variety of interfaces, we may develop and implement them using the notion of peripheral interaction, carrying out additional duties. But it's important to consider the proper design guidelines. Our comprehensive literature research on the safety features of IVISs (In-Vehicle Information Systems) has made several contributions to our knowledge of the intricate relationship between technology and driver safety, including:

Thorough Examination of Safety Issues: The review carefully examines a range of safety issues related to IVISs, including situational awareness, cognitive load, and driving distraction. Combining information from several research studies, it provides a comprehensive understanding of the diverse effects of these systems by highlighting how various IVIS technologies impact driving performance and driver emotional state.

2 Decision Making System for FCD-Epilepsy type-II Segmentation Using MRI

Rashad Ismail, Hariharan S, Hemalatha Karnan, Suganya K, and Balachandran S

2.1 INTRODUCTION

A seizure, which is also referred to as a convulsion, results from anomalous electrical brain activity and is also a form of epilepsy. It is a common brain ailment that is permanent and cuts across the entire population, with globally over 50 million people suffering from the disorder. It can produce several effects, including loss of consciousness, loss of control over certain bodily functions such as bladder or bowel control, as well as impairment of hearing or vision, and a reduction in the ability to coordinate movement. These symptoms may also lead to self-inflicted wounds, especially through trauma from falls that result from a lack of feeling and poor movement control. Most of them (about 80%) live in low- and middle-income countries. Although timely identification and management could leave between 60% and 70% of epilepsy patients seizure-free, a large segment, especially in poor-income countries, does not have access to primary care. This treatment gap reaches alarming levels, with up to 90% of affected individuals in certain countries unable to access necessary care. In addition to this, it is also prevalent that healthcare providers in many of these countries are not adequately trained to identify, assess, and even treat epilepsy properly. Worsening the problem, antiseizure medications are not readily available in impoverished regions and areas. There is stigma and discrimination against people with epilepsy and their families all over the world. Societal stigma and cultural stereotypes add another layer of fear and misunderstanding. Even where drug treatment fails to control seizures optimally, various operative interventions can offer relief. Epilepsy patients, along with the psychosocial assistance, might also have co-existing mental health comorbidities like anxiety or depressive disorders. The World Health Organization (WHO), along with health ministries and other stakeholders, is addressing multiple population-level issues, such as focal cortical dysplasia (FCD), which causes abnormal contour and distribution of the cerebral cortex in a manner that resembles a three-dimensional game. FCD type II [1] also features dysmorphic neurons, also known as balloon cells, which are arranged in a disorganized manner. Most of the time, this FCD subtype is detected using MRI, which is typically performed in early infancy. Focal means that each sequence of the epileptic seizure originates from a focal point, which is always a pathological focus of

 DOI: 10.1201/9781003561309-2

the brain tissue. Cortical features refer to the areas of the cortex where the first attack typically occurs. "Dysplasia" refers to the presence of abnormal or disorganized cells within the tissues of an organ, specifically the brain. Dysplasia in the brain can affect the type of seizure and symptoms experienced by the patient. Typically, tonic-clonic seizures, characterized by falling and shaking, or absence seizures, marked by staring into space and repetitive movements, are most common. Symptoms of FCD typically manifest within the first five years of life for approximately two-thirds of individuals, while most of the remaining cases develop seizures before reaching the age of 16. The onset of FCD in adults is relatively rare. While the interictal scalp electroencephalogram (EEG) may reveal focal-ictal-like activity localized to dysplastic lesions, highlighting their high epileptogenicity, there's a lack of clear correlation between interictal EEG findings and imaging features in FCD. However, patients with FCD show EEG evidence of persistent epileptiform discharges, which have been associated with a better outcome after surgery. Multiple studies have confirmed the intrinsic hyperexcitability of abnormal cortex in FCD, often leading to rapid propagation from the neocortex to mesial temporal regions. Ictal EEG investigations suggest that FCD represents a disorder of the neural network with secondary ictal zones. Intraictal activation is characteristic of FCD and can occur either adjacent to or distant from the primary epileptogenic area. Research indicates that surgical removal of the epileptic focus in the brain can result in seizure freedom for up to 67% of individuals. Diagnosing FCD requires a brain MRI that reveals specific characteristics of FCD. Key MRI findings include abnormal thickening and altered architecture of the gyri, potentially accompanied by changes in T2-weighted images of gray and white matter. Additionally, focal increases in T2 or FLAIR signals, as well as blurring between gray and white matter, may be present. The trans mantle sign, characterized by increased signal extending from the cortical surface to the ventricle, is also indicative. These changes may be localized or extensive, affecting multiple gyri or lobes. Achieving an accurate diagnosis often requires a high-resolution MRI with thin slices and multiplanar reconstruction, along with the simultaneous use of T2 and FLAIR imaging, to detect subtle FCD lesions. The architectures used to deploy the segmentation process are the U-Net and the Generative Adversarial Network (GAN). The U-Net is a widely used deep learning architecture in biomedical image segmentation [2]. It consists of a convolution layer, encoder, and decoder networks. This effectively leverages a smaller amount of data with speed and accuracy. It addresses the challenges of limited annotated data in the medical field. Then, the GAN architecture trains two neural networks to compete against each other, generating more authentic new data from the input data. It generates new data from the sample input, and the discriminator attempts to predict whether the generated output belongs in the original dataset, i.e., whether to describe the generated output as real or fake based on the original input data that was fed during the training process. Conditional GAN (CGAN) is primarily used for segmentation purposes, where the generator and discriminator receive additional information, such as class labels or other forms of conditioning data. With CGAN, the Pix2Pix architecture is used for segmentation purposes. Pix2Pix learns the mapping from input to output image using a loss function during the mapping process.

2.2 LITERATURE SURVEY

Epilepsy presents a significant health risk, and minimally invasive surgery offers effective treatment for refractory cases. However, localizing lesions in MRI-negative patients remains challenging. Studies focuses on segmenting and classifying the hippocampus, a crucial brain region implicated in epilepsy, using diffusion kurtosis imaging (DKI). DKI provides insights into tissue pathology at the molecular level. Using DKI parameters, a convolutional neural network (CNN) with transfer learning is employed to extract features for classification. The CNN, which uses a pre-trained VGG16 model, achieves a classification accuracy of 90.8% in distinguishing between epileptic patients and normal individuals. These results highlight the success of DKI in the forensic diagnosis of epilepsy, with FA and MK becoming the prominent features. This also underscores the need for further research on DKI for in-depth analysis [3] of the spatial structures of tissue pathology for clinical purposes. A recently developed segmentation architecture based on Generative Adversarial Networks (GANs) called Vol2SegGAN is presented in a study [4]. The objective is to delineate tissues, specifically cerebrospinal fluid (CSF), gray matter (GM), and white matter (WM) from 3D T1-weighted MRI images. Furthermore, the segmentation included nine regions, specifically identifying cortical gray matter (CGM), basal ganglia (BG), white matter hyperintensities (WMH), cerebellar fissures (CF), ventricles (VE), cerebellum (CE), and brainstem (BS). It can be suggested that the 3D-Edge Enhancing Gradient Echo MRI (EDGE) technique has high potential for diagnosing FCD due to its high contrast-to-noise ratio (CNR). However, due to the inhomogeneities of the transmit field (B1+) inherent in the application of 7T MRI, the application of the EDGE technique presents challenges. The authors [5] describe the first application of 7T EDGE MRI in the context of identifying FCD within the region of epilepsy, highlighting its efficacy in distinguishing fine details, SNR, and imaging contrast uniformity. The EDGE-MP2 RAGE sequence enhances the visibility of the alterations between gray and white matter that are characteristic of regions with FCD, making it a valuable and time-saving addition to 7T MRI protocols for focal epilepsy. A deep learning-based transformer model, titled Epilepsy Net, was trained using EEG signals from 35 channels and generated 1-minute-long recordings of each participant's activity. Each training repetition was limited to a case in which sample data were randomly drawn from revenue participants of EEG activities of 1-minute duration. Later, the 5-second epochs were combined with the MCC explored epoch matrices, which were initially combined in the upper triangles of the midpoint matrix that has a vectorized data input structure. This relationship of the observations was determined using PCC as a robust statistical analysis tool. This one-dimensional array of signals is created from EEG data using an embedding over 5 seconds of the participants' alternating activity across ten regions. Positional encoding was also included, where the parameters were learnt and incorporated into each correlation coefficient that corresponded to its embedding before the data was passed to Epilepsy Net for the analysis of the EEG signal for epilepsy. This model was trained, and its performance was tested using tenfold cross-validation. The Epilepsy Net Model performed remarkably, with classification accuracies, sensitivities, specificities, and positive predictive values of 85%, 82%, 87%, and 82%, respectively [6]. The labeling of "MRI-negative

TLE" was applied [7] when there was no gray matter (GM) loss in the temporal or limbic lobes, and when epileptogenic lesions or atrophy, as seen by an expert visually assessing MRI scans, were not available. The above study indicates a strong correlation between epilepsy lateralization in TLE patients with GM reductions detected by the algorithm and the epileptic zone identified by experts through conventional EEG recordings. Epileptic seizure detection relies on expert clinicians visually analyzing EEG signals, a process that is time-consuming, resource-intensive, and prone to errors and biases. Epilepsy diagnosis scheme can be improved by leveraging Tunable-Q factor wavelet transform (TQWT) and bootstrap aggregating (Bagging) techniques with EEG signals. The proposed method [8] demonstrates superior performance in terms of sensitivity, specificity, and accuracy. Recent advancements in colorectal cancer diagnosis have led to increased interest in less invasive endoscopy-based methods. Computer-aided diagnosis systems, leveraging deep learning, aim to enhance diagnostic accuracy. A study [9] proposes a novel data augmentation approach using Pix2Pix to generate polyp images from depth maps, thereby addressing the limitations of existing training datasets. Quantitative evaluation shows improved performance of the Single Shot Multibox Detector (SSD) in polyp detection. Incorporating generated images, particularly those with depth maps, enhances metrics such as precision, recall, and F-measure. Pix2Pix, coupled with depth maps, produces more natural and effective images for data augmentation in polyp detection. Future research will focus on optimizing Pix2Pix for clearer image generation and exploring the detection of different polyp types. The effectiveness of diffusion-weighted MRI methods in identifying the epileptogenic zone (EZ) was assessed in 25 patients with refractory epilepsy undergoing surgery. White matter (WM) asymmetry, as measured by mean kurtosis (MK), was analyzed [10] to identify the impaired lobe, followed by the utilization of the iDrArK metric for EZ detection. Results showed successful lobe and EZ detection in ten and nine patients, respectively, with 100% and 89% accuracy, respectively. Crack detection in bridges is crucial for ensuring structural safety, yet it requires extensive datasets of crack images for effective deep learning-based methods. This study introduces a GAN-based approach to synthesize crack images and annotations, supplementing traditional data augmentation techniques. By employing the DCGAN and Pix2Pix models, synthesized crack images and annotations were generated and evaluated for use in DNN training. Results demonstrated that DNNs trained with synthesized images achieved a Mean IoU of 74.34%, comparable to those trained with real images. Pre-training DNNs with synthesized images before fine-tuning with real data proved to be the most effective approach. This research contributes to the discussion on machine learning for crack detection and the use of GAN for generating a crack image dataset, thereby enabling DNN training for DNNs [11]. Magnetic Resonance Imaging (MRI) is a crucial diagnostic method for evaluating the heart, assessing heart function, and determining the size and shape of the ventricles. However, segmenting ventricle regions in the MRI images proved to be challenging due to low image contrast, blended boundaries, and the presence of noise in the images. To address this issue, we conducted cardiac MR imaging in 33 cases and employed the U-Net neural network architecture, incorporating high-resolution image information to enhance segmentation features. Furthermore, we attempted a transfer learning and a multi-dimensional multi-scale dissimulant Generative Adversarial Network (TLMDB GAN) approach to address a case of insufficient ventricle image data. The experimental results demonstrate that TLMDB GAN outperforms U-Net, as evidenced by the higher Dice coefficients for inner and outer ventricular wall segmentation compared to TLMDB. This demonstrates that TLMDB GAN [12] is effective in improving segmentation accuracy, and thus it has great potential in ventricle analysis during cardiac MRI diagnostics. Furthermore, a variety of neutrosophic-based image processing techniques—including thresholding, denoising, clustering, segmentation, and classification—have been reviewed across different medical imaging modalities [13].

2.3 METHODOLOGY

2.3.1 Workflow

In this research, the authors utilized the total workflow scheme presented in Figure 2.1. The study begins with the acquisition of volumetric 3D anatomical cerebral MRI images from the open-source "Open Neuro" repository. It concludes with the development of comprehensive MRI preprocessing techniques designed to enhance the overall quality of the data and address any existing flaws. Next, after preprocessing is complete, the MRI scans are subjected to two models of convolutional neural networks, namely UNet and CGAN, to determine the location of disease areas during segmentation processes. Subsequently, the models were assessed based on accuracy, model loss metrics, and mean Intersection over Union (mIOU), as well as other relevant metrics.

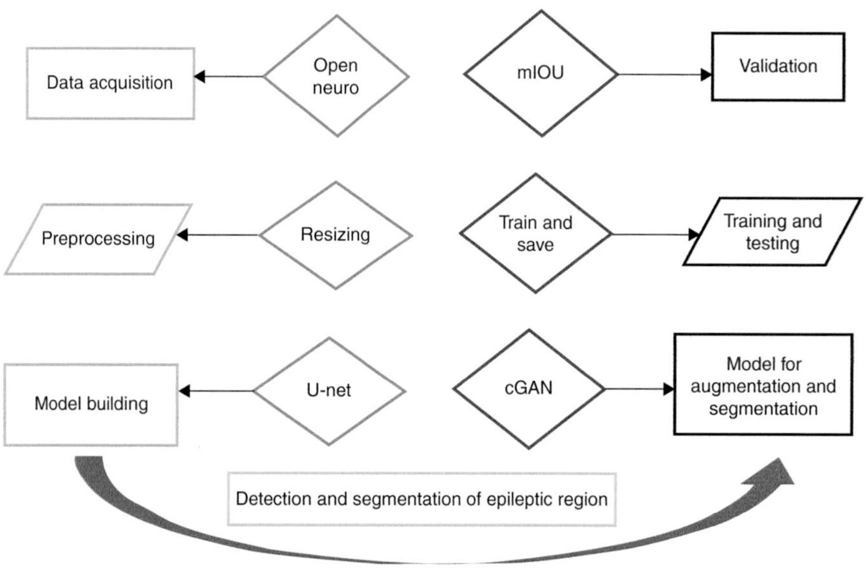

FIGURE 2.1 Workflow of MRI segmentation for FCD type II detection.

The workflow proceeds as follows:

- Data Acquisition: MRI brain scan images of patients diagnosed with FCD type II were sourced.
- Preprocessing: In this phase, enhancement and normalization procedures were performed on the data to enable a single input to be fed to the deep learning networks.
- Model Training and Testing: Both the UNet and CGAN models were fitted on the acquired data and their effectiveness in accurately segmenting the data with epileptic regions was assessed.
- Evaluation: The models were evaluated based on conventional standard metrics, including accuracy, loss, and mIOU.

2.3.2 Data Description

The dataset was obtained from "Open Neuro," and includes a collection of pre-surgery MRI scans of patients with FCD type II and seizures. It contains 170 MRI images in the Neuroimaging Informatics Technology Initiative (Nifty) format. Each subject enrolled in the dataset has a photo with no masking and with masking techniques applied. Such a dataset is of considerable help in understanding the structural brain malformations caused by epilepsy and FCD type II, thereby giving researchers a chance to evaluate and provide diagnostic and therapeutic measures to these conditions.

2.3.3 Anatomical plane

Figure 2.2 shows the anatomical planes showing the epileptic regions in a brain MRI. Coronal, transversal (commonly referred to as axial), and sagittal metplanes are critical orientations in medicine that assist in three-dimensional imaging of the brain in patients with FCD epilepsy. By utilizing all planes, structural deformations of the brain can be assessed, enabling the identification of the affected sites with FCD.

2.3.3.1 Coronal Plane

In the coronal plane, the brain is divided into two components: anterior and posterior regions. In the anatomical imaging, it is possible to view two-dimensional objects in three-dimensions, allowing stereological analysis of the structures in coronal section from the front to the rear and thus spotting such abnormalities as FCD lesions.

2.3.3.2 Transversal (Axial) Plane

The transverse or vertebral plane structure of the brain has its horizontal cross-sections taken above its horizontal base and below its horizontal cut. During scans performed in the axial plane,

the head-basis is sliced horizontally thereby leading to the identification of vulnerable regions with lesions. These lesions aid in detecting FCD epilepsy disturbed areas through a single semi-circle upright scan segment..

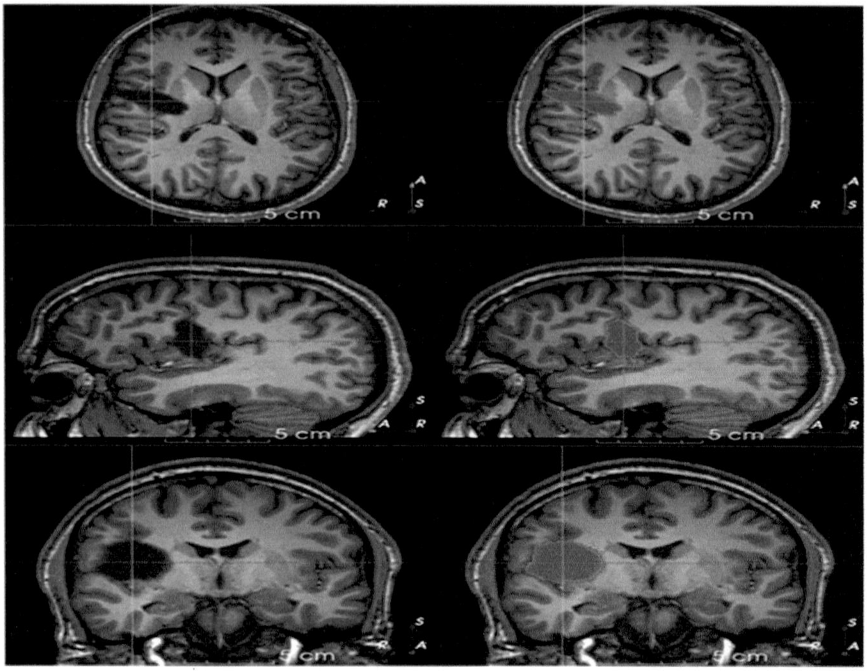

FIGURE 2.2 Anatomical planes showing epileptic regions in brain MRI.

2.3.3.3 Sagittal Plane

Figure 2.3 shows the MRI anatomical planes for FCD analysis. The sagittal plane is the vertical division of the brain into the left and right hemispheres. Head imaging scans yield one semi-sectional area perpendicular across the two humanoid frontal sections, subdividing the head into eight slices comprising six major cross-sections from the coronal and axial orientations. These scans are used to train the algorithm to detect areas of the structures affected by nodules using the CDF matrix.

The three perspectives—coronal, transversal, and sagittal—are essential in evaluating both the average and the distribution of FCD lesions in the brain's cortex. The integration of anatomical orientations and FCD lesions is highlighted by creating an MRI image where areas affected by lesions are colored red. The difference in color between lesions and normal tissues helps in establishing a diagnosis. This visual distinction between lesions and healthy tissue aids in diagnosis. By overlaying or highlighting FCD lesions in red on images obtained from each plane, clinicians can precisely localize and assess the impact of these lesions on brain function, guiding treatment strategies for individuals with FCD epilepsy.

2.3.4 MRI with Mask

A function is designed to segment lesion areas in MRI scans by utilizing a provided segmentation mask. The segmentation mask, typically represented as a binary image,

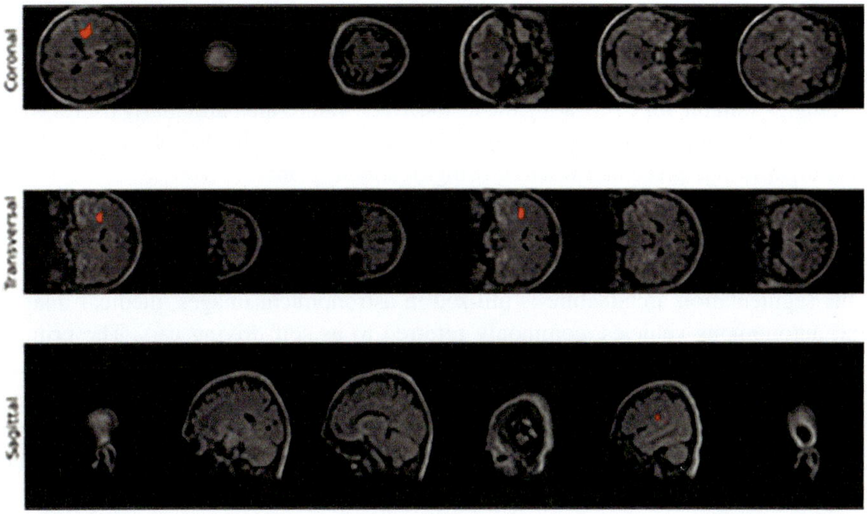

FIGURE 2.3 MRI anatomical planes for FCD analysis.

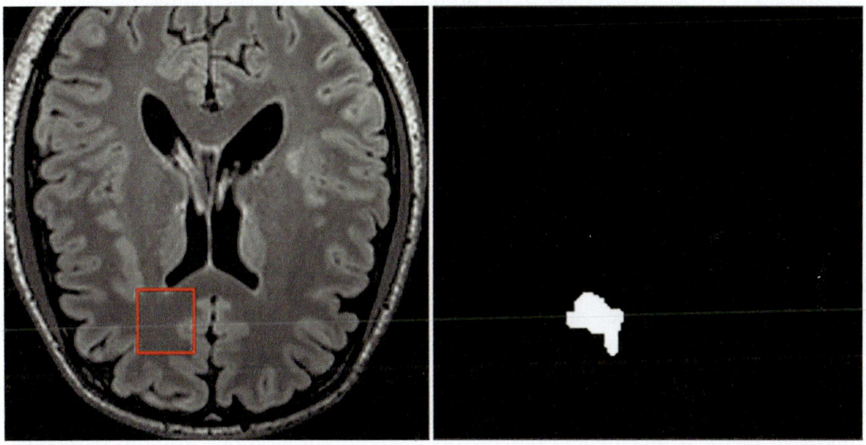

FIGURE 2.4 MRI image with segmented epileptic region.

is converted into a uint8 format for compatibility with OpenCV functions. OpenCV's find Contours function is employed to identify contours within the segmentation mask. Contours represent continuous regions of interest in the image. Among the contours detected, the function determines the largest one. Figure 2.4 shows the MRI image with the segmented epileptic region.

This contour is most likely to correspond to the lesion area in the MRI scan. From the most prominent contour, the function extracts the bounding box coordinates. These coordinates describe the rectangular region that encapsulates the lesion region. The last step involves retrieving the box coordinates, also known as bounding box coordinates, in the form of (x, y, width, height), to accurately describe the lesion area in relation to the MRI image. To conclude, the function efficiently handles large images using binary matrix representations and extracts the coordinates of bounding rectangles suitable for delineating the lesion. Such values are particularly useful when further diagnosing a patient, allowing for a clear outline of the disease stage and specific organs to be presented when drawing treatment plans.

2.3.5 UNET

This segmentation architecture is utilized in astronomical images, medical images, and autonomous vehicles, commonly referred to as self-driving cars. The primary distinguishing feature of this network is its architecture, which comprises two parts: an encoder and a decoder, as well as combinations of these parts that facilitate the isolation of specific objects. The first part comprises several components, primarily consisting of convolutions followed by max-pooling, which is sometimes referred to as a down-sampling operation that progressively reduces the spatial dimensions while increasing the number of feature maps. The decoder, in contrast, contains m layers for up-sampling, such as transposed convolutions, followed by additional convolutional layers. It is expected to reconstruct the spatial details that are missing due to encoding. Figure 2.5 shows the UNet architecture for MRI segmentation.

The UNet completes the connection of structures by introducing skip connections, which are connections that join encoder and decoder structures with similar spatial resolution, thereby linking the input layer and the output layer. With these skip connections, the decoder can utilize the encoded high-resolution feature maps for improved object segmentation, thereby enhancing the model's precision in segmenting regions of interest. By incorporating both low-level and high-level features, U-Net effectively combines local and global information, enhancing segmentation accuracy. During decoding, feature maps from the encoder are concatenated with those from the decoder. This feature fusion process enables the network to leverage both local context from the encoder and contextual information from the decoder, resulting in more accurate segmentation. Then, it employs pixel-wise loss functions, such as cross-entropy loss. Therefore, it takes an input image and produces a corresponding segmentation mask. The segmentation mask highlights regions of interest, such as tumors in medical images and objects on roads in autonomous driving, with pixel-level accuracy.

2.3.5.1 UNet Architecture

The architecture begins with an input layer of size $64 \times 64 \times 16 \times 1$. The contracting path (encoder) comprises multiple convolutional layers with ReLU activation and padding layers, which reduce spatial dimensions and extract features at different scales. Max-pooling layers are used to down-sample feature maps. The expansive path (decoder) begins by transposing convolutional layers to up-sample the feature maps. Concatenation layers combine feature maps from the encoder path and the decoder path. Convolutional layers are used in the decoder to refine the segmentation. The code continues this pattern of up-sampling and refining with additional layers.

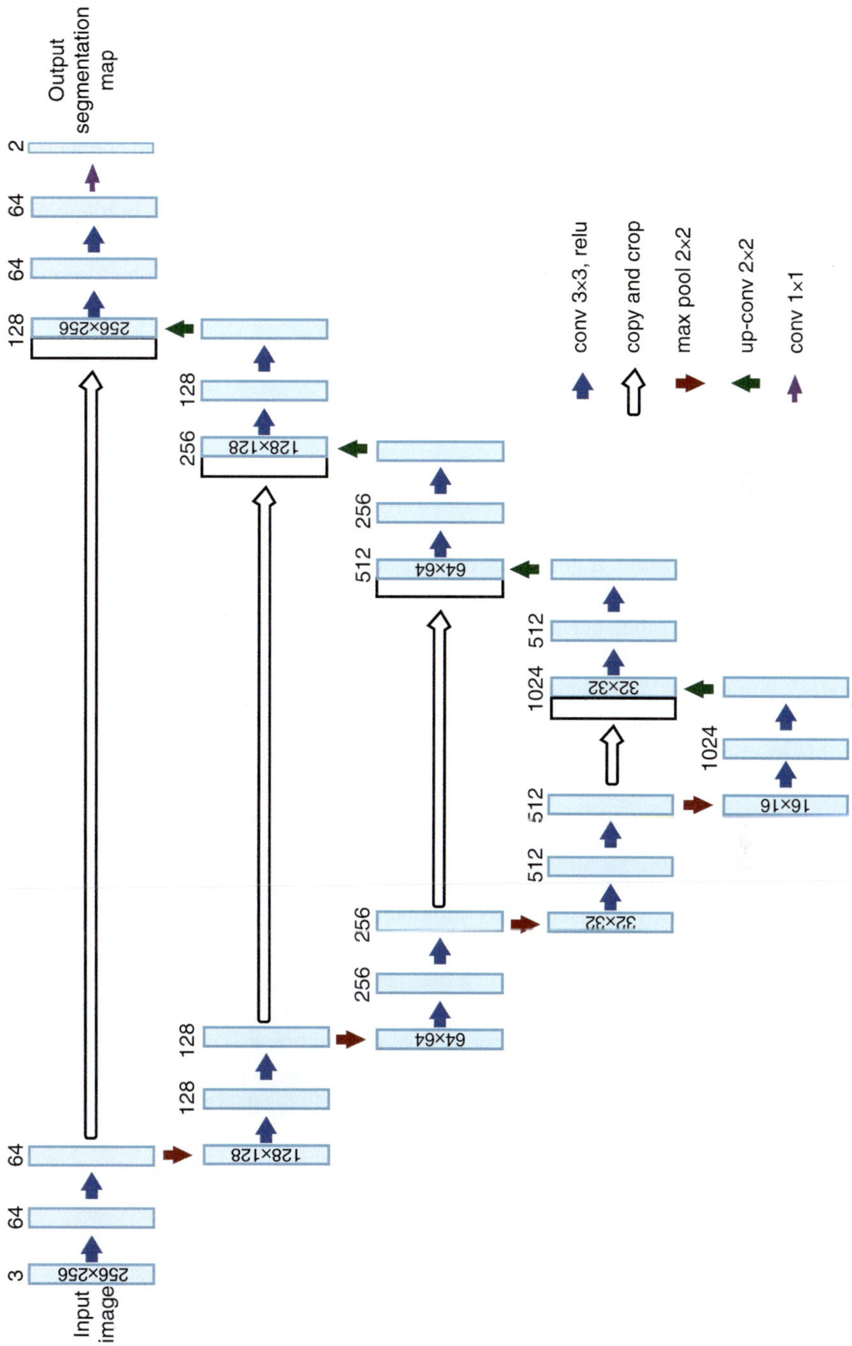

FIGURE 2.5 UNet architecture for MRI segmentation.

The decoder's output is flattened, followed by a dense layer with ReLU activation. The final output layer predicts the classification classes using the softmax activation function, and the U-Net model is instantiated. The down-sampling function defines a block in the encoder part. It consists of two 3D convolutional layers, followed by max pooling. These layers learn hierarchical features, while max-pooling reduces spatial dimensions. The up-sampling function defines a block in the decoder part of the U-Net model. It involves up-sampling followed by concatenation with skip connections from the corresponding encoder layers. Two 3D convolutional layers then process the concatenated feature maps. The bottleneck block function defines the bottleneck or central block of the U-Net model. It consists of two 3D conv layers with no down-sampling or up-sampling incorporated into the layers. The bottleneck block acquires high-level semantic features but loses the spatial outlines. GAN offers an option and a more domain-focused technique for data augmentation.

2.3.6 GAN

GAN has been reported to be effective in various generative tasks, including image generation, text generation, and music generation, among others. Saberi orients this concept within the context of games, where it is premised on adversarial training of two models: the ROC, a generator model; and its counterpart, the discriminator model. Now, through these competitive mechanisms, these models not only strive to outperform each other but also complement one another, leading to continuous improvements in the quality of the generated output. The Generator is a model that imitates other images and creates new, realistic examples from the particular domain for which it was trained. It takes random noise or input data as a seed and generates sensible examples. Its aim is to produce instances that cannot be differentiated from the genuine cases in that field. The Discriminator comes into play here as a sort of classifier, separating actual instances (from the field) from phony cases (through the Generator). It is intended to classify each of the raster into two binary classes: 'real' (where the raster originates from the field) and 'fake' (when the raster is generated). Pix2Pix is an extensively used GAN architecture for image-to-image translation tasks. These networks, termed as conditional adversarial networks, offer a versatile solution for various image translation challenges. In addition to acquiring the ability to map input images to corresponding output images, they possess the capability to learn a loss function to facilitate the training of this mapping. This unique characteristic enables the application of a unified approach to address problems that traditionally necessitate distinct loss formulations. Figure 2.6 shows the GAN architecture for MRI image generation.

2.3.6.1 Conditional GAN

Conditional GAN (CGAN) enables us to incorporate additional information, such as class labels, into the network. During training, images are provided to the network along with their corresponding labels, such as a mask image that locates the affected region of epilepsy in the brain MRI. This enables the network to distinguish between different classes. Consequently, we can instruct the model to generate images of specific flowers by specifying the desired class label.

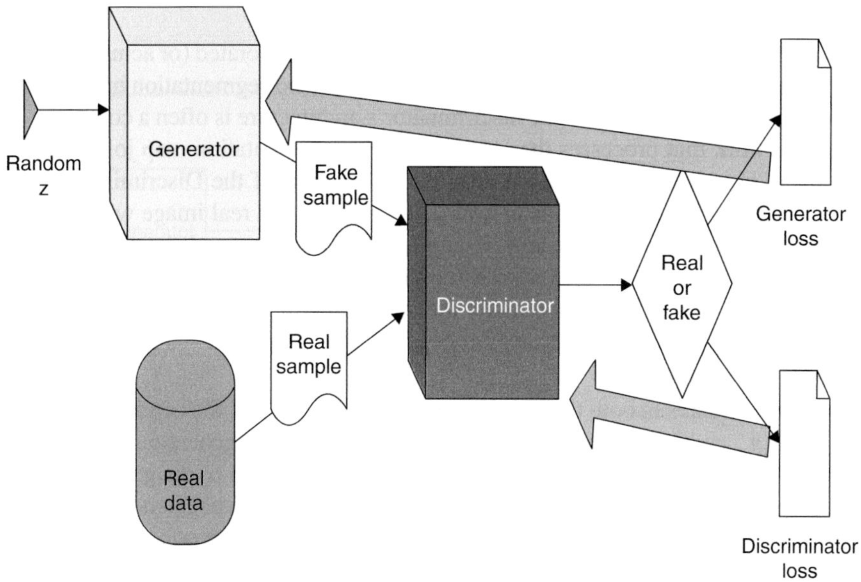

FIGURE 2.6 GAN architecture for MRI image generation.

2.3.7 CGAN Architecture

2.3.7.1 Loss Function

The loss function used in CGANs for segmentation typically consists of two components: adversarial loss and task-specific loss.

$$L_{GAN} = E_{x,y}[\log D(x,y)] + E_{x,z}[\log(1-D(x,G(x,z)))] \tag{2.1}$$

Adversarial Loss: This component encourages the generator to produce segmentation maps that are indistinguishable from real segmentation maps. It is formulated as a binary cross-entropy loss, where the discriminator tries to classify whether the segmentation map is accurate or generated.

$$L_{L1} = E_{x,y,z}[\|y-G(x,z)\|_1] \tag{2.2}$$

Task-Specific Loss: This component ensures that the generated segmentation maps accurately represent the objects in the input image. Common choices include pixel-wise loss functions such as Mean Squared Error (MSE) or Dice Loss.

$$G^* = \arg \min G (\min_D L_{GAN}(G,D) + \lambda L_{L1}(G)) \tag{2.3}$$

The overall loss function is a combination of these two components, often weighted according to the importance of each.

mIOU is a metric used to evaluate the performance of a segmentation model.

$$Mean\,IOU = \frac{1}{n}\sum_{k=i}^{n} IOU \tag{2.5}$$

2.4 RESULTS AND DISCUSSION

2.4.1 UNet Performance

The UNet model was observed to be highly effective in segmenting FCD type II regions from MRI images. The training accuracy was 99%, which suggests the ability of the model to understand and learn the pixel-wise labeling of epileptogenic areas. The model's performance was evaluated using the IoU metric. The performance in identifying epileptogenic regions among the adjacent cortex was also handled. Figure 2.9 shows the UNet performance in segmenting epileptic regions.

The results, as illustrated in Figure 2.10, also depict a steady increase in the IoU over successive epochs, culminating in a final mean IoU of more than 0.85 at the end of the validation phase, which again supports the reliability of the segmentation.

	epoch	acc	loss	mean_io_u	unet_loss	val_acc	val_loss	val_mean_io_u	val_unet_loss
0	0	0.998014	0.028771	0.499441	2.012249	0.999183	0.002420	0.499971	0.736983
1	1	0.998841	0.004237	0.499442	0.810860	0.999183	0.002196	0.499971	0.760245
2	2	0.998865	0.003589	0.499501	0.792611	0.999183	0.002257	0.499971	0.726909
3	3	0.998857	0.005152	0.499453	0.813887	0.999183	0.002861	0.499971	0.843373
4	4	0.998850	0.005082	0.499450	0.835808	0.999183	0.002358	0.499971	0.723533
5	5	0.999066	0.002868	0.499709	0.768509	0.999183	0.002214	0.499971	0.801150
6	6	0.998714	0.005898	0.499289	0.848994	0.999183	0.012171	0.499971	0.721289
7	7	0.998838	0.005305	0.499393	0.783660	0.999183	0.002587	0.499971	0.838868
8	8	0.998854	0.003303	0.499461	0.794753	0.999183	0.002077	0.499971	0.755023
9	9	0.999004	0.002751	0.499640	0.769336	0.999183	0.002062	0.499971	0.756626
10	10	0.998885	0.003250	0.499480	0.787316	0.999183	0.002521	0.499971	0.835813
40	40	0.998955	0.002650	0.499523	0.778535	0.999183	0.002076	0.499971	0.767425
41	41	0.998635	0.003548	0.499153	0.796421	0.999183	0.002076	0.499971	0.767425
42	42	0.998737	0.003310	0.499294	0.791190	0.999183	0.002076	0.499971	0.767425
43	43	0.998964	0.002659	0.499566	0.775730	0.999183	0.002076	0.499971	0.767425
44	44	0.998939	0.002704	0.499538	0.778636	0.999183	0.002076	0.499971	0.767425
45	45	0.998873	0.002906	0.499453	0.782213	0.999183	0.002076	0.499971	0.767425
46	46	0.998750	0.003218	0.499311	0.788843	0.999183	0.002076	0.499971	0.767425
47	47	0.998766	0.003212	0.499319	0.789227	0.999183	0.002076	0.499971	0.767425
48	48	0.998854	0.002951	0.499441	0.783302	0.999183	0.002076	0.499971	0.767425
49	49	0.998854	0.002938	0.499451	0.783138	0.999183	0.002076	0.499971	0.767425

FIGURE 2.9 UNet performance in segmenting epileptic regions.

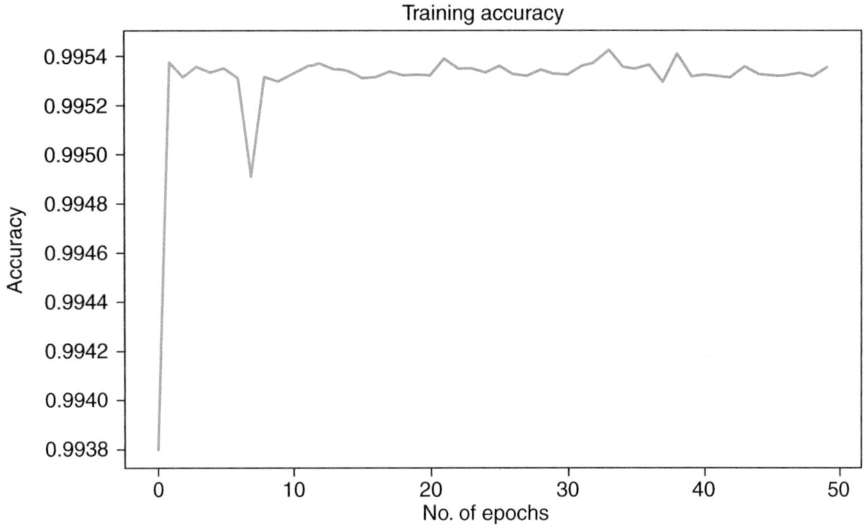

FIGURE 2.10 Training accuracy of UNet model over epochs.

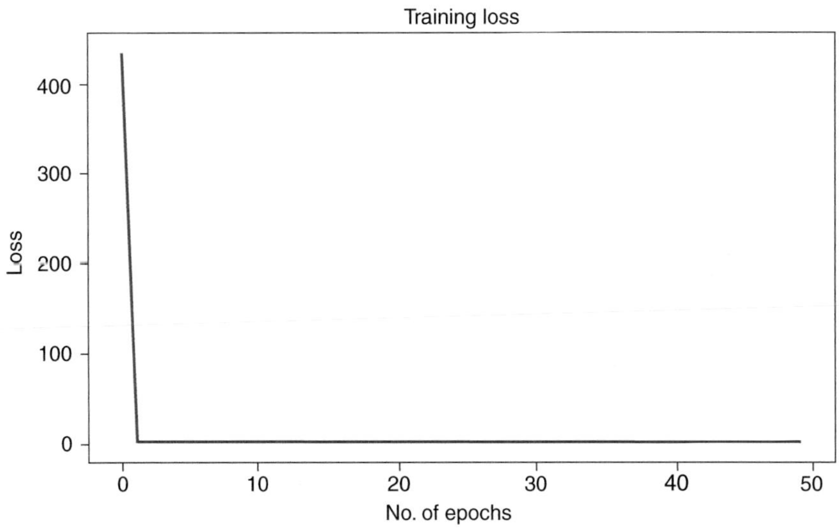

FIGURE 2.11 UNet training loss during segmentation model training.

Equally important, the loss function depicted in Figure 2.11 consistently showed a decreasing trend, indicating that the model was able to reduce errors during its training phase. These results highlight the UNet architecture's ability to extract subtle features from MRI images, which are crucial in delineating the abnormal contours of FCD. Much of the success of the UNet model can be attributed to the encoder-decoder architecture with skip connections.

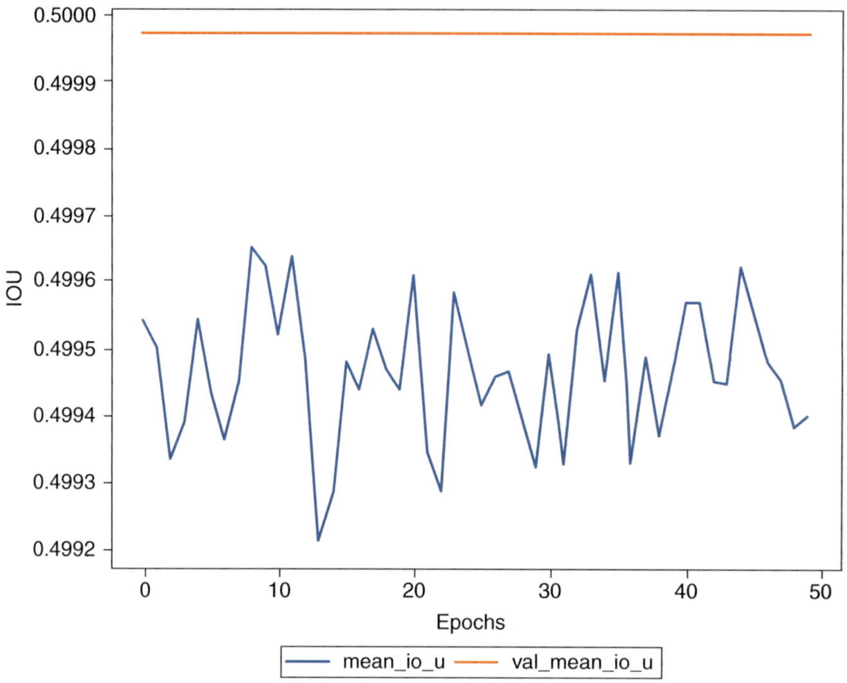

FIGURE 2.12 Mean intersection over union (IoU) scores for UNet model.

UNet has enabled the maintenance of high-resolution details, which is essential for accurate segmentation. This is especially true for medical images, which often contain small and delicate regions of interest. In addition, it is also worth noting that, due to the limited availability of annotated data, UNet is particularly useful for medical image analysis, including the current task, as annotated datasets are scarce.

Figure 2.12 provides an overview of the mIoU scores achieved by the UNet model across different epochs during both training and validation phases. This graph provides a visual representation of how the model's segmentation performance evolves during training. Figure 2.14 shows the mean IoU scores for the CGAN model.

2.4.2 CGAN

For the conditional Generative Adversarial Network (CGAN), usage of mIoU approach proved effective, although its performance on this specific project fell short of that of the UNet model. In terms of typical performance indicators, the CGAN achieved a lower IoU, with an average of 0.5, indicating that it had difficulties with muscle segmentation, particularly in distinguishing epileptic regions from other non-epileptic tissues.

The volumetric contraption of the CGAN, as observed in the generator and discriminator loss figures (Figure 2.13), resulted in delays in processing, as the CGAN demonstrated only reasonably good performance but was less effective compared

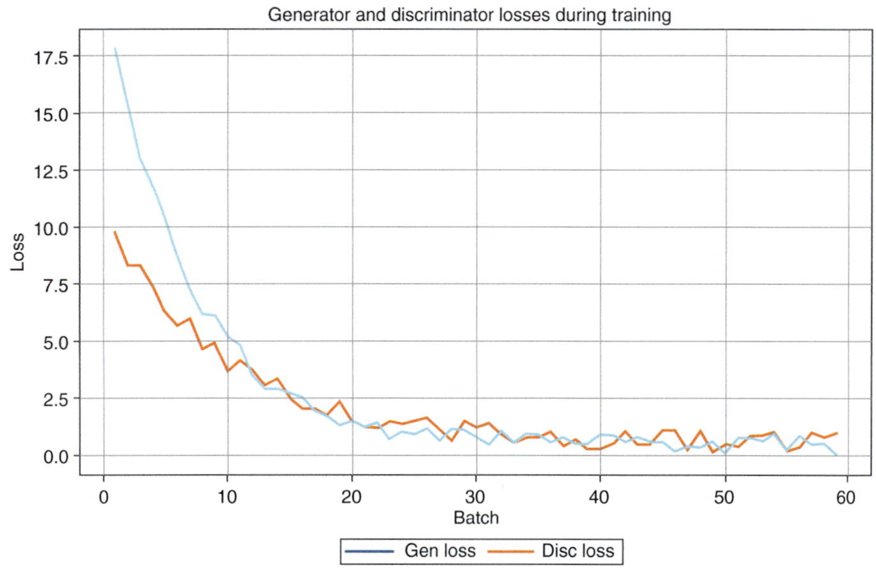

FIGURE 2.13 Generator and discriminator loss during cGAN model training.

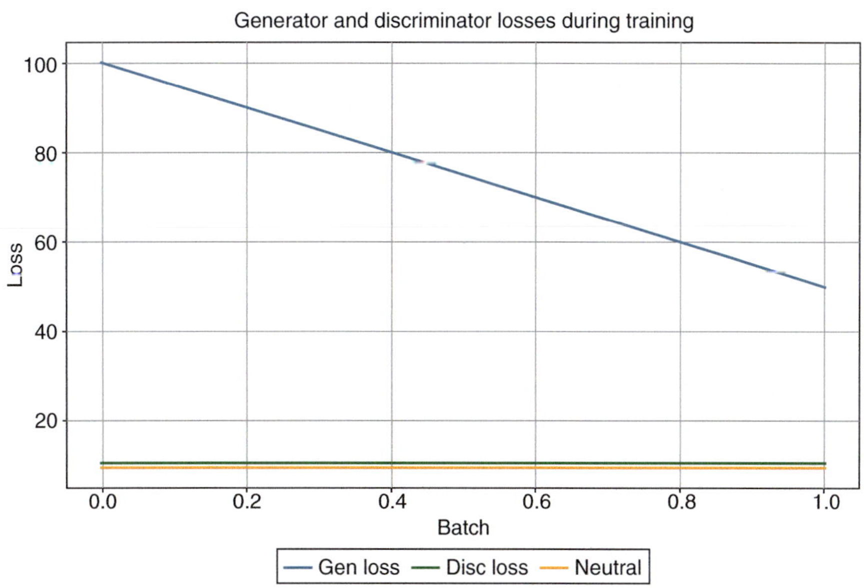

FIGURE 2.14 Mean intersection over union (IoU) scores for CGAN model.

to the UNet architecture. The concept of competing generators and discriminators, which improves performance for CGANs, is an excellent idea of an inclusive approach. Moreover, the CGAN's structure comprises the convoluted Generator and Discriminator models, which also incorporate surrounding contextual images, thereby leading to decreased accuracy in CT segmentation tasks. Despite the capabilities of CGAN and the absence of revolutionary changes in neural structures, CGAN frameworks take one step further in the quest for generalized image generation in specific tasks. However, they fail to be as effective on medical images, particularly in image segmentation tasks, due to the limitations of CGAN.

2.4.3 Discussion

Thus, the current study helps to understand the clear benefits of applying UNet compared to CGAN in segmenting FCD type II regions from MRI. The reason behind UNet's effectiveness in this task may be that it handles both local and global information efficiently, which is particularly useful in medical image segmentation. On the other hand, although the more sophisticated structure and longer training process of CGAN give more hope for other types of tasks, it still did not deliver as much accuracy/speed as required.

Additionally, the research highlights the rationale behind selecting models based on the type of data and the task requirements. While GANs have been proven to be quite flexible in generating images, medical image segmentation requires models that are detail-oriented and accurate, which is the case with UNet.

2.5 CONCLUSION

The chapter investigated issues related to the automated segmentation of FCD type II in MRI images using deep learning architectures, namely UNet and Conditional Generative Adversarial Networks (CGANs). Consequently, the paper demonstrated that the accuracy metrics, as well as the computation time, in using a UNet architecture were superior to those of CGAN approaches. Even though there were issues with the speed and accuracy of the UNet, the model achieved a mean IoU index of 0.85 and a training accuracy of 99%, thereby validating its efficiency in segmenting regions with epilepsy, making it a suitable algorithm in analytical radiology. By contrast, this aspect of a novel CGAN design did not perform satisfactorily, as the achieved IoUs consistently registered below 0.5, despite training and subjecting it to the correlations of the entire analysis series. The Barker and Instrumentation increased the degree of computing, both in hardware and software, as well as the time and space required for the performance of such activities. CGAN's chances of success were sufficiently reduced and thus CGAN's viability for this sort of work is improvised by using UNet. To achieve the objective of identifying the factors that hinder the patient's histopathological specificity in FCD epilepsy, the authors utilize the UNet architecture for medical image segmentation, which enables the capture of finer details without compromising accuracy. It is also suggested, on the other hand, that high-resolution pictures of FDN and FCD would help in boosting the performance of the algorithn.

REFERENCES

[1] Zohreh Ganji, Mohsen Aghaee Hakak, Seyed Amir Zamanpour, Hoda Zare. Automatic detection of focal cortical dysplasia type ii in mri: is the application of surface-based morphometry and machine learning promising?, Frontiers in Human Neuroscience, vol. 15, p. 608285 (2021).

[2] Oscar D. Pedrayes, Darío G. Lema, Daniel F. García, Rubén Usamentiaga, Ángela Alonso, Evaluation of semantic segmentation methods for land use with spectral imaging using Sentinel-2 and PNOA imagery. *Remote Sensing*, vol. 13, no. 12, p. 2292 (2021).

[3] Huang Jianjun, et al., Identifying epilepsy based on deep learning using DKI images, *Frontiers in Human Neuroscience*, vol. 14, p. 590815, ISSN=1662-5161 (2020).

[4] Loukas Ilias, Dimitris Askounis, John Psarras, Multimodal detection of epilepsy with deep neural networks, *Expert Systems with Applications*, vol. 213, no. Part B, p. 119010 (2023).

[5] Erik H. Middlebrooks, Elena Greco, Xiangzhi Zhou, Vivek Gupta, Brin E. Freund, Amit K. Agarwal, M. Erin, Edge-Enhancing Gradient Echo MRI at 7T for detection of focal cortical dysplasia in epilepsy, *Neuroimage: Reports*, vol. 3, no. 4 (2023).

[6] Oh Shu Lih, et al., EpilepsyNet: Novel automated detection of epilepsy using transformer model with EEG signals from 121 patient population, *Computers in Biology and Medicine*, vol. 164, p. 107312, ISSN 0010-4825 (2023).

[7] Cansel Ficici, Ziya Telatar, Osman Erogul, Localization of epileptic focus by gray matter reduction analysis from brain MR images for temporal lobe epilepsy patients, *Biomedical Signal Processing and Control*, vol. 83, p. 104716, ISSN 1746-8094 (2023).

[8] Mingkan Shen, et al., Real-time epilepsy seizure detection based on EEG using tunable- Q wavelet transform and convolutional neural network, *Biomedical Signal Processing and Control*, vol. 82, p. 104566, ISSN 1746-8094 (2023).

[9] Haruki Yamane, Shinji Fukui, Yuji Iwahori, Hiroyasu Usami, M.K. Bhuyan, Naotaka Ogasawara, Kunio Kasugai, Automatic generation of polyp image using depth map for endoscope dataset, *Procedia Computer Science*, vol. 192, pp. 2355–2364 (2021). https://doi.org/10.1016/j.procs.2021.09.011

[10] Michaela Bartoňová, et al., The benefit of the diffusion kurtosis imaging in presurgical evaluation in patients with focal MR-negative epilepsy, *Science Reports*, vol. 11, p. 14208 (2021).

[11] T. Jin, X.W. Ye, Z.X. Li, Establishment and evaluation of conditional GAN-based image dataset for semantic segmentation of structural cracks, *Engineering Structures*, vol. 285, p. 116058 (2023).

[12] Yongtao Zhang, Jianqin Feng, Xiao Guo, Yande Ren, Comparative analysis of U-Net and TLMDB GAN for the cardiovascular segmentation of the ventricles in the heart, *Computer Methods and Programs in Biomedicine*, vol. 215, Article 106614 (2022). https://doi.org/10.1016/j.cmpb.2021.106614

[13] Deepika Koundal, Bhisham Sharma, Challenges and future directions in neutrosophic set-based medical image analysis, In Y. Guo & A. S. Ashour (Eds.), *Neutrosophic Set in Medical Image Analysis* (pp. 313–343). Academic Press (2019).

3 Design and Optimization of a Multiaxial Knee Exoskeleton for Lower Limb Rehabilitation

Ravindrakumar Selvaraj, Justin Paul J, Kishore Kumar D.S, Sebasheela T, and Theivanai T

3.1 INTRODUCTION

Exoskeletons promise to revolutionize rehabilitation and assistive technology, especially for individuals with mobility impairments. Challenges in this area exist and must be addressed to unlock the full potential of exoskeleton designs. Most conventional approaches to exoskeleton design have yielded designs that are heavy and impractical to wear for extended periods. Construction materials, primarily metals and rigid plastics, add to the weight and inconvenience, making them less practical for everyday use. In addition, the cost of these materials, combined with the sophisticated technology used, often renders exoskeletons too expensive for those who are most likely to benefit from their use. The third problem with exoskeletons is mechanical failure. The modern exoskeleton, with its complex mechanical and electrical system, often collapses due to damage, which decreases reliability and results in enhanced maintenance costs. Such failures threaten the user's safety and are both costly and time-consuming to repair. Researchers continually assess new materials, designs, and technologies to overcome these challenges. Lightweight materials, such as carbon fiber and advanced composites, can significantly reduce the weight of exoskeletons, thereby improving comfort and usability. Meanwhile, soft exosuits incorporating flexible materials and inflatable elements are being developed to provide support while maintaining a non-bulky and flexible design. These soft alternatives can offer more comfort and flexibility than traditional designs, which are often stiff. Another strategy also being developed is modular design, which makes maintenance and customization easier. Because different modules can be easily replaced or upgraded, these systems can offer a longer lifespan for the devices, as well as reduced maintenance costs. This also means customization that allows the design of the exoskeleton to meet the user's needs, making this technology more effective in the long run. However, another area of emerging new developments is related to advanced control systems. However, by utilizing machine learning and artificial intelligence, such systems can learn from a user over time to become more accurately calibrated for their movements, thereby

DOI: 10.1201/9781003561309-3

becoming more attuned to the user's needs. Such systems begin to learn specific patterns. Additionally, such systems would enable more intuitive and personalized support, resulting in a significantly enhanced end-user experience. With innovations in materials and technology, these next-generation exoskeletons may become more effective, practical, and accessible by addressing key issues such as weight, cost, reliability, and adaptability. These advances will significantly enhance the quality of life for patients with mobility issues. Impairments give the individual more independence and functionality.

The aim here is to construct a lower-limb exoskeleton for rehabilitation in orthotic patients; in this aspect, the system must enhance biomechanical support, kinematic alignment, and dynamic stability, which are of utmost importance. The exoskeleton system must be integrated with advanced technologies, including adaptive gait correction algorithms, sensor fusion for real-time feedback, and motion capture systems to monitor the patient's progress. Integrating force distribution mechanisms and joint actuation systems ensures smoother joint mobility. Materials such as carbon fiber composites, thermoplastic elastomers like polyurethane, and lightweight aerospace-grade aluminum alloys should exhibit high strength-to-weight ratios, corrosion resistance, and fatigue resistance, ensuring long-term durability and patient comfort. With multi-degree-of-freedom actuators and soft wearable sensors, the wearable robots can offer the most ergonomic experience through faithful torque control and load-bearing support from head to heel. In this regard, active exoskeletal components, as well as smart textiles for pressure redistribution, could be achieved through a system that not only rehabilitates the patient's mobility but also ideally aligns with their posture and reduces the risk of pressure sores or discomfort. Furthermore, through the use of machine learning algorithms in adaptive control and personalized rehabilitation protocols, the exoskeleton would be able to adapt to the patient's specific needs and requirements. Thus, rehabilitation technology can provide patients with a personalized therapy experience tailored to their individual needs. Such is the trend in materials science, and Mechatronics will enable the construction of a lighter, stronger, yet more comfortable device for the patient, thereby allowing for optimal rehabilitation.

3.2 LITERATURE SURVEY

SETS, which is short for Smart Exoskeleton Tremor Suppression, demonstrated a notable reduction at the wrist level, recording a 61.39% drop in acceleration magnitude and a 56.22% decline in angular velocity, thereby indicating mechanical efficiency in this system [1]. That being the case, these numbers indicate the healing capabilities of the system using SETS, as tremors were considerably reduced. This determines the ability to cancel undesirable movements at the wrist. More specifically, the percentages highlight the system's capacity to handle the magnitude of acceleration and its angular velocity content. This level of performance underscores the reliability and functional capability of SETS to have a significant mechanical impact on patients affected by wrist tremors, making it an up-and-coming solution for tremor cancellation.

A study, titled "Biomimetic Exoskeleton Controller for Enhancing Gait Balance and Minimizing Muscle Activity During Walking" [2], involved developing a controller to stabilize gait while minimizing the effort exerted by muscles during walking. The newly devised, innovative controller was experimentally implemented on the developed bilateral ankle exoskeleton, which is based on a well-defined biomechanical model. The results, obtained from trials involving 12 subjects, revealed reduced calf muscle activation under the exoskeleton support during steady-state walking compared to a minimal impedance controller ($p < 0.001$). More importantly, when the controller was used without center of mass feedback, muscle activity decreased by 9% ($p = 0.026$) and 18% ($p = 0.002$) in response to muscle perturbations simulating push and pull conditions, respectively. These types of perturbations were considered to simulate some of the most challenging conditions of walking in the real world. Conclusions: The results show that the developed biomimetic controller exhibits a notable ability to reduce physical effort in the musculature while providing substantial support for balance during walking. The system's ability to adapt to various types of perturbation scenarios further emphasizes its effectiveness as an assistive device in impaired gait conditions. Such exoskeleton systems might enable individuals to walk, improve mobility, and reduce the physical burden on the users, thus marking an advancement in the world of assistive technologies.

As human-computer interaction devices, lower limb exoskeletons, have gained significant interest in the last few years with the aim of assisting, augmenting, treating, or protecting the human body [3]. Researchers have emphasized the need to improve these systems to establish more effective ones that enhance rehabilitation, mobility assistance, and other forms of physical improvement. A critical point of such devices is the contact between the exoskeleton and the user, which is primarily controlled by the exoskeleton's sensing and actuation systems. Those systems are of paramount importance in making the final difference between efficiency and comfort when using an exoskeleton for lower limb assistance or augmentation. However, it is still a long way from the broader application of lower-limb exoskeletons, as the sensing and control technologies do not yet meet the current standards. Effect sensing and precise control ensure smooth and responsive movement; however, popular techniques often fail to meet these needs due to the lack of real-time feedback and adaptability. The study examined how sensor type and control model affect the functionality of such devices and their impact on the user experience. The paper describes several complex problems related to exoskeleton control, primarily concerning stabilization and comfort for the wearer. Fundamental technical issues arise from the complexity of the real-time interaction between the exoskeleton and its wearer's body, compounded by the need for accurate movement control. Moreover, the paper identifies emerging technologies that may support future innovations in actuators, functional materials, invasive and epidermal electronic sensors, and data-driven deep learning approaches. The study will pave the way for future work in advancing sensing and control techniques that enhance the precision and adaptability of exoskeleton systems. Even by further introducing cutting-edge technologies and novel approaches, it would become possible to overcome its current limitations and, thus, facilitate the use of lower-limb exoskeletons to a significantly greater degree, ranging from actual applications to medical rehabilitation and physical enhancement.

Lower limb exoskeletons or wearable lower-body robots have emerged rapidly in the last decade, following Hao Lee's work [4]. There are three types of lower limb exoskeletons available: assistive, restorative, and augmentative exoskeletons. The first two types of exoskeletons are designed for use by the elderly or individuals with neurological disorders. Assistive exoskeletons are more focused on clients who will never walk again. These exoskeletons support or replace the user's disabled body parts, allowing the client to live and act like an able-bodied individual while wearing the device. Precise position control, typically achieved with electric motors, is the most common combination for this type of exoskeleton. On the other hand, restoration exoskeletons aim to assist patients with disabilities who can recover through treatment and preparation. These designs aim to facilitate patient contact, enabling recovery and ultimately achieving typical performance without the need for the device. An exoskeleton of this kind often employs impedance control to provide resistance during training. Augmentative exoskeletons, the third type, are designed to support healthy users performing tasks that would otherwise be difficult or impossible without assistance, such as lifting heavy loads or extended endurance activities. Positive feedback or force control is typical for this class because the device must accurately track the user's movement. Much more common for actuators in this class are higher power density types, such as pressure-driven, pneumatic setup flexible actuators. Several successful exoskeletons are described in the literature, although the evaluation of weight, stability, and user expectations are still evolving and require further improvement. Being light, strong, and capable of locking incessantly with the user will determine the course for future exoskeletons.

A fundamental aspect of exoskeleton research is adapting the device to different gait patterns as the user progresses. Determining the wearer's movement goal to control the stride preparation of the exoskeleton can effectively advance the human-machine interaction experience after using the exoskeleton [5]. A help vector machine (SVM) used for classification detects the sEMG signal on the human surface, classifying the wearer's movement posture. The location result forms the gait stride of the exoskeleton and controls its change through the interpreted intentional flag. At the same time, the validity of the designed gait was tested during locomotion. The tests demonstrate that the sEMG flag interpretation for human development and stride adjustment control in the exoskeleton robot exhibits high accuracy and real-time execution, enabling patients to complete their rehabilitation training more safely and efficiently [6].

This section reviews environmental perception technologies in lower-limb exoskeletons, including visual sensors, control systems, terrain detection, and adaptive gait planning, highlighting current challenges and future research directions [7]. The discussion begins with an overview of visual sensors and control systems, followed by a detailed examination of the key technologies involved in environmental perception, including relevant datasets, terrain detection, and adaptive gait planning tailored to the environment. The chapter concludes by surveying the current challenges that hinder the progress of environmental perception in exoskeletons and suggest future research directions [7].

Over the past few decades, although remarkable progress has been made in gait recognition for lower limb exoskeleton robots, persistent challenges still exist in their practical application within rehabilitation and clinical practice. For example, interactive information fusion technology presents a novel approach to addressing these shortcomings, suggesting a promising direction for future development. This section presents a structured review of current state-of-the-art methods applied to data acquisition, interaction, fusion, and gait recognition in lower limb exoskeleton robots [8]. To further explore this field, techniques for gait recognition based on interactive information fusion have been examined. Further, the paper outlines existing challenges, promising solutions, and future aspects. It provides valid insights for research on gait recognition and interactive information fusion in rehabilitation exoskeleton robots [8].

Robot-assisted rehabilitation and technology to support elderly populations are experiencing rapid growth. For the last three decades, lower limb exoskeletons have been at the forefront of engineering research in the context of rehabilitation and assistance [9]. However, most of them are still under research, although a few are commercially available today. The last two decades have witnessed continuous advances in technology, particularly in manufacturing techniques and materials, culminating in the development of various exoskeleton models designed to assist the elderly and individuals with disabilities in walking. Actuation and the method of actuation are critical considerations in designing such an exoskeleton. Actuation methods and the choice of actuators are critical considerations in designing lower-limb exoskeletons, as they directly influence the device's weight, performance, and overall fabrication strategy. While materials and manufacturing techniques are also important, proper actuator selection is equally vital for achieving an effective and efficient exoskeleton design. Different materials, manufacturing techniques, and actuators have been discussed in the literature. It appears that areas for improvement also exist in these areas. This paper discusses various robotic lower limb exoskeletons, examines their materials, manufacturing methods, and actuation systems, and provides a critical evaluation of their merits and demerits. The review also identifies potential future research directions for the engineering community, as well as materials, fabrication methods, and actuation systems [10].

Lower limb dysfunction has been associated with the most severe health issues and significant costs, not only in terms of human suffering but also economically [11]. Despite the efforts of experts in various fields to date, there is still no single treatment that can fully restore the lost functionality of a limb. With advancements in both biomechanics and engineering over the past 50 years, exoskeleton technology has led to significant improvements in prosthetic and orthotic support and rehabilitation for individuals with impaired limb function, and has therefore become an increasingly important area of interest for both medical and engineering communities. This chapter reviews key developments in the history of lower limb exoskeletons and examines neuromuscular interactions between users and exoskeletons over the last five decades. In the early phases, lower limb exoskeleton prototypes were still in the developmental stage. The chapter discusses some of these early designs, focusing on their structural components, sensors, and control systems. It then outlines significant landmarks in the development of modern lower-limb exoskeletons and discuss the strengths and limitations of these models. Lastly, the chapter reviews the state of the art in neuromuscular control systems and sensors, demonstrating the impact of these technologies on neuromuscular function in users. We conclude by highlighting the prospect of future innovations through the integration of diverse existing technologies to achieve various goals using lower limb exoskeletons.

Since the beginning of the 2000s, scientists have been developing lower limb exoskeletons that decrease the metabolic cost of walking and running compared to human locomotion without a device, while assisting with human mobility [12]. They first achieved this "metabolic cost barrier."

We undertook a literature search up to December 2019, selecting 23 studies that brought to our attention exoskeleton designs that have helped achieve improved efficiency during walking and running compared with humans. The following review synthesizes these studies, focusing on the core innovations and techniques that enabled overcoming the metabolic cost barrier across successive increments in improving user walking and running efficiency from 2003 up to nearly 2020. These advances include the physiologically informed targeting of lower-limb joints, the rapid prototyping of exoskeleton controllers using off-board actuators, mechatronic designs of both active and passive systems, as well as a renewed focus on optimizing the human-exoskeleton interface. Lastly, we outline emerging trends that are likely to propel wearable-device performance further, shaping the field and addressing future challenges for exoskeleton technology in enhancing human mobility [13].

3.3 EXISTING SYSTEM

Exoskeletons are advanced wearable devices that support and enhance human movement, particularly for patients with neurological injuries or undergoing rehabilitation. They can work either passively through mechanical means or actively use actuators in conjunction with control systems. The primary aim of exoskeletons is to augment the wearer's physical capabilities. Therefore, they prove highly significant for patients who are in the recovery phase of accidents or injuries due to neurological conditions or other debilitating health issues. Current models of exoskeletons present several significant challenges, despite their promising potential. To begin with, most exoskeletons are too heavy, thus affecting comfort and usability. The choice of materials for some of them has been inadequate, leading to questions about the strength and performance of the devices.

The high costs of development and production make them inaccessible, and problems associated with the device's life cycle may generally lower their effectiveness. These factors could limit the overall adoption of exoskeletons in both clinical applications and daily life. Here are some potential downsides to the use of exoskeletons:

Expensive: Exoskeletons are known to be very expensive, with a price range often ranging between tens of thousands and hundreds of thousands. The high initial cost may thus become a significant deterrent to the broader acceptance of this technology. High costs associated with implementing these innovations often prevent individuals from embracing the change, despite their potential to achieve significant benefits in the long run. Such financial constraints limit accessibility in areas or institutions with tight budgets. A few ideas could include cost reduction through technological advancements, subsidies, or alternative financing models. This could make the technology more economical and accessible to a larger population.

Weight and bulkiness: The exoskeleton is typically large and very heavy, making it cumbersome for the user to wear. Although these devices are intended for use in mobility and to compensate for weakness, their stiff structure can occasionally negatively impact mobility. The heaviness and bulk of these devices are indeed factors that pose a challenge to user comfort. However, they also pose a problem since they sometimes omit essential functionality over the long term or even in daily use. As such, miniaturization and lightening of exoskeletons present a primary scope in current research and development. Another important advance is in materials science, lightweight construction, and more compact designs. This is necessary for improving the wearability and practicality of exoskeletons, ultimately making them more user-friendly and suitable for a broader range of applications. More weight and larger dimensions make it difficult to maneuver in confined spaces or perform delicate tasks.

Power requirements: Exoskeletons require a power source, usually batteries, to operate. The power demands of exoskeletons can be very unforgiving in terms of duration, necessitating frequent recharges and limiting their overall use. Additionally, the dependence on an uninterrupted power supply also means that users may endure inconveniently long interruptions for extended periods of use, especially when continuous support is needed. Furthermore, this recurring need for recharging adds to the maintainability burden and could impede the device's portability, especially in areas where power sources are not readily available. Solutions to these power challenges would thus become inevitable in augmenting the practicality of exoskeletons. Further research into more energy-efficient systems, advanced battery technologies, and alternative power solutions, such as regenerative energy harvesting, could increase the device's usage time and reduce the need for constant recharging, thereby enhancing its reliability and usability experience.

Complexity and maintenance: Exoskeletons are composed of complex mechanical and electrical systems, which require frequent maintenance and necessitate technical expertise to identify and resolve fault conditions. Exoskeletons bear safety-related issues. They can break down or fail, which may result in damage to the users. The workplace is accompanied by safety and training. They equip employees with the necessary skills, reduce the likelihood of accidents, and enhance productivity. Updated safety measures protect employees and minimize the legal risks. Confident and fulfilled employees, along with a more efficient operation, are maintained through ongoing training and a healthy safety culture. There are continual improvements to provide a safe and productive work environment.

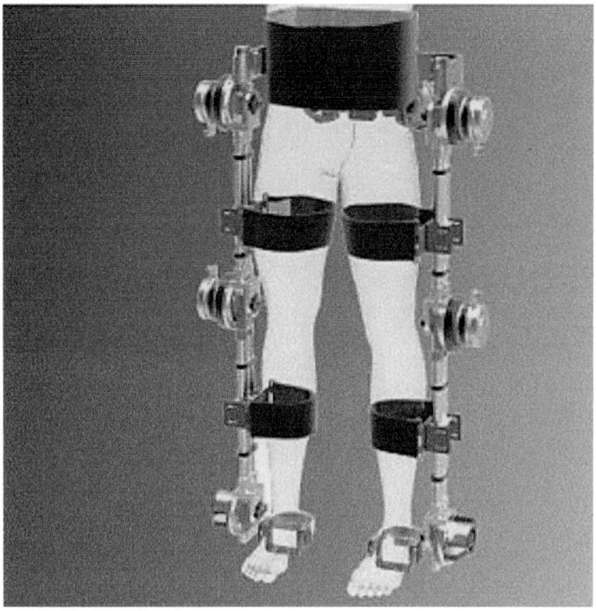

FIGURE 3.1 Mechanical lower limb exoskeleton.

Adaptation and comfort: Users must undergo a period of adaptation to become comfortable and coordinated with the exoskeleton, which can create a hurdle for immediate and effective use.

Environmental constraints: The exoskeletons may not be suitable for use in highly confined spaces, rugged terrains, or extreme temperatures, which could compromise the device's performance and dependability. The existing exoskeleton systems are illustrated in Figures 3.1, 3.2, and 3.3.

Existing systems are used as examples of the above:

ReWalk: An exoskeleton designed for the lower limbs, enabling patients to regain the ability to walk after suffering a spinal cord injury. It is motorized at the hip and knee.

Ekso Bionics: A rehabilitation exoskeleton applied to patients with paralysis or stroke, providing gait assistance through its sensors and adaptive control algorithms.

Indego: A wearable, modular exoskeleton designed for both rehabilitation purposes and personal use, providing partial or complete support based on the user's needs. These devices work to assist the user, either as a supplement to their regular movements or as a replacement for a function lost due to injury or disease. There are several reasons why lower limb exoskeletons have failed commercially and in the environment. Many of these can be classified as technical; the others fall under economic, social, or regulatory categories.

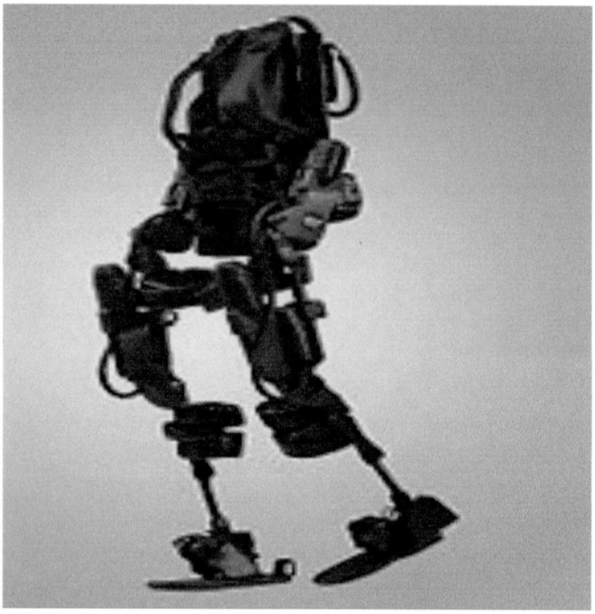

FIGURE 3.2 Robotic exoskeleton.

The following are some of the main challenges and limitations associated with the practical use of lower-limb exoskeletons:

1. Cost
   Development and Manufacturing: The cost of developing and manufacturing exoskeletons is very high, as it involves several advanced sensors, motors, and lightweight materials such as carbon fiber. This makes the product very expensive and only a few can afford it.
   Accessibility to Users: Many of the targeted users, such as individuals with spinal cord injury or stroke, cannot afford the high cost of the devices without adequate support from significant insurance.
2. Bulky and Uncomfortable Design, Weight and Size:
   Although significant progress has been made, many exoskeletons are still very heavy and bulky, making them difficult to wear for extended periods. Users are then exposed to discomfort and fatigue, thus limiting their usability in practical daily life settings.
   Fit and Customization Issues: There is a lack of flexibility in fitting exoskeletons for different body sizes and shapes, which can limit user comfort and make it more challenging to accommodate individuals with varying body types and needs.
3. Energy and Battery Limitations Short Battery Life:
   Most exoskeletons rely on batteries that have a limited lifespan, typically lasting only a few hours before needing to be recharged. In most cases, this

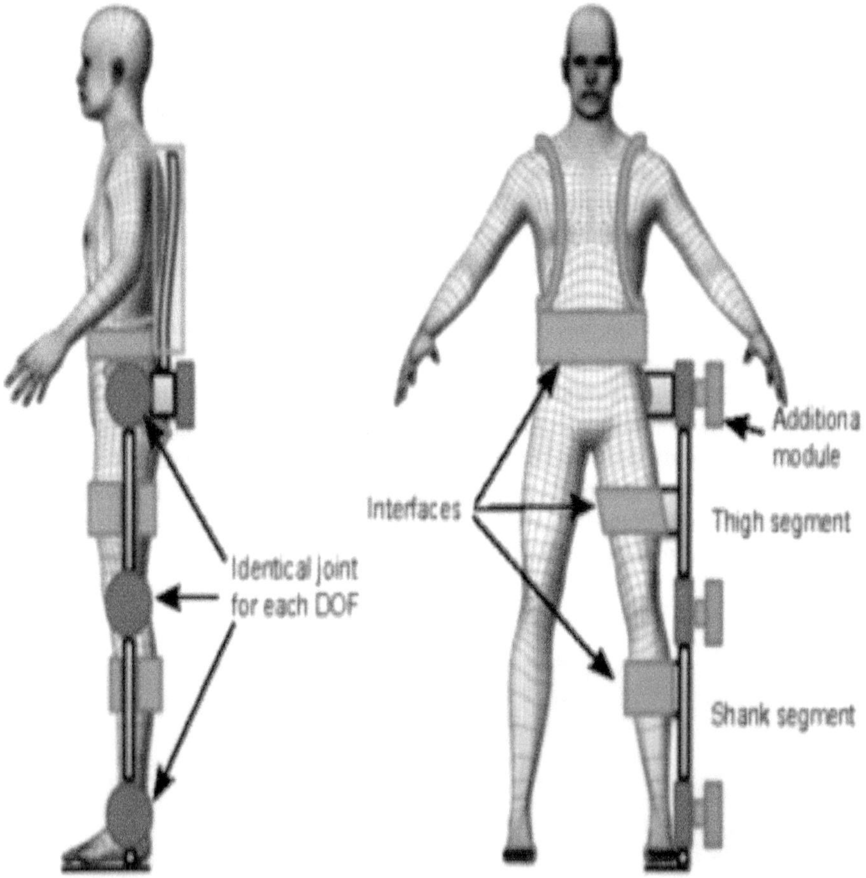

FIGURE 3.3 Modular lower limb exoskeleton.

may prove to be a significant limitation for users, especially those with all-day requirements.

Energy Consumption: Exoskeletons consume a considerable amount of energy due to the motors and sensors used for precise movement, making them relatively ineffective for long-term use unless the battery requires frequent recharging.

4. Safety Concerns

The Danger of Falling: If there is a failure or the exoskeleton needs to be stopped while the user is in action, the user may fall and sustain physical injuries. Users should be well-trained, and some systems would require supervision in their initial use.

Unforeseen Mechanical Failures: The failure of an actuator or motor can result in non-support or misalignment of movement, potentially causing harm

Technical Specifications and Design

The ReWalk exoskeleton is a lightweight, strong framework that supports the user's body, providing mechanical support while helping the user to move their legs. The over-clothing construction is well-supported by robust structures in the legs and lower back region, and its harness system secures the device to the human body. High-strength materials, such as aluminum and carbon fiber composites, are utilized to design a device that is both robust and lightweight. This system utilizes the movement of the hip and knee joints, leveraging the use of electric motors and actuators. In such a device, motors must be designed to allow for highly accurate movement, as this is required for simulating a natural gait while walking. A battery pack powers it to track the user's movement patterns to aid walking and standing. In addition to the sensors, ReWalk also features an array of gyroscopes, accelerometers, and tilt sensors that continuously monitor the user's body position and movement. The sensors provide instant feedback to the control system, allowing it to adjust immediately and maintain balance and coordination. The safety of the user and the smooth operation of the appliance depend on the proper functioning of feedback systems. The sophisticated computer system serves as the brain of the ReWalk exoskeleton, processing input from sensors and the user's commands to control the motors and actuators. The high-level algorithms are designed to interpret user intent and output the corresponding movements. For instance, as the user leans forward to initiate walking, the system detects this signal and activates the motors to move the steps. ReWalk operates from rechargeable lithium-ion batteries, which have hours of operation on a single charge. The battery pack is strapped to the belt or backpack and is designed to be easily replaceable, minimizing downtime. One of the key aspects of the system is power management, which ensures sufficient power to run the motors while maintaining a lightweight design to facilitate easy carrying. Users primarily interact with the ReWalk system through a wrist-mounted remote control, which allows them to switch between various operational modes, including walking, standing, and sitting. The interface is intuitive enough that it can be learned very quickly and used efficiently. The system can also be programmed and monitored by software, allowing healthcare professionals to customize settings and track patients' progress.

Functionality and Operation

ReWalk offers various modes, each designed to cater to different activities and user needs. When walking, the system helps the user take steps. It does this by activating motors in the hip and knee joints. In standing mode, the exoskeleton supports the user in maintaining an upright and balanced position. Sitting mode enables a smooth transition from a standing position to a seated position. Furthermore, ReWalk enables users to walk upstairs, which is yet another highly impactful mobility augmentation. The default control mechanism of the ReWalk is based on the movement of its user's body. The exoskeleton is based on a lean-based mechanism of control whereby the user tilts his upper body weight forward to indicate the need to move ahead.

Applications of ReWalk

- Clinical Rehabilitation: Programs and protocols utilize ReWalk in physical therapy and rehabilitation settings.
- Personal Mobility: It is used for daily mobility by patients with spinal cord injuries or other mobility disabilities.
- Military and Industrial Applications: Potential applications in military or industrial fields that enhance endurance and reduce fatigue associated with work.
- Research Applications: Research settings designed to study human gait, biomechanics, and their impact on human health through the use of robotic assistance.

Benefits of ReWalk

- Enhanced mobility: ReWalk aids in the rehabilitation of walking ability, rising, and integration into an environment.
- Health Benefits: Decrease in secondary health complications; improved cardiovascular strength, muscle tone, and bone density
- Psychological and Social Benefits: Improvement in independence, self-esteem, quality of life
- Rehabilitation Benefits: Aiding recovery and physical therapy, reactivating muscles, and promoting neuroplasticity.

Limitations and Challenges

- Cost: High acquisition and maintenance costs, as well as access costs for users and institutions.
- Learning Curve: The amount of time and effort required for a user to become proficient in using the device effectively.
- Physical Limitations: Accessibility for users with a wide range of injuries, varying weight and size requirements, as well as limitations on speed and range of motion.
- Battery Life: The duration for which the device can operate before needing to be recharged, and the implications for all-day use.
- Environmental Conditions: How it performs over rugged terrain, in adverse weather conditions, or over obstacles such as curbs and stairs.

Future Improvements

- Technological Innovations: New functionalities and enhancements in sensor technology, incorporation of AI, and energy efficiency.
- Applications in New Areas: Future applications in various fields, including entry into new markets.
- Interconnection with Other Devices: Potential interconnection with brain-machine interface technologies, virtual reality, and other support systems.

- Regulatory and Accessibility Issues: Strides in making the technology more accessible, reducing costs, and addressing regulatory issues.

Indego Exoskeleton

The Indego exoskeleton is one of the most up-to-date assistive technologies, primarily designed for individuals with spinal cord injuries and other conditions that may impair mobility. This wearable robotic device enables users to stand, walk, or perform various other movements that would otherwise be impossible without assistance. The primary objective of Indego is to enhance the quality of life for individuals with paralysis of the lower limbs. Apart from physical mobility, numerous psychological and physiological benefits accompany it. Figure 3.5 shows the Indego exoskeleton.

The Parker Hannifin Corporation-designed Indego exoskeleton is light, compact, mobile, and more flexible than many of its peers in similar classes. This particular device has dramatically impacted the line of rehabilitation robots and wearable technologies. Since its invention, it has evolved into various forms over the years and has proven to be a highly regarded tool for both rehabilitation purposes and personal use. The concept and development of the Indego exoskeleton trace their origin to early research into wearable robotic technologies. However, powered exoskeletons have been in development for several decades. Parker Hannifin is a leader in motion and control technologies, working on this device as part of a larger initiative to apply its technical excellence to healthcare and assistive devices. Research professor, Michael Goldfarb at Vanderbilt University, has been instrumental in the early design and

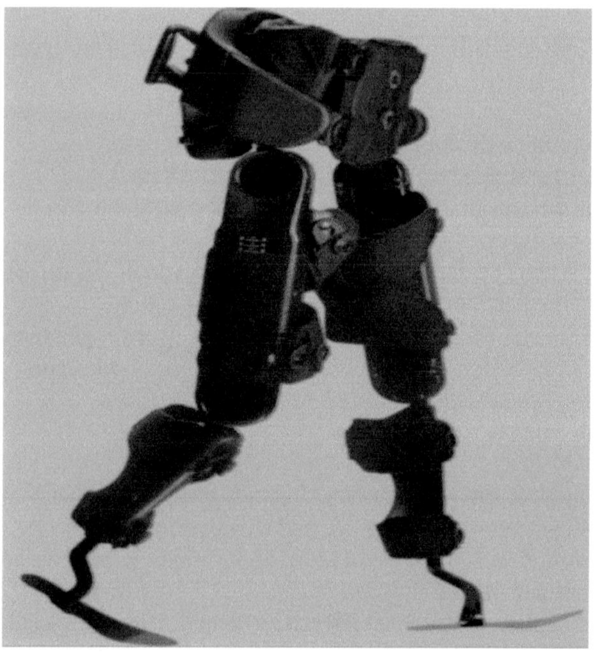

FIGURE 3.5 Indego exoskeleton.

conceptualization of the Indego exoskeleton. His work on wearable robots, which focuses on restoring the gait of patients with spinal cord injuries, contributed to the development of the Indego exoskeleton.

Several improvement stages and numerous tests comprised the product's history before its commercial release in the mid-2010s. Throughout the years, Parker Hannifin has continued to improve its functionality, making it easier to use and adaptable to diverse users.

One of the best features of the Indego exoskeleton is its lightweight design. Compared to other exoskeletons that weigh significantly more, making the user feel cumbersome, the Indego weighs approximately 12 kg. This certainly makes the user's experience effortless, allowing them to carry and control the device with ease, while also enhancing comfort during use. The main critical components combine to ensure efficient movement and smooth control for the user.

Key Features

1. Modularity:
   The exoskeleton is a modular structure, meaning it can be easily disassembled into constituent parts for reuse. That is an important feature in the exoskeleton design, as it dramatically aids transport and modification according to the user's needs. The modular aspect ensures its parts are relatively easy to repair and replace, compared with those in monolithic devices.
2. Power Supply:
   The exoskeleton is powered by a battery pack consisting of a lithium-ion battery, which is capable of storing sufficient energy to power the exoskeleton for several hours on a single charge. A power management system complements the lightweight design of the battery, ensuring the device delivers steady performance over extended periods.
3. Sensors and Actuators:
   Much of Indego's functionality is based on advanced sensors and actuators. The latter are equipped to sense where the user's body is headed and respond with an equivalent action, enabling the system to participate in walking and other movements in real time. Actuators are essentially small motors located at key joints, providing the mechanical forces necessary to move limbs.
4. Control System:
   The Indego system is both intuitive and sophisticated in its control. The device operates based on information gathered from the user's body movements. For instance, if a user leans forward, the device interprets this as walking, and when the user leans backward, the device stops working. This system enables a more natural walking experience, providing users with a greater sense of control and mastery over their movements.
5. Fitting and Adjustments:
   The exoskeleton is adjustable for the user. For instance, the adjustable length of its leg supports can be modified to fit the user's comfort and safety needs, as users have different heights and body types.

The Indego exoskeleton is designed to assist individuals with paralyzed or weakened lower limbs in walking. The piece has been designed with several sensors and actuators integrated to mimic a gait that almost feels like natural walking. It allows users to stand, walk, turn around, and sit without losing their balance and support.

Walking Capabilities

The most vital feature of the Indego exoskeleton is its ability to assist people in walking. The gadget is such a vital support system for people who have either spinal cord injuries or any other conditions that make one unable to walk. It does this by sensing the user's weight shift and body orientation. For instance, it detects the signal of leaning forward as a cue for initiating movement. Conversely, when the user leans backward, the exoskeleton stops moving. The weight-shifting control system provides intuitive operation, allowing users to efficiently utilize the device without requiring complex controls or buttons. The exoskeleton will also ensure that users maintain proper posture and balance while walking. Additionally, it will provide mechanical support to the lower limbs and work towards ensuring that movements are always smooth and consistent, thereby reducing the risk of falls and injuries.

User Control and Feedback

This allows the user to adjust their gait and posture in response to feedback from the device. The feedback system is thus of primary importance in enabling users to feel a sense of control during their movements. Significantly, health and well-being will be affected both physically and psychologically.

One of the key features of the Indego exoskeleton is its ability to be customized according to user-specific needs. It can be adjusted to accommodate different heights, weights, and body shapes, ensuring a comfortable and secure fit. This customization is significant because the exoskeleton can be utilized by large segments of users with varying degrees of mobility impairment. Additionally, the device is very portable and easy to assemble, allowing you to pack it up for travel or storage with ease when not in use. The Indego exoskeleton provides several different modes of operation, based on which someone may need to select:

1. Therapeutic Mode:
   This is primarily the mode for which the equipment is intended for rehabilitation purposes. Here, the therapist can control the equipment to assist the patient with specific movements or exercises. It is an excellent tool for individuals undergoing physical therapy after an injury to regain lost strength and mobility.
2. Personal use mode:
   With the exoskeleton, the user has greater independence outside the clinical environment if it is being used in personal use mode. In this mode, the user will have complete control over the device, allowing them to walk without requiring any assistance from a therapist.

3. Balance Mode:
   This mode is designed to help users with balance issues. It provides additional support and stabilization, ensuring that users can maintain their balance while walking or standing.

Applications of the Indego Exoskeleton

It is utilized in a wide range of applications, particularly in the fields of rehabilitation and personal mobility. Its versatility renders it useful for both clinical settings and individual use. It has thus been adopted in various rehabilitation centers and by individuals worldwide.

This exoskeleton, however, is primarily utilized in rehabilitation for people suffering from spinal injuries or conditions that tend to immobilize the individuals. In the rehabilitation facility, the device is used to help patients regain strength, coordination, and mobility. The device is significant for gait training, as it enables patients to practice walking in a controlled and supportive environment. The exoskeleton also provides benefits beyond mobility restoration. It can help patients to gradually improve their posture and enhance their muscular strength and cardiovascular well-being. Besides these, standing and walking with the exoskeleton is believed to offer psychological benefits by enhancing the patient's mood and subjective well-being. Rehabilitation specialists can modify the device to meet the individual patient's specific requirements. For example, the amount of force generated by the exoskeleton could be adjusted depending on the overall improvement of the patient. This adaptability makes it a valuable tool for long-term rehabilitation programs.

For patients suffering from spinal cord injuries or other mobility-related disabilities, the Indego exoskeleton can serve as a personal mobility aid. Users could go about their daily activities, such as walking within the house, visiting friends or colleagues, or going shopping. This level of independence is precious to users who are otherwise dependent on wheelchairs or other assistive devices. Portability is one of the most notable features of an Indego personal exoskeleton. Its entire unit can be easily broken down for transport, allowing users to carry it anywhere, and ensuring they are assured of mobility assistance whenever needed. The psychological benefits of using an exoskeleton like Indego cannot be overstated, especially when it enables a patient to stand up and walk again. It can enhance the mental and emotional well-being of individuals who have lost their ability to walk for any reason. Indeed, many users felt more confident and independent after using the device, which may lead to an improvement in their overall quality of life. In addition to the psychological benefits, the Indego exoskeleton offers numerous advantages related to physical health. For instance, standing and walking with this exoskeleton will enhance blood circulation, decrease pressure sores that many wheelchair users suffer from, and generally contribute to good cardiovascular health. Utilized in the Military and Industry, the primary focus of the Indego exoskeleton is to enhance people's mobility.

3.4 METHODOLOGY

A. Frame or Skeleton

The frame or skeleton essentially constitutes the backbone of the exoskeleton, providing the necessary support, resistance, and stability to the body. All the other subsystems are attached to this structure through sensors, actuators, and control systems. The skeleton must be both light and strong, providing comfort for the user while being rigid enough to offer structural integrity in safe and effective rehabilitation. These materials include carbon fiber composites, aluminum alloys, and polyurethane, which have high strength-to-weight ratios and are typically biocompatible. The design must be ergonomic so that prolonged usage would not create discomfort. At the same time, it should allow proper anatomical alignment to ensure biomechanical support.

B. Non-Mechanical Actuators (Gas Pumps)

Non-mechanical actuators, such as gas pumps in pneumatic systems, provide power for joint movement in the exoskeleton. These actuators convert compressed air into mechanical energy, providing smooth and controlled assistance to the lower limbs during walking or other lower limb movements. Gas pumps are chosen for exoskeletons due to their compact size, lightweight nature, and constant torque output with minimal energy consumption, thereby reducing the total weight of the exoskeleton while increasing efficiency, particularly in gait assistance and balance control. In rehabilitation, these actuators are primarily helpful for enabling controlled movement that mimics the natural biomechanics of walking.

C. Sensors

Sensorial devices play a crucial role in the feedback loop of the exoskeleton's control system. These provide real-time data on movement, balance, and interaction with the exoskeleton, thus enabling dynamic adjustments. A variety of sensors are used:

Gyroscope: Measures the angular position of limbs as well as the exoskeleton, providing information for joint alignment and correcting posture.

Accelerometers: Instantaneous acceleration values enable the identification of phases within the gait cycle. The recorded data, therefore, triggers responses from the actuators to ensure that the exoskeleton assists in the correct gait cycles, such as during stance and swing.

Force/Pressure Sensors: These measure the distribution of load across the limbs, which helps adjust the supports and the strain across weakened muscles or joints.

This feedback system ensures that the exoskeleton adapts to the wearer's movement, providing both stability and mobility.

D. Servo Motors

These are the gears that form the heart of an exoskeleton's movement, offering precise control over joint movement. These motors are selected for their high torque, reliability, and lower price; these are essential demands for any lower-limb exoskeleton, where accurate and controlled motion is required. Servo motors offer broad movement ranges with multi-degree freedom, providing smooth transitions between different phases of gait cycles. With the ability to generate finely graded movements, they are instrumental in rehabilitation processes, where controlled assistance is required to help rebuild standard walking mechanics. They are integrated with the sensor system to enable real-time adjustments based on the user's movement patterns.

E. Power Supply

The exoskeleton's power supply is provided by a Lithium-ion rechargeable battery (11.1V, 5000mAh, 2A), chosen due to its high energy density and lightweight properties. The power for actuators, sensors, and control systems can thus be utilized for an extended period without the need for frequent recharging, thanks to the stable and reliable power supply. The battery power can enable the device to last for a sufficient period during therapy sessions as well as for day-to-day mobility aid. Battery management systems are integrated into this exoskeleton, ensuring that charge levels are maintained to optimize performance and minimize downtime, thereby maximizing the overall efficiency of the exoskeleton system. This hybrid actuator, sensor, advanced materials, and power source, assisted by the proposed lower-limb exoskeleton, aims to provide better support, mobility, and stability for patients undergoing rehabilitation and those requiring assistive technologies to maintain their quality of life.

3.5 PROPOSED SYSTEM

Exoskeletons designed for use by individuals with mobility impairments hold great promise for restoring functional mobility and independence. The existing designs are more characterized by their weight, cost, and usability deficits rather than overcoming the limitations. The developed lower limb exoskeleton system aims to address the existing shortcomings in terms of efficiency, user adaptability, and improved accessibility, providing a more practical and economical solution. Figure 3.6 shows the lower limb exoskeleton.

1. Light structural design

   One of the significant disadvantages of currently existing exoskeleton designs is that they are too heavy, resulting in significant user discomfort and limiting their use for extended periods. To alleviate this problem, the current system has extensively incorporated advanced lightweight materials, including carbon fiber composites and high-strength aluminum alloys. Carbon fiber is known to have a dramatically high strength-to-weight ratio, thereby providing the structural integrity necessary while significantly reducing the overall weight of the system. High-strength aluminum alloys offer additional strength without a significant weight burden, enabling a design that can support a person's weight with sufficient material while applying minimal pressure to the human body. This reduction in weight leads to improvement in comfort while also reducing the energy spent by the actuators to perform their specific functions, thus giving rise to an efficient system.

resume their routine activities independently. The system can be modified for military and industrial use, such as helping laborers to carry loads of heavier weights or to reduce fatigue when performing specific physical tasks for long periods. Future versions of the system, however, will explore neural interface control to enable direct brain-computer communication for individuals with severe disabilities. This will be a fully thought-controlled exoskeleton that enables the highest autonomy and ease of use.

3.6 WORKFLOW

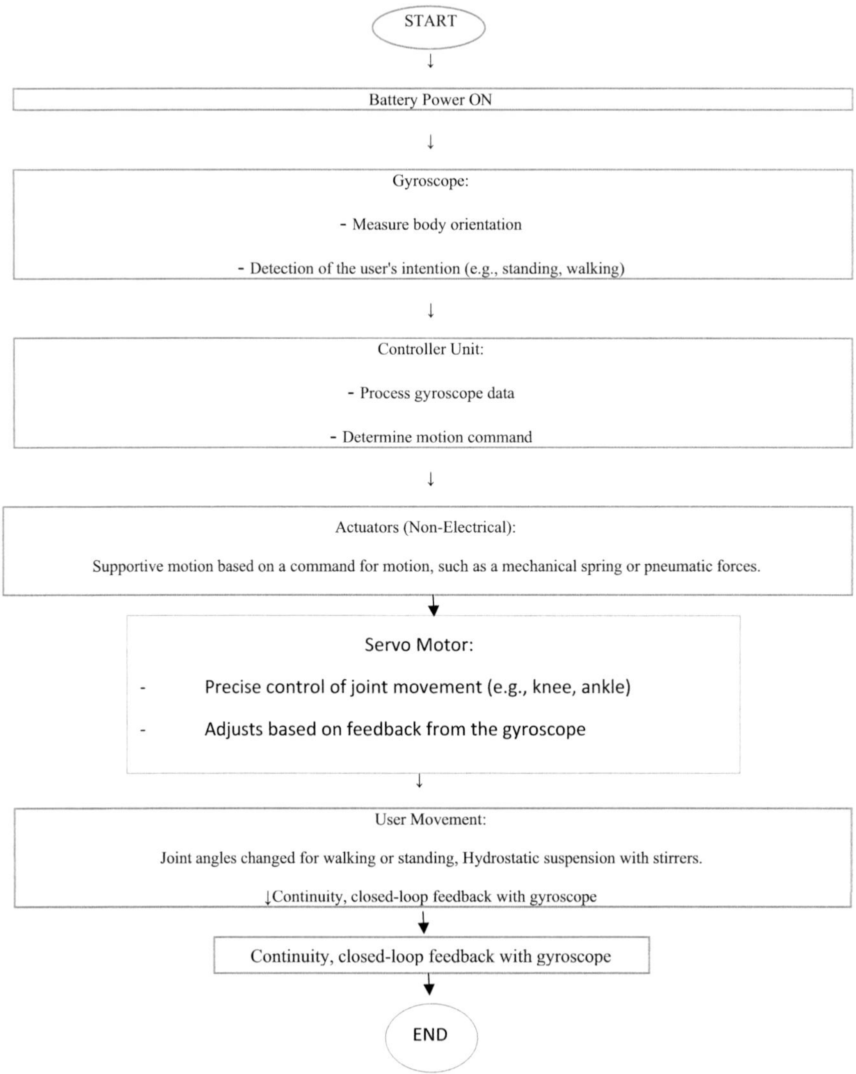

This new system details the functionality of a hybrid assistive mobility device, blending electronic sensors with mechanical assistance. It could represent an evolution in assistive technology, the device being an advanced exoskeleton, say, or a sophisticated mobility aid. Essentially, it is based on a smart power management strategy. Once activated, the device's battery powers the electronic equipment, primarily consisting of a high-precision gyroscope. This sensor must be understood to grasp the user's physical state and intentions. It continuously tracks the body's orientation in space while attempting to interpret slight changes that may signal the user's desire to stand, walk, or perform any other movement. The retrieved gyroscopic data feed into a highly advanced controller unit. This computational heart of the system processes information in real time, translates raw sensor data into actionable motion commands using advanced algorithms, and represents what makes a controller powerfully adept at the fast and accurate interpretation of user intention. It is the innovative approach to actuation that separates this system from anything previously built. There isn't a reliance on the traditional power-hungry electric motors instead; it relies on non-electrical actuators to assist movement. For instance, they can take the form of carefully calibrated mechanical springs that store and release energy in an efficient way or pneumatics by means of compressed air to generate the force. The efficiency of this kind of passive or semi-passive system greatly reduces the power needs of the device. The actuators work in tandem to change the angles of the user's joints to provide just enough support and assistance in walking or holding a standing position. This mechanical support is optimized to the commands of the controller, so that the support offered can be an appropriate response according to the needs and intentions of the user at the current time. Drawing upon this hybrid approach—electronics-based sensors and decision-making systems, but non-electrical physical support—the machine achieves remarkable levels of energy efficiency. This design approach should thus also allow the achievement of at least considerably longer running times than fully motorized systems, since the power-expensive operation of movement assistance is offloaded to mechanical systems.

3.7 BLOCK DIAGRAM

This is an integrated control system. It has likely application in a mechatronic or robotic component. The heart of this system with the Arduino UNO is the central control system working as the central processor and controller. In this system, the Arduino is orchestrating and controlling many components so that it will be able to function well and in harmony.

A servo motor is one of the key components in this system. This system uses a servo motor as the main actuator in motion control. This motor can be driven to such-and-such angles or hold its position as commanded from the Arduino. With an angle sensor, this motor is directed towards perfect alignment and movement according to desired instructions. The sensor is important for the Arduino because it updates it on real time whether or not there is running movement of the motor. Having this in mind, the angle sensor data is critical to the closed-loop control system configuration within the Arduino so that it can always adapt in such a way that it attains or maintains a specific position or movement. Although there is no visible feedback loop shown in the diagram, one would have intuitively expected continuous feeding back of sensor information into the Arduino for improving the control strategy.

On the output side, there exist actuators of any kind of electromechanical devices capable of doing physical work through operation on the commands issued by the system. The application could call for additional motors, linear actuators, grippers, or any other mechanical device designed to perform some action. The system is powered entirely by a battery, which supplies electrical energy to both the Arduino and the servo motor. This design makes the setup independent of a fixed power supply, ensuring greater flexibility for portable or remote applications.

The module can be made scalable and modular. It can be applied to numerous projects related to motion control. Such applications include:

Robotic arm systems: They are used a lot in industrial automation and other research projects which specifically require very high-end multi-axis motion control.

Automated camera tracking systems: Servo motors provide smooth motion controls to achieve the smoothness of movement, and can be applied for the control of camera mounts, with obtaining real time data responses.

Self-balancing devices: This would be realized by using gyroscopes and accelerometers as sensors. Theoretically, personal mobility devices or even robots can self-balance.

Smart home automation: The same motorized control principles used in exo-skeleton joints can also be applied in home automation systems. For example, motorized mechanisms may adjust the slat positions of window shades or doors to regulate light entry, illustrating how similar actuation and control strategies are transferable across domains.

This is a dynamic sculpture, where actuation is part of this installation with moving parts that interact with the environment, perhaps through sound or motion.

This modular design supports easy extension and augmentation in this modularity. As an example, it is possible to add as many servo motors and sensors as needed to control more complex motions, for instance in robotic arms. It might even be constructed to look for additional peripherals like accelerometers or gyroscopes to enhance its spatial awareness and perform stabilization or object-tracking tasks. Figure 3.7 above illustrates the block diagram of the control system.

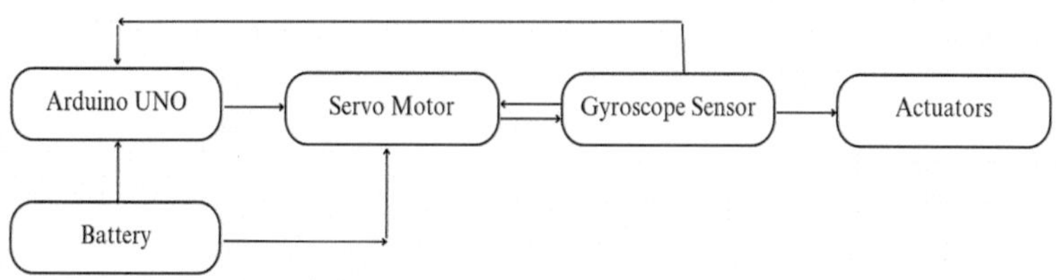

FIGURE 3.7 Block diagram of integrated control system for motion control.

3.8 CONCLUSION

In conclusion, the development and integration of lower limb exoskeletons form a transformative step forward in the domain of assistive technology. Such a device is full of promise to not only move people more safely but to promote rehabilitation and enhance the quality of life for people with movability impairments. The lower limb exoskeleton would bring back or supplement the walking ability for people, hence promoting independence and participation in everyday practices. However, realization of the full value of these lower limb exoskeletons is also accompanied by its own set of challenges. One of the major stumbling blocks remains in terms of relatively high upfront costs that may prohibit access to the technology for many of the users who could benefit from it. The significant size and weight of such exoskeleton models mean that they can also be cumbersome to handle, thus affecting the comfort and practicality of the user. Additionally, their power requirements may limit the time during which they can be used effectively and require frequent recharging, an activity that may break constant use and limit the convenience of movement. Of course, to overcome these challenges, research and development in these areas need focused efforts. The innovations in newer materials for the bodyweight, and designs would help create less cumbersome exoskeletons, thus making them more wearable and portable. Advances in battery technology and energy-efficient systems are important factors to extend the operational duration as well as decrease the cycle count between recharges. Secondly, aggressive comprehensive training programs and proper safety protocols should be instituted to allow the efficient and safe use of the devices by the users thus reducing the dangers of injuries and maximizing benefits. The future of lower limb exoskeletons is bright, considering efforts that will continuously be channeled towards making such devices easier to access, functional, and effective in performance. Indeed, this will be instrumental in collaborative research among researchers, developers, and users in filling in the gaps to further continue advancing this technology. So, in working towards a near-term practical and accessible lower limb exoskeleton, we're moving towards a future where the technology will increasingly hold value and benefit more people, leading towards greater independence and a higher quality of life.

REFERENCES

[1] Ahmad Zahedi, Andong Yi, Dingguo Zhang, and Bin Zhang. (2020). "A Soft Exoskeleton for Tremor Suppression Equipped with Flexible Semiactive Actuator." *Soft Robotics* 8 (4), 432–447.

[2] M Afschrift, M van Mierlo, C Bayon, A Keemink, L D'Hondt,, E van Asseldonk, H van der Kooij, F De Groote (2023). "Assisting Walking Balance using a Bio-Inspired Exoskeleton Controller." *Journal of Neuro Engineering and Rehabilitation* 20, 82.

[3] Yuanxi Sun, Yuntao Tang, Jia Zheng, Dianbiao Dong, Xiaohong Chen, and Long Bai. (2022). "From Sensing to Control of Lower Limb Exoskeleton: A Systematic Review." *Annual Reviews in Control* 53: 83–96.

[4] Hao Lee, Peter Walker Ferguson, and Jacob Rosen. (2020). "Lower Limb Exoskeleton Systems Overview." *Wearable Robotics, Systems and Applications* 207–229.

[5] Ziming Guo, Can Wang, and Chunning Song. (2020). "A Real-Time Stable-Control Gait Switching Strategy for Lower-Limb Rehabilitation Exoskeleton." *Plos One* 15 (8): 1–19.

[6] V. M. Senthilkumar, S. Ravindrakumar, D. Nithya, and N. V. Kousik. (2019). "A Vedic Mathematics Based Processor Core for Discrete Wavelet Transform using FinFET and CNTFET Technology for Biomedical Signal Processing." *Microprocessors and Microsystems* 71: 102–115.

[7] Chen Wang, Zhongcai Pei, Yanan Fan, Shuang Qiu, and Zhiyong Tang. (2024). "Review of Vision-Based Environmental Perception for Lower-Limb Exoskeleton." *Biomimetics* 9 (4): 254–274.

[8] Wei Chen, Jun Li, Shanying Zhu, Xiaodong Zhang, Yutao Men, and Hang Wu. (2022). "Gait Recognition for Lower Limb Exoskeletons Based on Interactive Information Fusion." *Applied Bionics and Biomechanics*. 9933018, 19.

[9] Fahad Hussain, Roland Goecke, and Masoud Mohammadian. (2021). "Exoskeleton Robots for Lower Limb Assistance: A Review of Materials, Actuation, and Manufacturing Methods." *Proceedings of the Institution of Mechanical Engineers, Part H: Journal of Engineering in Medicine* 235 (12), 1375-1385.

[10] V. M. Senthil Kumar and S. Ravindrakumar. (2019). "Design of an Area-Efficient Finfet-Based Approximate Multiplier in 32-Nm Technology for Low-Power Application." In V. Bhateja, S. C. Satapathy, H. Satori, & N. Nguyen (Eds.), *Soft Computing and Signal Processing*, 505–53. Singapore: Springer.

[11] Yu-Ning Chen, Yi-Ning Wu, and Bing-Shiang Yang. (2023). "The Neuromuscular Control for Lower Limb Exoskeleton- A 50-Year Perspective." *Journal of Biomechanics* 158: 11338.

[12] Gregory S. Sawicki, Owen N. Beck, Inseung Kang, and Aaron J. Young. (2020). "The Exoskeleton Expansion: Improving Walking and Running Economy." *Journal of Neuro Engineering and Rehabilitation,* 17 (1), 25.

[13] M. A. Guptha, S. Rao and R. Selvaraj. (2023). "An Efficient Discrete Wavelet Transform Architecture with Low Power and Multiplier-Less Structure for Pervasive Biomedical Image Processing Application." *EAI Endorsed Transactions on Pervasive Health and Technology* 9 (1): 1–8.

4 Comprehensive Examination of Biomedical Robotics

Shalini Kumari and Chander Prabha

4.1 INTRODUCTION

Biomedical robotics is a multidisciplinary field that integrates concepts from engineering, computer science, and medicine to create robotic systems for healthcare applications. These robots are specifically designed for medical procedures, rehabilitation, prosthetics, and patient care. The area has experienced exponential expansion in recent decades due to technological advancements and a growing need for more effective and accurate medical treatments. Robotics has transformed numerous aspects of human life. Robots have evolved beyond manufacturing and are now utilized in various fields, including agriculture, aerospace, and education [1]. Over the past decade, robots have been used in operating rooms worldwide to develop and improve minimally invasive surgical techniques. Minimally invasive surgery reduces patient pain, costs, and hospital stay. Robotic surgery enables precision operations, easy-to-understand interfaces, and remote surgical access with minimal devices. Thus, robotics can improve minimally invasive surgery and offer new methods. Traditionally, robots are made of rigid materials, such as metals and alloys, performing complex and repetitive tasks for people, delivering real-time information, and providing accurate feedback [2]. Due to advancements in science and technology, industrial robot control has made significant strides in Computer Vision (CV), Deep Learning (DL), imitation learning, and other related domains. However, diverse working situations necessitate ongoing improvements in robot control operation for reliability, flexibility, adaptation, and user-friendly interface [3]. Limited uses exist for delicate or soft targets in severe conditions due to their stiffness and limited adjustability. Soft robots are gaining popularity due to their flexibility and adaptability, which sets them apart from stiff robots. Soft robots typically utilize materials such as gels, functional polymers, and other flexible materials with moduli similar to those of soft creatures (e.g., fat, cartilage, and skin), ranging from 10^4 to 10^9 Pa [4]. Soft robots typically exhibit safe human-robot interaction and offer various degrees of freedom. Soft robots show potential for biomedical applications, bionic movements, camouflage, and smooth electronic devices [5]. Soft robots aid in exploring confined spaces, navigating uneven terrain, and mitigating toxic conditions following natural disasters and the collapse of structures.

DOI: 10.1201/9781003561309-4

Surgical robots have gained popularity over the last decade. The da Vinci robotics, developed by Intuitive Surgical Inc., are the most widely used for minimally invasive surgery. Currently, 3,398 da Vinci Xi systems are installed worldwide, representing the fourth generation of the da Vinci system. According to [6] and [7], da Vinci is a remotely controlled robotic system that enables surgeons to control 3D vision systems (endoscopes) and laparoscopic surgical instruments through a central input device in an intraocular imaging environment, known as a surgical console. Robotically controlled surgery offers improved instrumentation and enhanced mobility through small incisions, all controlled by the physician. Most surgical robots have large operating chambers and use rigid instruments and articulated tips. The trend towards minimally invasive surgery is evident, and robotics has improved performance in minimally invasive abdominal surgery. Managing fragile cycle areas remains challenging, and certain procedures still necessitate a more open invasive approach. The historical developments in medical robots are shown in Table 4.1.

Surgical robot systems (SRS) have gained popularity, drastically changing the surgical procedural paradigm. Traditional surgery relies on the surgeon's expertise and clinical experience but might be limited by imaging limitations, visual field restrictions, and subjective biases. Physical restrictions, such as hand tremors or fatigue, can exacerbate surgical planning and execution errors. In contrast, SRS enhances surgical precision, reduces operator fatigue, shortens procedure time, and lowers radiation exposure. Robot-assisted surgery (RAS) reduces trauma, pain,

TABLE 4.1
Historical Developments

History	Year	Description
Early Foundations	1960s-1970s	In the 1960s, the concept of utilizing medical robots emerged. The PUMA 560 was one of the first; it was developed for industrial use but modified for neurosurgical biopsies in 1985.
Surgical Robots	1980s-1990s	The first generation of surgical robots emerged in the 1980s. Hip replacement procedures used the ROBODOC system, which first appeared in 1992. To operate an endoscopic camera, the AESOP system made history in 1994 as the first surgical robot to receive FDA approval.
Minimally Invasive Surgery	Late 1990s-2000s	In 2000, minimally invasive surgery was transformed with the introduction of the da Vinci Surgical System. It gave surgeons more control, accuracy, and dexterity.
Rehabilitation and Assistive Robots	2000s-present	Robots and exoskeletons for rehabilitation were added to the scope. One of the earliest gait rehabilitation robots was the Lokomat, which debuted in 2001.
AI and ML Integration	2010s-present	Thanks to advancements in AI and ML integration, more advanced, self-governing robots are now within reach.

TABLE 4.2
Comparison between Surgeon and SRS

Classification	Merits	Demerits
Surgon	• Perfect hand-eye coordination. • Flexibility and exceptional judgment. • Enhanced manual coordination.	• Restricted visual perception and measurement. • Not enough stability and accuracy. • Exposure to radiation and viral infection during surgical procedures.
SRS	• Visual aid. • Accuracy, quantification, and stability • Capacity to combine data from many sources	• Poor coordination between vision and motion • Inadequate judgment and lack of flexibility. • Capacity to combine data from many sources

complications, and recovery time with a minimally invasive method. SRS aims to provide access to high-quality medical care, allowing more people to benefit from improved surgical techniques. Standardizing training and usage guidelines reduce reliance on specialist skills and experience. Essentially, SRS aims to enhance human surgeons' abilities, precision, accessibility, and surgical quality and safety. SRS has improved surgical precision and reduced surgeon fatigue, but it still faces substantial obstacles [8]. The main issue is their lack of judgment and adaptability, similar to human surgeons, especially in complex or unexpected scenarios. While capable of performing precise, pre-programmed tasks, they need to develop the subtle decision-making skills that come with experience [9]. Despite its fast-processing capabilities, SRS requires assistance to handle dynamically unstructured data. While minimally invasive surgery is less traumatic than traditional procedures, it has downsides, such as limited working space and vision. Significant opportunities exist for development in technology and functionality. Table 4.2 shows the comparison between the surgeon and SRS.

4.1.1 Gaps in Biomedical Robotics

In the field of biomedical robotics, several critical challenges and gaps exist that this chapter aims to address as follows [10]:

Precision and Control: Achieving high levels of accuracy in complex biological environments is a significant challenge. The intricate nature of human anatomy requires robotic systems to perform precise movements, which can be difficult to attain in real time during surgical procedures.

AI and Autonomy Integration: The integration of artificial intelligence (AI) into robotic systems is essential for enhancing their functionality. Developing intelligent systems capable of making real-time decisions during medical procedures can significantly improve outcomes. This includes the ability to learn from vast datasets and adapt to varying surgical conditions

Human-Robot Interaction: Enhancing the interfaces between surgeons and robotic systems is crucial for improving usability and efficiency. Current systems may not provide intuitive controls, which can hinder the surgeon's ability to operate effectively. Addressing this gap can lead to better collaboration between humans and robots in the operating room

Cost and Accessibility: The high costs associated with advanced robotic systems can limit their accessibility in various healthcare settings. Finding ways to reduce costs while maintaining quality and effectiveness is a crucial challenge that must be addressed to ensure widespread adoption.

The chapter reviews biomedical robotics, their historical perspective, classification, rehabilitation, medical applications, surgical procedures, and so on.

4.1.2 Organization of Chapter

The rest of the chapter is organized as follows: Section 4.2 gives an historical perspective of SRS. Section 4.3 deals with how medical robotics is classified in biomedicine. Section 4.4 presents the rehabilitation concept in robotics history. Section 4.5 briefly describes some of the medical applications of surgical systems. Section 4.6 presents AI-assisted SRS emphasizing control strategies and surgical planning. Section 4.7 gives insight into some examples of successful surgical SRS implementation using AI. Section 4.8 presents revolutionary tools and their impact on modern medicine. Section 4.9 briefly describes the challenges faced, followed by a conclusion and future scope in section 4.10.

4.2 HISTORICAL PERSPECTIVE OF SRS

The word "robot" comes from the Czech word "robota," which refers to the artificial worker in Karel Capek's play "Rosum's Universal Robot." The term now refers to mechanical or artificial objects having human-like characteristics that perform tasks for humans. Robotic surgery began in the 1980s. In 1985, researchers used the PUMA robot to perform 0.05 mm neurosurgical biopsies. ROBODOC works well in orthopaedic hip replacement. In 1992, Computer Motion Inc. developed the Automated Endoscope System for Optimal Setup (AESOP), which received FDA approval in 1994.

The first version, AESOP 1000, featured a mechanical arm with laparoscopic optics controlled by pedals. It was enhanced in 1996 with the.HERMES system, which introduced voice control and haptic feedback. The original goal of AESOP was consistent video images with minimal help. Allowing small camera changes during surgery was later found to be necessary. In 1998, ZEUS debuted. It included dual handles and a TV monitor for 2D instrument control. In 1998 and 1999, this procedure was used for fallopian tube anastomosis and CAG. The first successful transatlantic operation, Operation Lindbergh, occurred in 2001.

The ZEUS robot and SOCRATES telecollaboration system helped a New York surgeon operate on a Strasbourg patient in an error-free 54-minute operation. Founded in 1995, Intuitive Surgical Inc. invented the da Vinci SRS in 1998 while developing the ZEUS system. Due to its ergonomics, seven degrees of freedom, two axes of rotation, stereoscopic viewer, and control pedal, the SRS platform has been successful.

To focus on newer models, Computer Motion Inc. combined with Intuitive Surgical and discontinued the ZEUS systems after a year of rising usage of these technologies. 2000, the Food and Drug Administration (FDA) authorized the da Vinci robotic system for abdominal surgery. In 2006, Intuitive Surgical introduced the da Vinci S system, which included easier handling and improved 3D endoscopic vision. The da Vinci Si system, modified in 2009, uses dual-console technology for cooperative surgical treatments and training. This version integrated the Firefly system, enabling real-time fluorescence imaging for improved surgical visualization [11]. The da Vinci Xi surgical robot debuted in 2014 has an adjustable exoskeleton and integrated table movements, reducing intraoperative repositioning and setup times. The smart tissue autonomous robot (STAR) system was developed in the same year. A new technology featuring real-time visual and tactile feedback and autonomous machine learning (ML) algorithms may conduct small intestinal suturing without human involvement, advancing RAS.

SRS ia advancing rapidly, resulting in discoveries and developments across numerous indications. In 2021, Advanced Osteotomy Tools Inc. introduced CARLO, the first approved laser osteotome [12]. CARLO enables precise, personalized bone cuts, enhancing surgical outcomes and recovery. EndoQuest Robotics introduced the first flexible SRS in 2022 to revolutionize minimally invasive procedures. The technique allows for endoluminal and single-incision surgery using natural orifices or trans umbilical incisions, reducing external incisions and problems. This new method differs from typical open, laparoscopic, or RAS methods that entail incisions through healthy tissues.

In 2023, Levita Magnetics launched MARS, the first minimally invasive surgical platform combining magnets and machines, which got FDA approval. Magnetic technology improves surgeon precision and control during abdominal surgeries. Proprio revolutionized spine surgery navigation using light-field technology with real-time 3D anatomy and operative scene representation. The system uses modern sensors to collect high-definition, multi-modal intraoperative images. This data is incorporated with preoperative images to improve spine surgical precision and visualization. Rossum Robot introduced the R-Universal orthopaedic SRS for difficult pelvic fracture procedures in trauma surgery. The system offers high-quality care for patients with complex trauma fractures through 3D real-time navigation, AI-based planning, and automated surgical operations. This technology is the first clinical application for complex pelvic fracture procedures. Table 4.3 shows the evolution of SRS. Table 4.4 presents some robotic systems and their uses, features, and limitations.

TABLE 4.3
SRS Evolution with Images

Year of Evolution	Surgical System Image	Name of Robotic System
1980	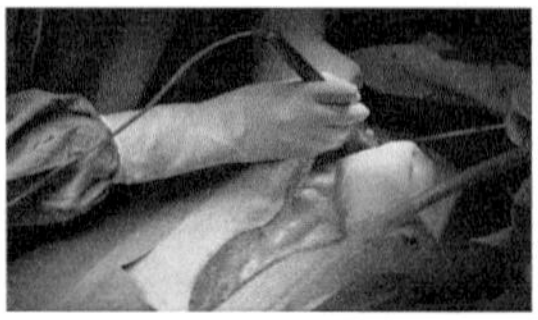	Open surgery robotic system
1990	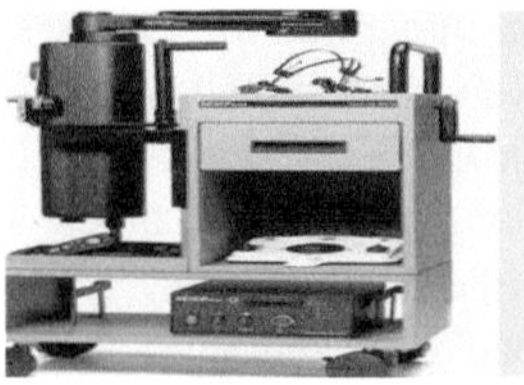	AESOP robotic system
2000	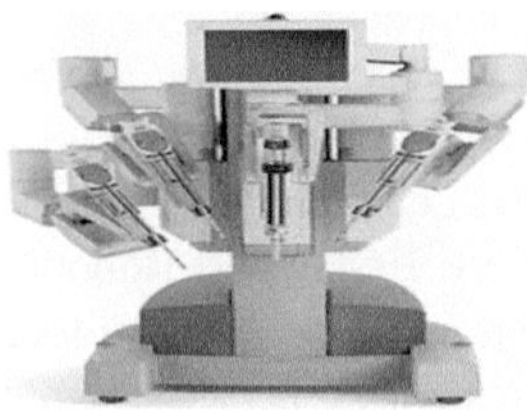	da Vinci robotic system
2010	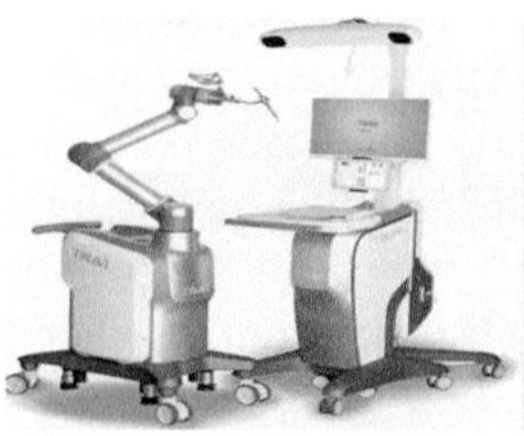	Ti-robotic system
2022	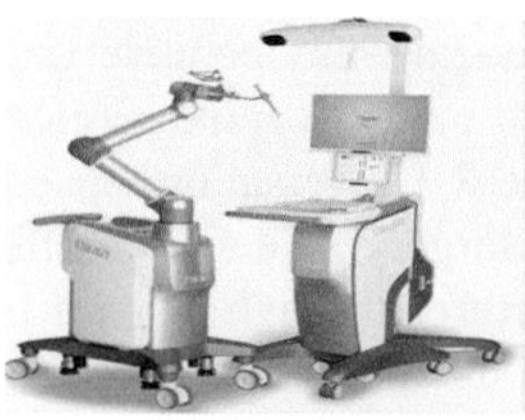	Endo quest robotic system
2024	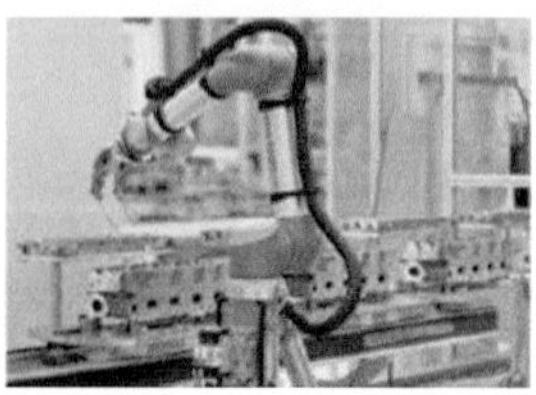	R Universal robotic system

TABLE 4.4
Robotic System Features, Uses and Limitations

Robotic System	Features	Uses	Limitations
da Vinci Surgical System	High precision, multi-joint arms, AI-assisted control	Minimally invasive surgeries, urology, gynaecology	High cost, requires extensive training for surgeons
RFA Surgical Robot	Focused on radiofrequency ablation, specialized tools	Tumor treatment, localized therapies	Limited to specific procedures, and less versatile than general surgical robots.
KUKA LWR4b	Lightweight, flexible, capable of collaborative tasks.	Rehabilitation and assistive tasks in patient care	The precision required for delicate surgeries may be lacking

4.3 CLASSIFICATION OF MEDICAL ROBOTICS IN BIOMEDICALS

Robots can be classified and analyzed using several taxonomies [13]. Robots can be divided into two main groups based on their application: robots designed to help doctors and nurses, and robots designed to help people with health problems [14]. The first phase includes surgical robotics, research missions, diagnostics, and treatment. The second category includes assistive technologies such as robots that improve the lives of the disabled and the elderly, promote personal independence, and robotic medical devices that people with motor disabilities use due to dementia. Figure 4.1 shows the functional classification of medical robots.

Medical robots are divided into three categories based on size: (1) macrorobotics, (2) microrobotics, and (3) biobotics.

Macrobotics refers to larger robotic systems used in various medical applications, including surgical and rehabilitation manipulators, as well as mobility aids like wheelchairs. These robots are typically designed for more extensive procedures and can assist in surgeries or rehabilitation processes.

Microrobotics encompasses robots for minimally invasive surgery (MIS) and small mechatronics devices utilized in routine surgical procedures. These robots are designed to perform delicate tasks within the human body, enabling precision and reducing recovery times. They can also include miniature mechatronics tools that assist in traditional surgical procedures.

The biobotics category focuses on simulating biological systems to enhance our understanding of human physiology. Biobotics can involve robots that mimic biological functions or assist in studying biological processes, contributing to advancements in medical research and treatment.

The classification of surgical robots is based on their role in clinical applications. These robots are classified as tools that can collaborate with doctors to perform surgical procedures. This system divides the system into five parts: (1) intraoperative

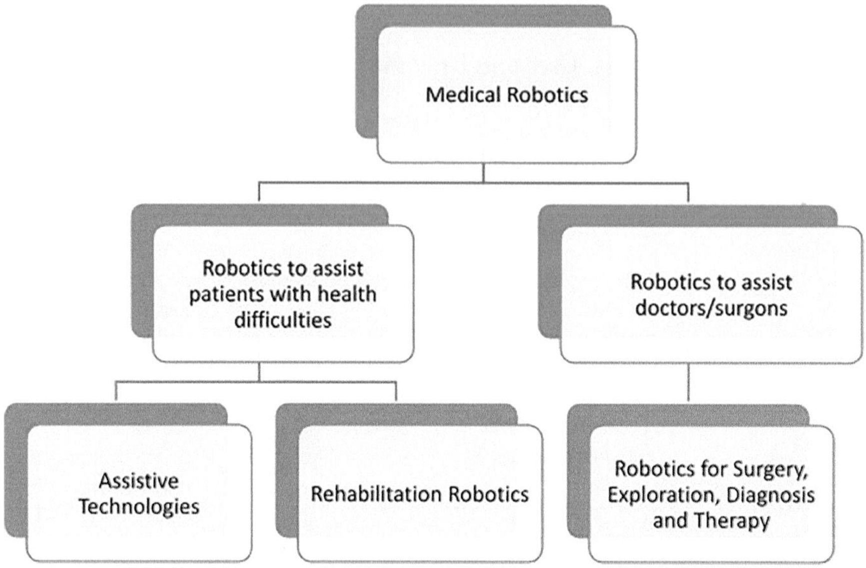

FIGURE 4.1 Classification-based applications of medical robotics

transfer, (2) telesurgical system, (3) navigation devices, (4) standard coordination system, and (5) standard control system [15].

Robotic surgery is based on a computer-integrated system (CIS). Procedures are divided into two categories: (1) CAD/CAM surgery and (2) specialist surgery. A classification system for medical robots based on their role. The three roles that a robot can play in a process are: (1) a passive role, where the robot is not involved, and the risk is low; (2) limited responsibility, where the robot is responsible for many tasks involving the highest risk, but still limited by the importance of the process; and (3) critical responsibility, where the robots participate in the process and take the pressure, responsibility, and risk [16].

In addition to the primary classifications, here are examples of surgical robots categorized by their specific types:

- Automated Arms (Mako Robotic-Arm Assisted Surgery): This system is used for orthopaedic surgeries, particularly in knee and hip replacements, allowing for precise bone cutting and implant placement.
- Mobile Devices (RoboCup): A mobile robotic system designed for telemedicine, enabling remote consultations and examinations by healthcare professionals.
- Mills (Surgical Robots for Bone Milling): These robots are used in orthopaedic surgeries to mill bone surfaces accurately, ensuring a proper fit for implants.
- Telerobotic Devices (Remote Surgery Systems): The Remote Presence Robot (RP-VITA) allows doctors to conduct remote examinations and consultations, providing care to patients in distant locations

These examples illustrate the diverse applications and capabilities of medical robotics across various classifications, highlighting its significance in modern healthcare.

They classify medical robots according to their type of practice, including neurosurgery, ophthalmic surgery, otolaryngology (ENT), general surgery, thoracic surgery, cardiac surgery, gastrointestinal surgery, colorectal surgery, and urological surgery. This type of work is classified based on mechanical design and robotic technology.

Rehabilitation robots are primarily categorized into two types: auxiliary and therapeutic. Assistive robots can help people with mobility issues, such as aging, disability, or stroke, perform daily tasks efficiently and effectively. Robots cannot prepare a patient's nervous system to regain control of a damaged or inflamed limb, nor can they provide feedback on the rehabilitation process. Careful planning is critical for patients' long-term or permanent use of these robots. A common example of this group is measles. However, medical procedures can aid patients in their recovery. These devices are used for a short period of time to support the patient's work. Medical robots can help caregivers and patients, making treatment faster and less stressful for both parties.

4.3.1 Technological Limitations in Early Biomedical Robotics

The evolution of biomedical robotics has been marked by significant technological limitations in its early stages, particularly in computational power and AI capabilities. Table 4.5 presents these limitations.

The early stages of biomedical robotics were hindered by significant technological limitations, particularly in terms of computational power and AI capabilities. However, modern advancements have successfully overcome these obstacles, leading to more sophisticated, efficient, and safer robotic systems in healthcare. This evolution underscores the importance of continuous research and development in the field of biomedical robotics.

4.4 REHABILITATION ROBOTICS HISTORY

This section introduces early technologies that have gained clinical and commercial significance.

4.4.1 Assistive Robotics

Assistive robots with complex systems and virtual reality monitors are used in healthcare and other fields. Fifty years ago, robotics played no role. Master/enslaved person tuners were used until 1960. Tuners were initially designed for radio equipment. Master/slave control is made easier with the simulated human hand. Engineers chose humanoid animals for expressions to make control easier. Integrated circuits were developed in the early 1960s, coinciding with the emergence of minicomputers. This new computer-controlled orthosis allows paralyzed patients to move their arms as needed. Many paralyzed patients lost feeling in their legs due to trauma and the lack

TABLE 4.5
Limitations and Advancements

Early Limitations		Overcoming Obstacles with Modern Advancements	
Key	**Description**		
Computational Power	Early robotic systems were limited by their processing capabilities, which hindered their ability to perform real-time, complex calculations. This limitation hindered the robots' responsiveness during surgical procedures, making them less effective in dynamic environments where quick decision-making is crucial	Enhanced Computational Power:	Today's biomedical robots are equipped with powerful processors that enable real-time data processing and the execution of complex algorithms. This advancement allows for more precise control and quicker responses during surgeries, improving patient outcomes
AI Capabilities	The initial stages of biomedical robotics lacked sophisticated AI algorithms, which meant that robots could not learn from data or adapt to new situations. This rigidity made it challenging for early robotic systems to handle the variability of human anatomy and the unpredictability of surgical scenarios.	Advanced AI Integration:	The integration of machine learning and AI has revolutionized biomedical robotics. Modern systems can analyze vast datasets, learn from previous surgeries, and adapt their techniques based on real-time feedback. This capability enhances the robots' decision-making processes, making them more effective in unpredictable surgical environments
Sensor Technology	Early robots often relied on basic sensors that provided limited feedback about the surgical environment. This lack of advanced sensory input restricted the robots' ability to interact safely and effectively with delicate tissues, increasing the risk of complications during procedures.	Improved Sensor Technology	The development of advanced sensors, including 3D imaging and haptic feedback systems, has greatly improved the interaction between robots and human tissues. These technologies enable more precise navigation and manipulation of delicate structures, thereby reducing the risk of damage during procedures.

of early warning systems, leaving operators desperate. Engineers have developed internal or remote manipulators to support the complex structure of the injured upper limbs. The Rancho Los Amigos telemanipulator, a seven-degree-of-freedom (DOF) robotic arm, utilizes bidirectional translation for remote control. In vertical medical rehabilitation, a human-machine interface is unnecessary for a telemetrically-actuated wheelchair. Engineers recognize that effective human-centered design relies entirely on the hands-on operator.

In the 1980s, wheelchair manufacturers used autonomous navigation systems as the first vision systems. Ultrasonic sensors can measure the distance of objects within their field of view by emitting sound waves. Several sensor rings are installed on the wheelchair, allowing a comfortable ride. Vision servo systems utilizing laser distance sensors were developed in the 21st century to enable wheelchair navigation. Although expensive, they are faster, more accurate, and more effective in finding the most suitable routes. The Hephaestus system led to smart wheelchairs with sonar navigation in the 21st century [17].

Before 2000, many assistive robots, in addition to arms and wheelchairs, were introduced to the market. Oxford Intelligent Machines (OxIM) developed a range of robotics for recovery in the late 1980s and 1990s, including the RT series, the RAID project, and the MASTER system. A vertical support system is designed to organize various professional tasks for a working person. One of the most popular work-assistance machines of the 1990s was the Handy-1 feeding robot, developed by British researcher Mike Topping. Handy-1, sold by Rehab Robotics (UK). The product was initially created as a nutritional aid for people with disabilities, such as children with cerebral palsy (CP). Later improvements allowed robots to paint, shave, and wash.

4.4.2 Automated Diagnostic Systems

Biomedical robotics is an advanced technology that integrates robotics, artificial intelligence, and medical expertise to independently identify, examine, and diagnose health issues. These systems originated in the late 20th century, initially used for image analysis and rudimentary decision assistance. Since then, the field has undergone tremendous evolution, driven by advancements in machine learning, sensor technology, and robotics. There is a growing trend of incorporating automated diagnostic systems into various medical equipment and platforms. These include advanced imaging systems that utilize artificial intelligence to identify tumors and wearable devices that track vital signs and predict potential health issues. The present research focuses on enhancing the precision and immediacy of diagnostic capabilities, refining the interaction between humans and robots in medical environments, and designing systems that can adapt to each patient's specific needs. As these technologies advance, they hold the potential to enhance the delivery of healthcare, improve patient outcomes, and reduce healthcare expenditures [18].

4.5 MEDICAL APPLICATIONS OF SURGICAL SYSTEMS

This section summarizes notable research on continuum robots and commercial systems relevant to surgical applications.

Neurosurgery: Neurosurgical methods involve delicate and intricate procedures targeting vital brain architecture. Neurosurgery should be performed less invasively to improve treatment success and feasibility, as current practices include risks such as wide cranial openings, tissue pushing, and proximity to vital functional structures. Image guidance is commonly used in operating rooms worldwide, enabling neurosurgeons to target brain targets precisely. Surgical robots like Rosa and Renaissance assist surgeons in frameless stereotactic and spine surgeries. Current systems only use straight and rigid instruments. Continuum robots can access nonlinear routes within the brain, enabling new surgical treatments.

Otolaryngology: They provide access to many target areas through natural environments, thus facilitating various operations. Surgeons often use a flat or flexible endoscope and instruments to access the nose, mouth, or ear canal. However, these tools only offer a limited number of routes, making some areas inaccessible or difficult to navigate. Traditional open surgery is used to treat infections in these areas. Continuous and controlled robots can provide flexibility that is not available otherwise.

Cardiac Surgery: Heart surgeries such as valve replacement/repair or septal defect closure often require open heart surgery. Special surgical procedures can be performed while the heart is still beating, allowing for targeted treatment of specific areas that require attention. In recent years, cardiac surgery based on sterile cardiac surgical catheters has become available. However, catheter-based surgery has two significant challenges: 1) the limited ability to apply and control the forces required for this procedure, and 2) the difficulty in correctly inserting the catheter into the heart. This has prompted research into robotic operators for heart surgery.

Vascular Surgery: Minimally invasive procedures typically use catheters and guidewires for injections, irrigation, and device placement. Typical uses include angioplasty, the treatment of aneurysms, and the treatment of embolisms. During catheter placement, control is the biggest challenge for motorists using cables and guidewires. This is because friction between the catheter and the vessel wall may impede the transmission of pressure and torque to the head [19]. This is especially true when the catheter tip extends beyond the vascular access. During intraoperative medical diagnosis using fluoroscopy, it is challenging for physicians to coordinate catheter push/pull and guidewire rotation with the movement of the imaging area. Automated robotic catheters aim to address these barriers. Hansen Medical's Magellan Endovascular Robotic Catheter System comprises a lead, a controllable internal guide, and an external guide, all connected to the proximal end where insertion, withdrawal, and exposure occur.

The specification is achieved by placing four coaxial cables at the conductor's end, green. The distal part of the guide is 2 cm long and can bend up to 180◦ °, with a bending radius of 7 mm. Both the Magellan and Sensei X systems use tendon displacement. The main difference between them is their purpose: radiofrequency cardiac ablation (Sensei) or minimal endovascular surgery.

Abdominal Interventions: In addition to laparoscopic surgery, small advanced robots can deliver needles through small incisions for invasive surgery. The success of central resection of abdominal tumors using repeated ablations and radiography depends on the surgeon's skill. The challenge is to move the graft from the tissue to the surgical site and control the necrotic area. Webster and colleagues developed the ACUSITT device, a central ultrasound ablator connected to an acoustic medical system with a two-tube robot (active cannula). The working cannula is guided through the peripheral wound to gain access to the liver. This allows an indirect insertion procedure to avoid the sizable hepatic artery and vein. In addition to robotic devices, manual insertion units have been proposed. The accuracy of this method has been tested in vitro and ex vivo using 3-D freehand ultrasound. Elastography is used to evaluate ablation procedures in a clinical setting.

Urology: The Da Vinci System, developed by Intuitive Surgical Inc., is widely used in urological procedures such as prostatectomy and hysterectomy surgeries. Future urological surgical platforms will need to have a single port to make the procedure less invasive, or through the urethra to treat prostate or bladder disease. The suitability of continuous robots for this application stems from their exceptional flexibility, scalable size, and stable positional movement.

4.6 AI-ASSISTED SRS

Alan Turing created AI in the 1950s with the concept of model intelligence and the Turing test, "Can Machines Think?" In 1956, the Dartmouth Conference established AI, marking its inception and laying the groundwork for its development and widespread adoption. AI research expanded from 1957 to 1974 due to advances in computer storage and processing and increased funding. Initial AI programs, such as Newell and Simon's General Problem Solver and Weizenbaum's ELIZA, demonstrated problem-solving and language interpretation capabilities. But the AI journey remains a hurdle. Funding and interest in AI declined during "AI winters" due to disappointed expectations and technological limits, particularly in data storage and processing speed. The AI comeback in the 1980s was driven by advances in DL technologies and expert systems that mimic human decision-making. Despite obstacles, the field advanced in the 1990s and 2000s. Advancements in computer storage and processing speed have led to significant breakthroughs, such as IBM's Deep Blue defeating Garry Kasparov and Google's AlphaGo defeating Ke Jie [20].

The past decade has witnessed exponential growth in AI capabilities, driven by advancements in computer power and increased data availability. This period has seen the rise of deep neural networks (DNNs), advancements in machine translation, language models like OpenAI's GPT-3, and innovative developments in picture and speech recognition. Recent advancements, such as OpenAI's DALL-E, GPT-4's text and image processing capabilities, and Meta's Segment Anything, demonstrate the field's rapid advancement. AI has expanded to include other disciplines that aim to simulate or enhance human abilities. Critical areas of AI research include data-driven algorithmic learning (ML), deep learning (DL), natural language processing (NLP), robotics, expert systems, visual data interpretation, and reinforcement learning (RL). These disciplines contribute to the expanding range of AI applications across various industries.

4.6.1 Features of AI-Assisted SRS

AI can be utilized in SRS to analyze patient data, design surgical procedures, and enhance the motion control of surgical actuators. Surgeons, SRS, and AI-aided SRS may offer diverse solutions for surgical challenges. AI-aided SRS aims to improve information analysis, surgical planning, and robot execution under physician control. In SRS, AI applications can be classified as algorithmic or physical [21]. The computational component involves ML algorithms that learn from extensive medical data over time. Generalized machine learning (ML) algorithms in medicine utilize supervised and unsupervised learning, as well as reinforcement learning (RL) and transfer learning techniques, to improve model accuracy and resilience. These strategies are commonly employed to address challenges in managing multi-source information and surgical planning. The physical component involves sophisticated control algorithms that enable SRS to adapt to unexpected events during surgery and make real-time decisions. This real-time decision-making capability assesses the robot's intelligence. Autonomous decision-making is a typical difficulty in designing robotic systems, such as surgical robots. While fully autonomous surgical robot decision-making is still a distant goal, AI has advanced semi-autonomous and collaborative research. In this section, we examine how AI is utilized in perception, navigation, planning, and control modules to enhance the functionality of AI-aided SRS.

4.6.2 Perception and Navigation Improve with AI

AI has significantly enhanced perception and navigation modules in complex medical information processing. Combining medical data analysis with AI can significantly enhance patient treatment outcomes. Surgical data and surgeon experience are essential for analyzing complex medical information. Researchers have extensively studied picture segmentation, object identification, disease classification, signal processing, and multi-source information fusion utilizing classic ML and DL approaches [22]. Image segmentation accuracy has improved thanks to AI, enhancing the objectivity and automation of surgical procedures. Medical images are more complex than natural images, making classic segmentation methods, such as thresholding, region growing, and max-flow algorithms, less precise. According to current research, AI algorithms like FCN and U-Net are practical for medical image segmentation [23]. Achieved a Dice coefficient of 0.9376 using a fully convolutional Dense-Net and U-Net for semantic segmentation of spinal cord ultrasound images, enabling automatic analysis and autonomous laminectomy procedures. A cascading 3D-Unet was utilized to segment the left and right hip bones and sacrum from massive datasets, achieving a Dice coefficient of 0.987 and outperforming previous approaches in both accuracy and flexibility. Using an iterative deep learning labelling technique reduces data labelling expenses.

The use of AI in pathological classification has improved lesion recognition and categorization. It helps diagnose diseases quickly and accurately and enhances SRS procedures through standardization and automation. Machine Learning (ML) techniques, including random forest and gradient boosting trees, have been utilized in conjunction with Raman spectroscopy, to classify gliomas with an accuracy of 0.83 for normal tissue and 0.82 for malignant tissue. Using a dense convolutional LSTM algorithm, [24] improved breast tumor classification accuracy from 0.625 to 0.847, distinguishing between benign and malignant tumors. AI can provide objective, autonomous, and pre-sequential subprocesses for standardized surgical image diagnosis in SRS. AI excels at multisource information fusion, including image registration, which is crucial for pre- and intraoperative medical imaging. Traditional registration approaches align multi-source data using metrics and minimize them through parameter modifications. Faster and more accurate DL algorithms are outperforming previous methods. Transfer learning-based pseudo-Siamese multi-view registration framework effectively addresses the 2D–3D rigid registration issue. The technique uses feature-based transfer learning to extract characteristics from fluoroscopic pictures. In a research study with three participants and fewer than 100 fluoroscopic images, the mean registration success rate was 40%. The system can produce accurate and dependable findings even with minimal real-image datasets. A CNN-based system for real-time localization of target organs and posture in endoscopic videos attained an average intersection-over-union score above 80% and excellent segmentation precision in all tests [25].

In conclusion, AI has improved SRS perception and navigation modules. AI improves diagnosis and navigation by improving image segmentation, surgical tool tracking, pathology classification, signal processing, and multi-source integration. The system enables precise diagnostics, surgical execution, and clinician decision support, thereby enhancing surgical standardization and consistency within the healthcare system.

4.6.3 AI Enhances Surgical Planning

Identifying patterns in surgical planning entails quantifying and simplifying the intangible "feel" of a plan. AI enhances surgical planning by recognizing trends based on surgeons' clinical experience. AI improves surgery planning using CAD/CAM and helpers. AI is improving surgical CAD/CAM autonomy, going from manual to computer-assisted planning by surgeons. Traditional computer-assisted planning often involves human intervention, which can lead to uncertainty and bias. AI is used to learn surgical planning from surgeons and extract techniques based on their experiences, addressing this issue objectively. AI-aided planning has applications in puncture path planning, reduction trajectory planning, tissue tracking, and implant planning. Wang et al. [26] built an atlas-based system to automate pelvic resetting reduction paths, mirror clinical patterns, and ensure secure techniques. This method used a statistical shape model (SSM) for patient-specific planning on a dataset of 40 patients. It has a positive prediction value of over 90% for safe trajectories within bone corridors. Additionally, cadaver research has demonstrated the effectiveness of enhanced fluoroscopy in ensuring accurate trajectory accuracy in safe corridors. This method is compatible with regular fluoroscopic surgery workflow and does not require additional hardware. It may reduce surgery time and radiation exposure, simplifying percutaneous screw placement in pelvic trauma surgery. Yadav et. al [27] developed algorithms to extract crucial information from CT scans for automated grinding trajectory planning in robot-assisted laminectomies. This method utilizes a DNN optimized for precise lamina positioning, achieving 95.7% recognition accuracy and a positioning error of 1.12 mm. Their innovative trajectory generation and grinding-speed modification procedures, integrated into a system, permitted precise and automated surgical planning.

Utilizing AI in surgical planning represents a significant shift from manual to AI-aided methods. AI-aided SRS enhances surgical planning precision, speed, and safety by using surgeons' clinical experience. Patients benefit from more accurate and safer surgical procedures, which in turn reduce the risk of complications. AI-aided SRS also minimizes surgeon burden, enhances surgical precision, and enables them to focus on more intricate patient care.

4.6.4 AI Improves Control Strategies

Combining control strategies with AI can automate and standardize surgical processes. Optimizing surgical control involves considering the interactions among humans, robots, and the environment. AI enhances actuator dynamic control performance, particularly in HRI and REI. AI algorithms make HRI more innovative and more accessible. Surgeons can use intuitive means to regulate SRS, including body movements, voice, and vision. This method demands a robust control and feedback system, which is challenging for standard algorithms. ML and AI algorithms enhance HRI by enhancing processing efficiency and decision-making for control and feedback information. Recently, research groups have improved surgeon decision-making and navigation accuracy.

The authors in [28] propose eye-gaze-based technologies that utilize DenseNet and transfer learning to guide surgical robots intuitively. DNN training data difficulties were solved by automating gaze image capture and categorization. A DenseNet-22 variant makes the model computationally efficient and suited for memory-limited devices, such as field-programmable gate arrays. The 10 kb variant processes 64 pictures per second and has 82% accuracy across 36 categories, making it suitable for mobile computing devices and thus broadening its application reach. A RAS head-mounted master interface (HMI) improved continuous operation flow through head motions. This surgical robot-integrated system features a Human-Machine Interface (HMI), four degrees of freedom endoscopic control, and a da Vinci Research Kit. HMI reduced job completion time and system time delay to 0.72 s using SVM classification with 92.28% accuracy. This solution addresses discontinuous surgical operations, improving surgical efficiency and communication.

4.6.5 AI Techniques in Surgical Robotics

Artificial Intelligence (AI) plays a crucial role in enhancing the capabilities of surgical robots (Table 4.6). Various AI techniques, particularly deep learning architectures and

TABLE 4.6
Applications and Suitability of AI Techniques

Deep Learning Architectures	Application	Suitability
Convolutional Neural Networks (CNNs):	CNNs are widely used for image analysis in surgical robotics. They can process and analyze medical images, such as CT scans or surgical videos, to identify anatomical structures and assist in planning surgical procedures.	Their ability to learn spatial hierarchies of features makes them ideal for recognizing complex patterns in medical imaging, which is essential for accurate surgical navigation and planning.
Recurrent Neural Networks (RNNs)	RNNs, particularly Long Short-Term Memory (LSTM) networks, are used for analyzing sequential data, such as the movements of surgical instruments over time	They are effective in capturing temporal dependencies, which is crucial for understanding the dynamics of surgical procedures and predicting the next steps in real-time
Reinforcement Learning Algorithms	This technique allows surgical robots to learn from expert surgeons by observing their actions during procedures. For instance, the da Vinci surgical system utilizes imitation learning to enhance its capabilities in suturing and segmentation tasks.	By mimicking expert behavior, robots can acquire complex skills without extensive programming, making them adaptable to various surgical scenarios
Q-Learning and Policy Gradient Methods	These reinforcement learning techniques can be used to optimize the decision-making process of surgical robots, allowing them to learn optimal strategies for performing tasks based on feedback from their environment	They enable robots to improve their performance through trial and error, which is particularly useful in dynamic surgical environments where conditions can change rapidly.

reinforcement learning algorithms, are employed to improve surgical precision, efficiency, and decision-making. This section underlines these techniques and their suitability for surgical robotics.

These mentioned techniques are suited for surgical robotics due to their precision and adaptability, data-driven decision-making, and automation of complex tasks. Combining deep learning and reinforcement learning allows surgical robots to perform tasks with high precision while adapting to the unique challenges of each surgical procedure. AI techniques leverage vast amounts of surgical data to enhance decision-making processes, improving outcomes and reducing patient complications.

These AI methods enable the automation of intricate surgical tasks, reducing the cognitive load on surgeons and allowing them to focus on more complex aspects of patient care.

4.7 EXAMPLES OF SUCCESSFUL SRS IMPLEMENTATION WITH AI

AI-assisted surgical robotic systems (SRS) is best advanced by examining four exemplary instances: autonomous soft tissue suturing via the STAR robot, autonomous navigation of an intracardiac catheter, robotic pelvic fracture reduction with the R-Universal system, and autonomous operations on the da Vinci platform. Table 4.7 shows the examples of successful SRS implementation with AI.

The table above presents data on various robotic and automated surgical systems. The STAR (Smart Tissue Autonomous Robot) system is a robotic device capable of autonomously performing suturing procedures. It has been demonstrated to exhibit superior precision compared to human surgeons. The graphic also references a Catheter Autonomous Robot designed for heart interventional operations, which utilizes artificial intelligence and machine learning to enhance navigation and force control. Additionally, it examines the topic of fracture reduction using an unidentified robot that utilizes machine learning to realign segments. Lastly, there is a concise reference to automated da Vinci surgery, which utilizes artificial intelligence to assist in surgical tasks typically performed by skilled surgeons. The table generally showcases

TABLE 4.7
Classic Cases with AI and its Summary

Classic Cases Names	Summary
Soft Tissue Suture by STAR	With autonomous anastomosis, soft tissue surgery is hard. In 2014, the author claimed STAR improves laparoscopic suture surgery. Developed a three-dimensional NIRF imaging system and autonomous suturing algorithm for open-supervised autonomous soft tissue surgery in 2016. Developed and tested STAR-based shared control for human-robot surgery. In 2021, STAR added a second robot manipulator to manage loose sutures and introduced near-infrared fluorescent sutures for autonomous job segmentation and delimitation. In 2022, STAR demonstrated increased imaging, tissue deformation tracking, machine vision, learning algorithms, and real-time control for surgical planning and execution. Inconsistency and accuracy, STAR beat professional surgeons' manual methods and RAS. STAR had more consistent suture spacing at 3.05 × 0.8 mm and bite depth at 3.05 × 0.91 mm than LAP (2.28 × 1.04 mm, 2.02 × 1.10 mm) and RAS (1.58 × 0.65 mm, 1.69 × 0.55 mm). The simulation models and in-vivo research show that autonomous SRSs like STAR can improve surgical uniformity, patient outcomes, and procedure standardization.

TABLE 4.7 (Continued)
Classic Cases with AI and its Summary

Classic Cases Names	Summary
Catheter Autonomous Robot	Heart interventional procedures are difficult. An autonomous intracardiac catheter robot used haptics and vision to achieve wall-following and visual feature reproduction. Positive thigmotactic algorithm wall-following provides low-force feedback to reach the heart wall goal. Merging visuals and touch with a haptic vision sensor, endoscope, ML models, and image-processing algorithms. When an interventional catheter tip hits an object, picture, kind, and pressure force are recognized automatically. The autonomous navigation method obtained 95% success rate for paravalvular leakage, averaging 39 ±17 s, compared to 34 ± 29 s for teleoperation and 31 ±27 s for manual navigation. An average distance of 2.9 × 1.5 mm for autonomous estimating and 3.0 × 2.0 mm for operator-based registration was achieved for catheter tip positioning above leaks. The technique uses haptics and vision for fully autonomous navigation, according to experiments. Animal trials suggest that the autonomous robotic catheter can match clinical practitioners. A millimetre-scale soft robotic platform that guides interventional equipment to heart entrance targets was developed in 2023. This platform showed flexibility, stability, and Newton-level forces in two right atrial operations.
Fracture Reduction via R-Universal Robot	Trauma orthopaedics recognizes displaced pelvic fractures as complex, requiring accurate and efficient reduction during surgery. The R-universal robot system, featuring an optical tracking device, automated reduction planning, navigation software, and a UR16e manipulator, addresses the challenge by developing a UNet-based learning model for segmenting fracture fragments in large datasets and automating target position planning using an SSM-based method. With a segmentation accuracy of 0.998 Dice coefficient and a reduction precision of 3.07 mm, this methodology outperformed previous methods in accuracy and flexibility. An asymmetrical pelvis-specific automatic reduction path planning method was included to aid in fracture reduction. Implementing autonomous SRS decreases surgeon workload, and operating time, and provides X-ray radiation protection. Robot-assisted autonomous closure reduction of a pelvic fracture reported for the first time.

(*continued*)

TABLE 4.7 (Continued)
Classic Cases with AI and its Summary

Classic Cases Names	Summary
Automated da Vinci surgery	AI-aided surgical assistants have made significant progress in automating surgical planning. A unique imitation learning system enables SRS to learn crucial procedures by analyzing videos of skilled surgeons' surgeries. This method combines Motion2Vec, a Siamese network, and an RNN to train deep-embedding feature spaces from the surgical film efficiently. Using a da Vinci robot, they addressed challenges in surgical suturing segmentation and position imitation in simulation and reality, utilizing representation learning to replicate motion. Applying this method to the public JIGSAWS dataset yielded a mean accuracy of 85.5%, significantly improving over prior methods. This achievement highlights the potential of AI to enhance surgical precision and efficiency.

progress in self-governing and AI-supported surgical methods across several medical fields.

4.7.1 Medical Significance

The function of AI in healthcare settings is reviewed by examining cutting-edge intelligent SRS technologies and their novel applications. Medical research, including SRS, requires empirical evaluations in clinical or similar conditions. There are few recent clinical investigations on AI applications in SRS, with few involving human individuals. Most studies examined the performance of the AI component in AI-aided SRS. Ex vivo, animal, and cadaver experiments are the primary methods for verifying AI's practicality. The system uses a universal distributional Q-learning AI algorithm for robot planning and control. The method was tested in silico and ex vivo using a synthetic liver phantom, demonstrating its ability to address multiple targets with a single insertion point [29]. Studies indicate variations in accuracy and stability across AI-aided robotic procedures, traditional surgeries, and simple robotic surgeries [30]. Table 4.8 displays recent representative studies. Similar assessments demonstrate the superiority of AI techniques over conventional methods in surgical procedures.

The above table provides a concise overview of the various uses of robotic platforms and AI in medical procedures. The tasks encompassed in this field include estimating the force between tools and tissue, calculating the path for needle insertion, performing vascular catheterization, determining the trajectory for handling objects, localizing tumours, and segmenting CT images. Various robotic systems, including da Vinci, RFA surgical robot, and KUKA LWR4 b, are utilized alongside artificial intelligence techniques such as LSTM, UDQL, Rec-FNN, RNN, SVM, and Cascaded U-Net. The results column displays the performance data for each application,

TABLE 4.8
Current studies on Artificial Intelligence (AI) for SRS

Objective	Robotic Platform used	Type of AI Used	Results
Estimation of Tool-Tissue Force	da Vinci	LSTM	Accuracy: 90%
Path planning for the insertion of flexible needles.	Radiofrequency ablation (RFA) surgical robot	UDQL	Improved precision and durability Target error: 2.3 mm
Autonomous robotic vascular catheterization	6-DOF robot and 3-DOF manipulator	Rec-FNN	Vessel identification means dice: 0.70; Surface reconstructed error: 2.52 × 0.87 mm; Tracking error: 1.65 × 1.07 mm. In vitro: consistent; in vivo: decreased cannulation failures.
Handling trajectory	KUKA LWR4þ	RNN	RCM constraint: within 3 mm, End effector error: 4 mm.
Identification and rectification	da Vinci	EHNN	Improved precision in compensation: 78.64% is about equal to 93.32%.
Tumor localization estimation	URS	SVM	The registration error is around 0.20 mm, with a needle insertion error of 2.29 ± 0.68 mm. To enhance accuracy and repeatability, improvements are required.
CT image segmentation	UR16e	Cascaded U-Net	The dice score was 98.7%, indicating a high level of success. The procedure successfully produced an anatomic reduction, and no complications were experienced.
Assessment and analysis of surgical abilities	da Vinci	Domain-Adapted Machine Learning	The system's accuracy is 95.2%, with a margin of error of 2.98%. It is capable of effectively representing skill level, abnormality, and hidden information.

* LSTM: Long Short-Term Memory, *UDQL: Universal Distributional Q-Learning, *RNN: Recurrent Neural Network, *EHNN: Elastic Hysteresis Neural Network, *SVM: Support Vector Machine.

average absolute value, zero-crossings, and waveform length in mind, robots amplify EMG signals from seven arm muscles. This upper limb rehabilitation robot utilizes a splint to instruct patients on how to reach for objects. Seven-DOF ARMiN robots are notable breakthroughs in upper limb rehabilitation robots. Three shoulder rotation freedom levels are elbow, wrist, and forearm supination and pronation. The Wilmington Exoskeleton (T-Wrex) is a five-DOF ULRER that targets arm weakness in patients. The robot's upper arm and forearm have two connections. T-Wrex's antigravity effect enables patients to experience floating arms [33].

4.8.1.2 Lower Extremity

LLRERS utilize mechanical power devices and AI to enhance muscle mobility and address physical abnormalities in patients with lower limb dysfunction. Knees are among the most fragile joints in the human body, and their performance significantly impacts walking and daily activities. Knee exoskeleton robots enhance leg movement and provide lower limb mobility. Recently, a knee exoskeleton robot was developed using a linkage mechanism and an inverse dynamic model to predict the sit-to-stand trajectory. This robot is handy and efficient for patients with knee injuries during sitting-to-standing activities, as both clinical and experimental results demonstrate. Wearable soft knee exoskeletons are new in this sector. The IMU control system of this robot measures knee joint angles, reducing energy expenditure by 6.8% by aiding knee movement during walking. The robot's development highlights the discrepancy between lower limb movement and patient intention, improving knee exoskeleton function and patient safety.

4.8.1.3 Evaluation Standards

When evaluating a rehabilitation service provider, financial considerations are a crucial factor to consider. Due to considerations including accessibility, safety, material, and design criteria, robot costs vary. Also, cost impacts the audience's size and the type of service. Some items are only available to rehabilitation and medical institutes, while others are inexpensive for the general public. In this sense, third-party providers like health insurance firms can help reduce customer costs. Cost is not the sole factor influencing market and buyer size. Customers will be less likely to use an economical item requiring special maintenance or specialized knowledge to operate. Thus, accessibility is another important factor. A device used at home or local hospitals is considered conveniently accessible. A rehabilitation system or robot that requires frequent repairs or calibrations might be expensive and inaccessible, especially if it takes too long to be replaced. Maintainability is a concern; therefore, systems must be designed to reduce the frequency and duration of repairs and calibrations. Due to the COVID-19 pandemic and global isolation, new rehabilitation systems aim to provide remote assistance, supervision, assessment, and other services to stroke patients and the elderly, encouraging neural plasticity training.

4.8.1.4 Safety Assessments

A two-stage safety assessment for rehabilitation robots is possible. The first occurs during product development, while the second occurs during patient use. The latter is assessed by clinical trial monitoring and adverse event reports, whereas the former confronts challenges due to limited criteria for safety assessments of rehabilitation robots during development. When designing safety for robots that work with humans, common approaches include model-based systems using software packages, which examine the system, environment, and user knowledge. The recommended safety evaluation standards vary based on the application and domain. Safety measures in industrial and agricultural systems may include biosensors to prevent soil and water contamination. At the same time, rehabilitation robots require sensors to monitor pressures and patient weight and prevent falls. Different scopes and unsynchronized domains can hinder roboticists from applying proper standards to their systems. Proposing safety protocols for numerous domains and applications is a promising solution to this difficulty [34].

The goal is to reduce the likelihood of a hazard by recommending the appropriate safety protocol, also known as a safety skill. This method provides engineers with a clear framework for reducing account risk, including principles and norms applicable to diverse domains. Validating risk-lowering methods begins with hazard identification. The most common adverse events are soft tissue injuries such as skin abrasions, lesions, irritations, reddening, bruising, and discomfort. The second most common adverse effects are musculoskeletal, including lower back pain, muscular soreness, joint pain, tibia fracture, and tendinopathy.

4.9 CHALLENGES IN BIOMEDICAL ROBOTICS

Biomedical robotics is a dynamic and rapidly evolving field with numerous significant challenges. Here is a brief overview of several significant barriers [35]:

- **Miniaturization:** Creating miniature robots for minimally invasive medical operations.
- **Biocompatibility:** Ensuring the materials utilized are non-toxic and pose no harm to the human body.
- **Power supply:** Developing durable and secure energy sources for implanted devices.
- **Precision and control:** Attaining highly accurate motions within intricate biological surroundings.
- **Soft robotics:** Developing adaptable, regulatory-compliant robots that can securely engage with fragile tissues.
- **AI and autonomy:** Creating intelligent systems to make real-time decisions during procedures.
- **Human-robot interaction:** Enhancing interfaces for surgeons and healthcare providers
- **Regulatory approval:** Managing intricate regulatory procedures for medical gadgets.
- **Cost-effectiveness:** Enabling the affordability and accessibility of sophisticated robotic systems.

- **Ethical considerations:** Addressing issues related to the ability to make independent decisions, safeguarding personal information, and ensuring appropriate human supervision.

4.10 CONCLUSION AND FUTURE SCOPE

Biomedical robotics is a rapidly advancing and disruptive field in modern medicine, offering unparalleled possibilities in diagnosis, therapy, and patient care. Incorporating artificial intelligence and machine learning has significantly enhanced surgical robotic systems' accuracy, effectiveness, and autonomy. Significant progress has been made in minimally invasive robotic surgery, robotic-assisted rehabilitation, and automated diagnostic systems. Nevertheless, numerous obstacles must be addressed to achieve the full potential of biomedical robotics. These factors encompass reducing device size for less intrusive treatments, ensuring compatibility with living organisms and safety, advancing durable energy sources for implanted devices, achieving accurate manipulation in intricate biological environments, and fabricating flexible robots capable of securely interacting with delicate tissues. Furthermore, there are persistent obstacles to authorization by regulatory bodies, including cost efficiency and ethical concerns surrounding autonomous decision-making in healthcare facilities.

The field of biomedical robotics exhibits significant potential. Promising areas for expansion include the advancement of nanorobots for precise medication delivery, sophisticated robotic prosthetics with enhanced sensory input, and increased integration of artificial intelligence for real-time guidance in surgical operations. Advancements in soft robotics and biocompatible materials have the potential to result in medical devices that are more versatile and secure. With the increasing collaboration of engineers, computer scientists, and medical specialists, we can expect a rise in developing creative solutions to existing problems. Ultimately, the continuous advancement of biomedical robots can significantly transform the way healthcare is delivered, enhance patient outcomes, and improve the overall well-being of individuals worldwide.

REFERENCES

[1] Ahn, C., Liang, X., & Cai, S. (2019). Bioinspired design of light-powered crawling, squeezing, and jumping untethered soft robot. *Advanced Materials Technologies*, *4*(7), 1900185. doi:10.1002/admt.201900185.

[2] Arents, J., & Greitans, M. (2022). Smart industrial robot control trends, challenges, and opportunities within manufacturing. *Applied Sciences (Basel, Switzerland)*, *12*(2), 937. doi:10.3390/app12020937.

[3] Attanasio, A., Scaglioni, B., De Momi, E., Fiorini, P., & Valdastri, P. (2021). Autonomy in surgical robotics. *Annual Review of Control, Robotics, and Autonomous Systems*, *4*(1), 651–679. doi:10.1146/annurev-control-062420-090543.

[4] Battaglia, E., Boehm, J., Zheng, Y., Jamieson, A. R., Gahan, J., & Majewicz Fey, A. (2021). Rethinking autonomous surgery: Focusing on enhancement over autonomy. *European Urology Focus*, *7*(4), 696–705. doi:10.1016/j.euf.2021.06.009.

[5] Bergeles, C., & Yang, G.-Z. (2014). From passive tool holders to microsurgeons: Safer, smaller, more innovative surgical robots. *IEEE Transactions on Bio-Medical Engineering*, *61*(5), 1565–1576. doi:10.1109/TBME.2013.2293815.

[6] Choi, Y., Bae, M. S., Oh, Y., & Lee, S. (2024). Predictive Geogenic Radon Potential (P-GRP): A novel approach for comprehensive hazard assessment and risk modeling in subsurface environment. *The Science of the Total Environment*, *944*(173721), 173721. doi:10.1016/j.scitotenv.2024.173721.

[7] Curran, N. M., Sun, J., & Hong, J.-W. (2020). Anthropomorphizing AlphaGo: A content analysis of the framing of Google DeepMind's AlphaGo in the Chinese and American press. *AI & Society*, *35*(3), 727–735. doi:10.1007/s00146-019-00908-9.

[8] Daneshmand, M., Bilici, O., Bolotnikova, A., & Anbarjafari, G. (2017). Medical robots with potential applications in participatory and opportunistic remote sensing: A review. *Robotics and Autonomous Systems*, *95*, 160–180. doi:10.1016/j.robot.2017.06.009.

[9] Gu, G.-Y., Zhu, J., Zhu, L.-M., & Zhu, X. (2017). A survey on dielectric elastomer actuators for soft robots. *Bioinspiration & Biomimetics*, *12*(1), 011003. doi:10.1088/1748-3190/12/1/011003.

[10] Gumbs, A. A., Frigerio, I., Spolverato, G., Croner, R., Illanes, A., Chouillard, E., & Elyan, E. (2021). Artificial intelligence in surgery: How do we achieve autonomous actions? *Sensors (Basel, Switzerland)*, *21*(16), 5526. doi:10.3390/s21165526.

[11] Gupta, U., Qin, L., Wang, Y., Godaba, H., & Zhu, J. (2019). Soft robots based on dielectric elastomer actuators: A review. *Smart Materials & Structures*, *28*(10), 103002. doi:10.1088/1361-665x/ab3a77.

[12] Han, R., Uneri, A., De Silva, T., Ketcha, M., Goerres, J., Vogt, S., … Siewerdsen, J. H. (2019). Atlas-based automatic planning and 3D-2D fluoroscopic guidance in pelvic trauma surgery. *Physics in Medicine and Biology*, *64*(9), 095022. doi:10.1088/1361-6560/ab1456.

[13] Liu, Y., Wu, X., Sang, Y., Zhao, C., Wang, Y., Shi, B., & Fan, Y. (2024). Evolution of surgical robot systems enhanced by artificial intelligence: A review. *Advanced Intelligent Systems*, *6*(5), 2300268.

[14] Khan, R., Rehman, N. U., Ilyas, N., Sfina, N., Barhoumi, M., Khan, A., … Khan, A. (2023). Threshold switching in nickel-doped zinc oxide based memristor for artificial sensory applications. *Nanoscale*, *15*(4), 1900–1913. doi:10.1039/d2nr05257a.

[15] Khullar, V., R.M, V. M., Muthukumarasamy, S., Prabha, C., Singh, H. P., & Pavankumar, V. (2023). Hybrid of DNN feature extraction and ensemble classification for identification of esophagitis and barretts in upper gastrointestinal tract images. In 2023 International Conference on Computer, Electronics & Electrical Engineering & their Applications (IC2E3), Srinagar Garhwal, India (pp. 1–7). Institute of Electrical and Electronics Engineers (IEEE). doi:10.1109/IC2E357697.2023.10262774.

[16] Kim, Y., & Zhao, X. (2022). Magnetic soft materials and robots. *Chemical Reviews*, *122*(5), 5317–5364. doi:10.1021/acs.chemrev.1c00481.

[17] Kumar, V., Prabha, C., Sharma, P., Mittal, N., Askar, S. S., & Abouhawwash, M. (2024). Unified deep learning models for enhanced lung cancer prediction with ResNet-50-101 and EfficientNet-B3 using DICOM images. *BMC Medical Imaging*, *24*(1), 63. doi:10.1186/s12880-024-01241-4.

[18] Leonard, S., Opfermann, J., Uebele, N., Carroll, L., Walter, R., Bayne, C., … Krieger, A. (2021). Vaginal cuff closure with dual-arm robot and near-infrared fluorescent sutures. *IEEE Transactions on Medical Robotics and Bionics*, *3*(3), 762–772. doi:10.1109/tmrb.2021.3097415.

[19] Li, Z., Li, S., & Luo, X. (2021). An overview of calibration technology of industrial robots. *IEEE/CAA Journal of Automatica Sinica*, 8(1), 23–36. doi:10.1109/jas.2020.1003381.

[20] Maier-Hein, L., Vedula, S. S., Speidel, S., Navab, N., Kikinis, R., Park, A., … Jannin, P. (2017). Surgical data science for next-generation interventions. *Nature Biomedical Engineering*, *1*(9), 691–696. doi:10.1038/s41551-017-0132-7.

[21] Olfa, B. (2020). Medical robotics. In *Control Theory in Biomedical Engineering* (pp. 153–204). Elsevier. https://doi.org/10.1016/B978-0-12-821350-6.00008-1

[22] Saeidi, H., Opfermann, J. D., Kam, M., Wei, S., Leonard, S., Hsieh, M. H., … Krieger, A. (2022). Autonomous robotic laparoscopic surgery for intestinal anastomosis. *Science Robotics*, *7*(62), eabj2908. doi:10.1126/scirobotics.abj2908.

[23] Sreedevi, A. G., Nitya Harshitha, T., Sugumaran, V., & Shankar, P. (2022). Application of cognitive computing in healthcare, cybersecurity, big data and IoT: A literature review. *Information Processing & Management*, *59*(2), 102888. doi:10.1016/j.ipm.2022.102888.

[24] Taylor, R. H., & Stoianovici, D. (2003). Medical robotics in computer-integrated surgery. *IEEE Transactions on Robotics and Automation*, *19*(5), 765–781. doi:10.1109/tra.2003.817058.

[25] Tovar-Arriaga, S., Pérez-Soto, G. I., Camarillo-Gómez, K. A., Aviles, M., & Rodríguez-Reséndiz, J. (2024). Perspectives, challenges, and the future of biomedical technology and artificial intelligence. *Technologies*, *12*(11), 212. doi:10.3390/technologies12110212.

[26] Ureel, M., Augello, M., Holzinger, D., Wilken, T., Berg, B.-I., Zeilhofer, H.-F., … Mueller, A. A. (2021). Cold Ablation Robot-guided Laser Osteotome (CARLO®): From bench to bedside. *Journal of Clinical Medicine*, *10*(3), 450. doi:10.3390/jcm10030450.

[27] Wang, C., Xie, S., Li, K., Wang, C., Liu, X., Zhao, L., & Tsai, T.-Y. (2021). Multi-view point-based registration for native knee kinematics measurement with feature transfer learning. *Engineering (Beijing, China)*, *7*(6), 881–888. doi:10.1016/j.eng.2020.03.016.

[28] Yadav, P., Chaudhari, K., Dave, A., & Sindhu, A. (2024). Exploring the evolution of robotic surgery in obstetrics and gynaecology: Past, present, and future perspectives. *Cureus*, *16*(3), e57155. doi:10.7759/cureus.57155.

[29] Yibulayimu, S., Liu, Y., Sang, Y., Zhu, G., Wang, Y., Liu, J., ... & Wu, X. (2023). Pelvic fracture reduction planning based on morphable models and structural constraints. In Greenspan, H. et al. (Eds.), *Medical Image Computing and Computer Assisted Intervention – MICCAI 2023. MICCAI 2023. Lecture Notes in Computer Science* (Vol. 14228). Springer. doi:10.1007/978-3-031-43996-4_31.

[30] Zhang, K., Wang, X., Chang, Y., Wu, Y., Wang, S., & Wang, L. (2023). Carbazole-decorated organoboron emitters with low-lying HOMO levels for solution-processed narrowband blue hyperfluorescence OLED devices. *Angewandte Chemie (Weinheim an Der Bergstrasse, Germany)*, *135*(47). doi:10.1002/ange.202313084.

[31] Zhang, M., & Li, J. (2021). A commentary of GPT-3 in MIT Technology Review 2021. *Fundamental Research*, *1*(6), 831–833. doi:10.1016/j.fmre.2021.11.011.

[32] Zhang, Xin, Lv, S., Lu, X., Yu, H., Huang, T., Zhang, Q., & Zhu, M. (2020). Synergistic enhancement of coaxial nanofiber-based triboelectric nanogenerator through dielectric and dispersity modulation. *Nano Energy*, *75*(104894), 104894. doi:10.1016/j.nanoen.2020.104894.

[33] Zhang, X., Beeraka, N. M., Sinelnikov, M. Y., Glazachev, O. S., Ternovoy, K. S., Lu, P., … Chen, K. (2024). Breast cancer-related lymphedema: Recent

updates on the clinical efficacy of therapies and bioengineering approaches for personalized therapy. *Current Pharmaceutical Design*, *30*(1), 63–70. doi:10.2174/0113816128269545231218075040.

[34] Zhang, Z., Shi, Y., Fu, J., Liu, D., Zhu, D., Liu, X., … & Fan, H. (2022). Customized three-dimensional printed prosthesis as a novel intercalary reconstruction for resection of extremity bone tumours: A retrospective cohort study. *International Orthopaedics*, *46*(12), 2971–2981. doi:10.1007/s00264-022-05559-y.

[35] Zheng, H., Gu, Y., Qin, Y., Huang, X., Yang, J., & Yang, G. Z. (2018). Small lesion classification in dynamic contrast enhancement MRI for breast cancer early detection. In Frangi, A., Schnabel, J., Davatzikos, C., Alberola-López, C., Fichtinger, G. (Eds.), *Medical Image Computing and Computer Assisted Intervention – MICCAI 2018. MICCAI 2018. Lecture Notes in Computer Science* (Vol. 11071). Springer. doi:10.1007/978-3-030-00934-2_97.

5 Data-Driven Models for the Prediction of the COVID-19 Transmission

M. Vijayakarthick, S. Meyyappan, N. Vinoth, A. Ganesh Ram, and C. Meenakshi

5.1 INTRODUCTION

A novel coronavirus disease was discovered in the province of Wuhan, China, in December 2019 [1]. The disease can be transmitted from person to person and can lead to a range of illnesses, from mild to severe, and it is a novel virus for humans. The World Health Organization, WHO, named the new virus COVID-19. On March 11, 2020, the WHO assessed that the coronavirus contained all the attributes to become a pandemic [2] by looking at its spread and risk to human life.

Since October 7, 2020, due to this epidemic, a whopping 35,664,048 infected cases and 1,044,296 deaths have been reported to the WHO from 216 territories [3]. Scientists and global health professionals worldwide collaborated to accelerate research and development efforts aimed at containing the transmission of the COVID-19 pandemic [4]. The first affected case of COVID-19 in the Republic of India was recorded on January 30, 2020 [5]. The Indian government implemented numerous actions to control the spread of COVID-19. In its report, the WHO stated that several vaccines are in the research phase and are suitable for entering the test phase, with primary results expected within 3–6 months after entering the test phase [6]. In the early stages of the pandemic, the Indian Government enforced a nationwide lockdown, effective from March 25, 2020 [7], and extended it until May 31. As of the end of May, 182,143 affected cases and 5,164 fatalities had been officially reported nationwide [8]. However, lockdowns are not a permanent solution to this epidemic and cannot be sustained for extended periods, especially for a country like India. As soon as the Government of India lifted the lockdown, the affected population abruptly increased to 6,757,131, including 104,555 deaths and 5,744,693 recoveries as of October 7, 2020. According to the Ministry of India website [9], India's COVID-19 cases had crossed four crores on January 25, 2022. A total of 4,46,73,392 confirmed cases were reported in India on December 03, 2022. In addition, it is found that the recovery rate increased to 98.8% (44,138,235), and the total death rate is very low, at 1.19% (530,628). Due to the lower-case load rate and high recovery rate, there is expected to be a decline in COVID-19 cases in India. The federal government is still functioning strongly by coordinating all

DOI: 10.1201/9781003561309-5

state health departments and other public health partners to address the prevailing difficult situation.

The first case of coronavirus was reported on March 7, 2020, in Tamil Nadu, India. According to the state government's report dated 3 December 2022, the number of COVID-19 patients has increased to 3,594,186, comprising 38,049 deaths and 3,556,137 recoveries [10]. The state government has initiated several constructive steps to curb the transmission of the pandemic, including statewide lockdowns, creating social awareness, screening suspected individuals, and identifying COVID-19 clusters.

Mathematical frameworks play an important role as they serve the purpose of forecasting pandemic situations and suggest effective control methods. In this work, efficient Deep Neural models are developed for COVID-19, which can be used to estimate the number of infected populations, fatality rates, and requirements of COVID beds in hospitals.

The remainder of the paper comprises three additional sections. Section 5.2 presents the strategy behind the development of DNN infectious models, while Section 5.3 displays and analyzes the results obtained from the estimated models, and Section 5.4 concludes the research work.

5.2 MATHEMATICAL MODELLING OF COVID-19

Mathematical models and data analysis methods are practical tools for examining and predicting the spread of COVID-19. Mathematical models become essential as they assist decision-makers in obtaining medical supplies, assigning hospital beds, allocating human resources, and ensuring the sustainability of the health system throughout the entire epidemic period [11]. Moreover, the forecasting models are used to predict disease tendency, fatality rate, hospitalizations, and the impacts of intervention measures. Mathematical modelling-based analysis has been conducted by fellow researchers on the pandemic, considering its rapid spread [12,13]. The work proposes dynamic mathematical models for estimating the transmission of coronavirus using a DNN approach, considering the cases reported by the Government of Tamil Nadu, India. In the subsequent section, we present the proposed method and discuss the outcomes, with a primary focus on predicting the number of infected populations, the death rate, and live cases of COVID-19 in Tamil Nadu ahead of time.

5.3 DEEP NEURAL NETWORK MODEL USING LEVENBERG–MARQUARDT BASED BACK-PROPAGATION NEURAL NETWORK

A Deep Neural Network is a typical feedforward structure of neural network with at least three hidden layers (refer to Eq.5.1) as shown in Figure 5.1. The DNN is one of the spirits of Artificial Intelligence, and it is rapidly growing in medical analysis research [14].

Consider, the dimension of input layer in the Artificial Neural Network is $d \in N$

And the non-linear function (rectifier) $\beta = \mathbf{R} \rightarrow \mathbf{R}$

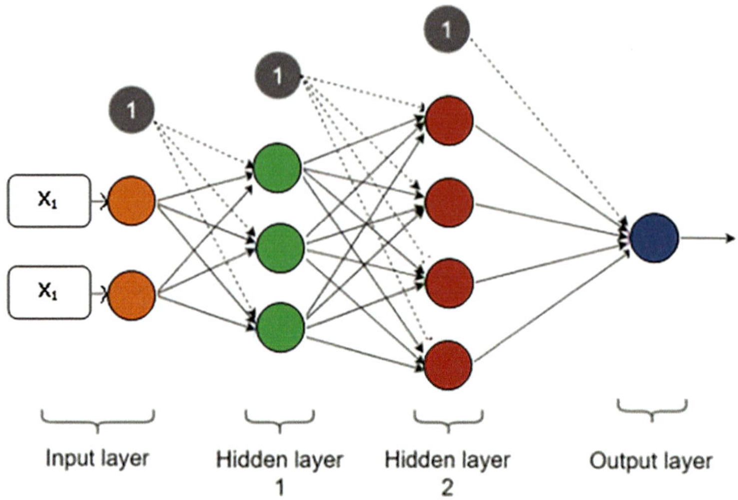

FIGURE 5.1 Deep Neural Network (DNN).

$$W_n = R^{N_{n-1}} \rightarrow R^{N_n}, n = 1....L:$$

The affine linear map A_n is defined by a matrix $W_n \epsilon\ R^{N_{n-1} * N_n}$ and $b_n \epsilon\ R^{N_n}$ by means of

$$A_n(x) = W_n x + b_n$$

Then $\Phi = R^d \rightarrow R^{N_n}$ given by

$$\Phi(x) = W_L \beta\left[W_{L-1}\beta(.....\beta(W_1(x))\right], \quad x \epsilon\ R^d \tag{5.1}$$

where,

N: Number of neurons
L is the Number of layers
Bn is the bias vector
A_n is the Pre-activation function
W_n is the Weight matrix
$\Phi(x)$ consists of a weight matrix of W_n and biases a vector of b_n

In recent years, the Back-Propagation Neural Network (BPNN) with learning capabilities has been widely used in Deep Neural Network (DNN) methods. The back-propagation algorithm consists of two passes through different layers of the neural network. The forward pass is the first one, in which the inputs are applied to the network, and it is trained with the back-propagation algorithm. During the forward pass, the weights are stable. The second one is the backward pass in which the network parameters are varied. Regarding the gradient steepest descent method, the backpropagation neural network trains and updates the weights, then reduces the cost function. To improve the convergence of the BPNN, a Levenberg–Marquard (LM) optimization method has been integrated.

5.3.1 Levenberg–Marquard Method

The LM method [11] is actually an integration of the gradient steepest descent and the Gauss–Newton method.

The fundamental step of Newton's method is:

$$\Delta x_m = A_m^{-1} g_m \tag{5.2}$$

where,

x_m is the weight vector and bias $= \nabla^2 F(x)$
A_m is the Hessian matrix and g_m is the present gradient $= \nabla F(x)$

The performance function F(x) of the Gauss–Newton method is given as

$$F(x) = \sum_{i=1}^{q} e_i^2(x) = e^T(x)e(x) \tag{5.3}$$

And its gradient is represented as

$$\left[\nabla F(x)\right]_j = \frac{\partial F(x)}{\partial x_j} = 2\sum_{i=1}^{q} e_i(x)\frac{\partial e_i(x)}{\partial x_j} \tag{5.4}$$

$$\nabla F(x) = 2J^T(x)e(x) \tag{5.5}$$

where,

e is the error vector
J is the Jacobian matrix

$$J(x) = \left[\frac{\partial e_1}{\partial x_1}\frac{\partial e_1}{\partial x_2}\cdots\frac{\partial e_1}{\partial x_n}\frac{\partial e_2}{\partial x_1}\frac{\partial e_2}{\partial x_2}\cdots\frac{\partial e_2}{\partial x_n}:::\frac{\partial e_q}{\partial x_1}\frac{\partial e_q}{\partial x_2}\cdots\frac{\partial e_{q1}}{\partial x_n}\right] \tag{5.6}$$

The Hessian matrix can be written as

$$\nabla^2 F(x) = \left[\frac{\partial^2 F}{\partial x_1^2} \frac{\partial^2 F}{\partial x_1 x_2} \cdots \frac{\partial^2 F}{\partial x_1 x_n} \frac{\partial^2 F}{\partial x_2 x_1} \frac{\partial^2 F}{\partial x_2^2} \cdots \frac{\partial^2 F}{\partial x_2 x_n} ::: \frac{\partial^2 F}{\partial x_n x_1} \frac{\partial^2 F}{\partial x_n x_2} \cdots \frac{\partial^2 F}{\partial x_n^2} \right] \quad (5.7)$$

$$\left[\nabla^2 F(x)\right]_{mj} = \frac{\partial^2 F(x)}{\partial x_m x_j} = 2\sum_{i=1}^{q} \left(\frac{\partial e_i(x) \partial e_i(x)}{\partial x_m \partial x_j} + e_i(X) \frac{\partial^2 e_i(X)}{\partial x_m \partial x_j} \right) \quad (5.8)$$

where,

$$\nabla^2 F(x) = 2J^T(x) J(x) + p(x) \quad (5.9)$$

and

$$p(x) = \sum_{i=1}^{q} e_i(x) \nabla^2 e_i(x) \quad (5.10)$$

Assuming p(x) is negligibly small, Eq. (5.9) is approximated as

$$\nabla^2 F(x) = 2J^T(x) J(x) \quad (5.11)$$

Substituting Eq. (5.11) in Eq. (5.2), the relationship for the Gauss–Newton method is then obtained by

$$\Delta x_m = -\left(\left[2J^T(x_m) J(x_m) \right]^{-1} \left[2J^T(x_m) e(x_m) \right] \right) \quad (5.12)$$

$$\Delta x_m = -\left(\left[J^T(x_m) J(x_m) \right]^{-1} \left[J^T(x_m) e(x_m) \right] \right) \quad (5.13)$$

The Gauss–Newton method, which is actually derived from Newton's method, has certain imperative benefits over its originating algorithm. In the Gauss–Newton method, the term $\left[J^T(x_m) J(x_m) \right]^{-1}$ does not exist, and the correction factor μ_m is included to address the numerical value problem that arises during the calculation of the inverse matrix. Therefore, Eq. (5.13) can be written as,

$$\Delta x_m = -\left(\left[J^T(x_m) J(x_m) \mu_m I \right]^{-1} \left[J^T(x_m) e(x_m) \right] \right) \quad (5.14)$$

Eq. (5.14) shows the Levenberg–Marquardt algorithm, which exhibits a significantly better convergence rate compared to the gradient steepest descent method when μ_m is large enough. However, if it is small, it may follow the footsteps of the Gauss–Newton method, exhibiting an appreciable convergence mechanism [15].

5.3.2 DNN Models

The proposed feedforward DNN architecture is fully associated with four layers, which include two hidden layers with ten hidden neurons in each, and it is trained with the Levenberg–Marquardt based back-propagation learning algorithm. Both hidden layers and output layers are configured with a tanh sigmoid activation function, and all neurons in the layers are fully interconnected. The accuracy of the DNN epidemic models is evaluated using the Mean Squared Error (MSE) and R-squared (R^2) values.

5.4 DATA SOURCES

The epidemiological data is fetched from the Health & Family Welfare Department, Government of Tamil Nadu [10] and the website authorized by the Government of India [9]. This website provides information on the total COVID-19 population, including active cases and deaths.

5.5 TRAINING AND MODEL VALIDATION

The recorded data used for training must be sufficiently rich to ensure a stable process, as no further learning occurs after training. During training, the DNN learns the dynamics of the epidemic process by mapping the input-output data, which is accomplished through the LM-based back-propagation algorithm.

Based on the reported data from the state of Tamil Nadu, India, simulations were executed in MATLAB software using a DNN model for COVID-19-affected individuals. The predicted output obtained through the DNN model for COVID-19-affected cases in Tamil Nadu, India, from March 9, 2020, to December 3, 2022, is shown in Figure 5.2. It is clear from Figure 5.2 that the forecast model output precisely fits the reported data. Figure 5.3 illustrates the training pattern of the MSE during model validation, where the error goal is achieved after 124 epochs. The training regression is also computed and depicted in Figure 5.4.

Likewise, two additional experiments are performed using the proposed DNN models, considering the total number of coronavirus live cases and mortalities. The forecasted outputs, performance of the validation in terms of MSE, and training regression are computed and presented in Figures 5.5 to 5.10. The calculated values of MSE and training regression value (R^2) are provided in Table 5.1.

From Table 5.1, it is observed that the proposed DNN models achieved high regression values, with R2 scores of 0.9959 for the confirmed cases, 0.99932 for the active cases, and 0.99997 for the total number of deaths. Ultimately, it is clear from the R^2

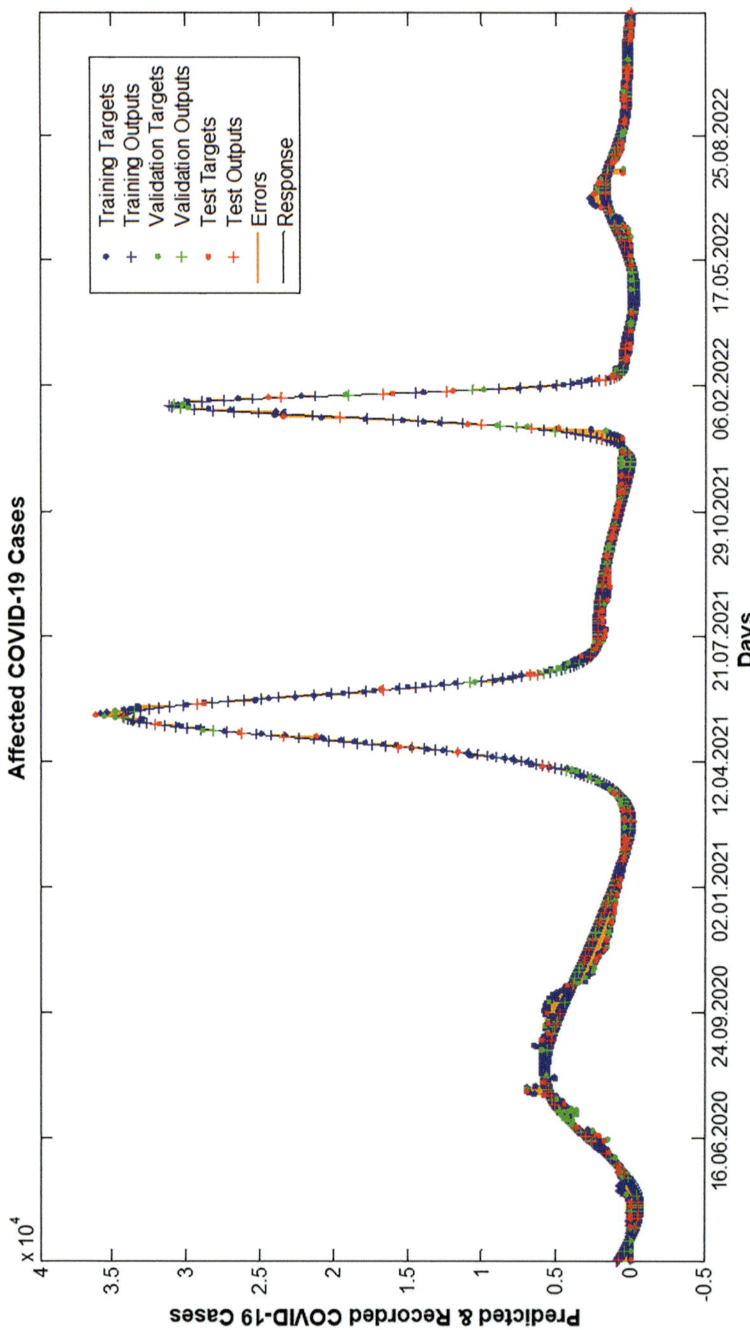

FIGURE 5.2 Response of the total COVID-19-affected populations in Tamil Nadu state.

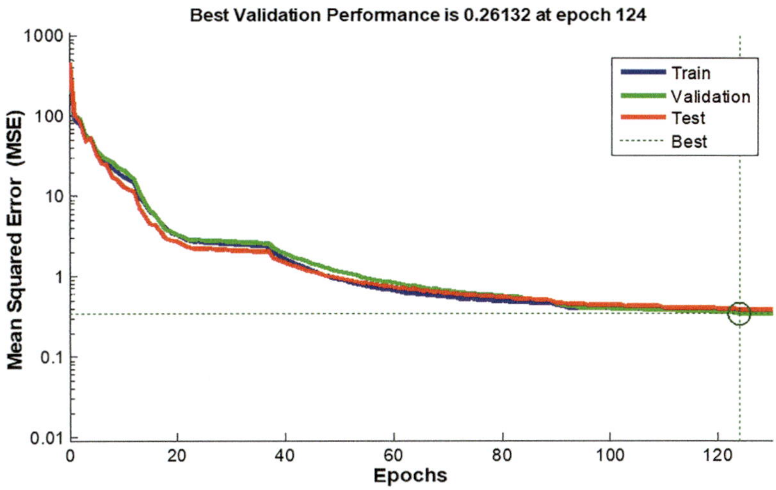

FIGURE 5.3 Validation performance (MSE) for total affected COVID-19 populations.

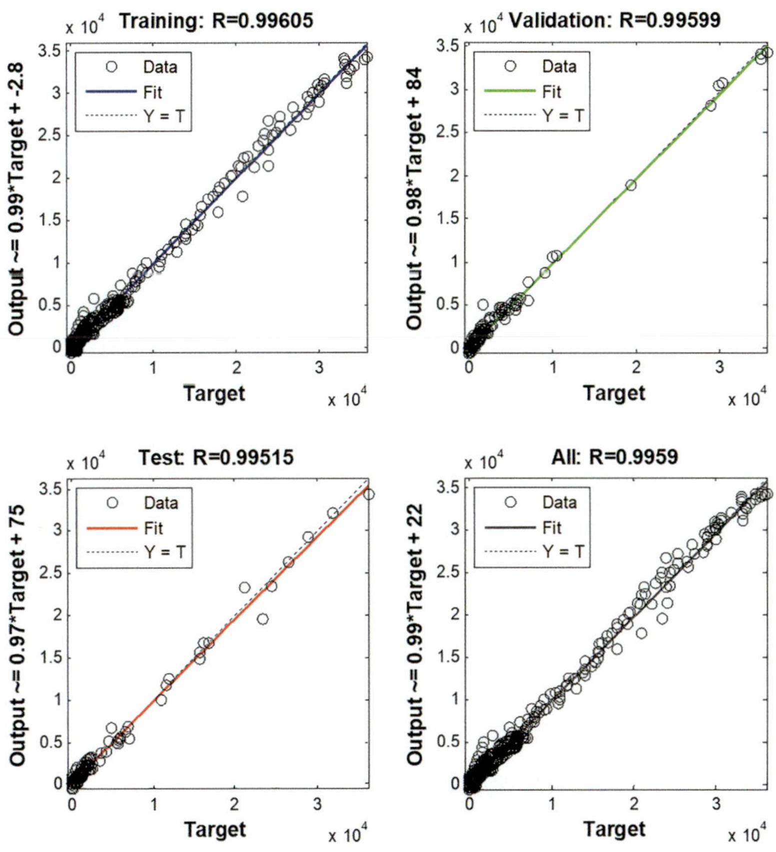

FIGURE 5.4 Regression map for total affected COVID-19 populations.

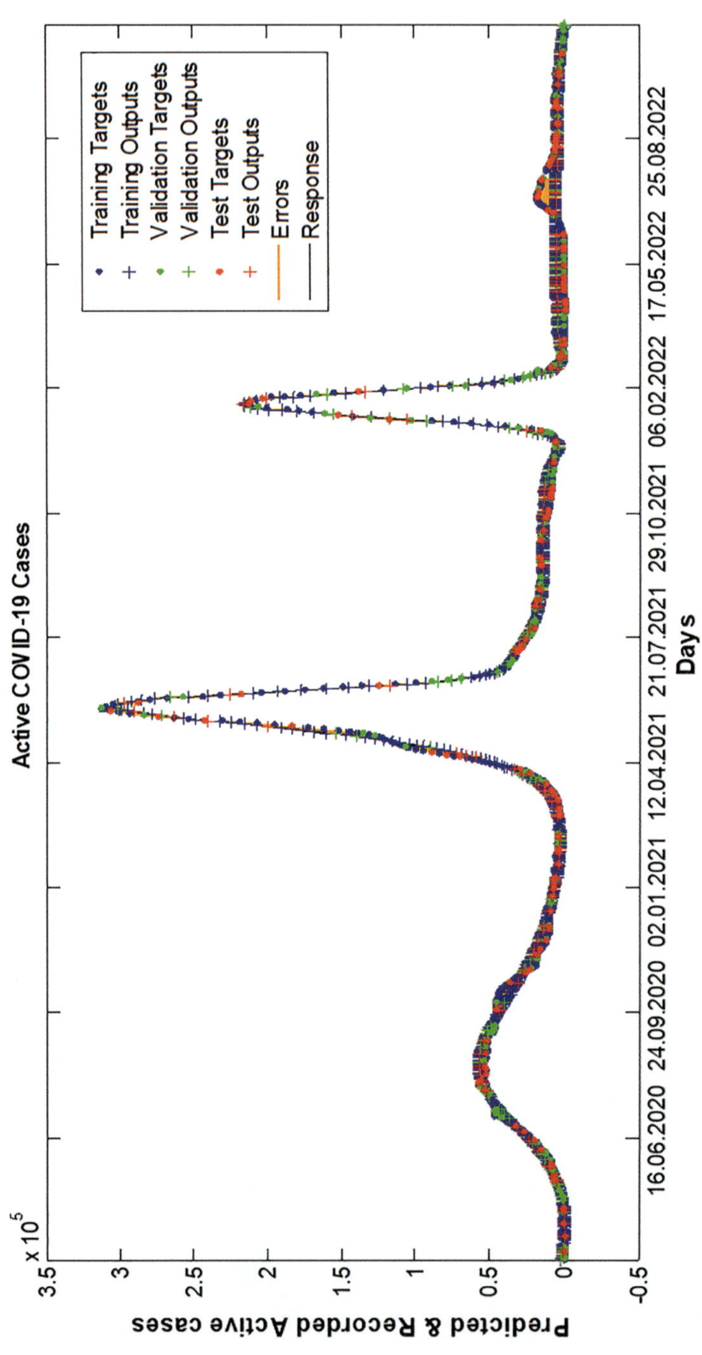

FIGURE 5.5 Response of the total number of active cases in Tamil Nadu.

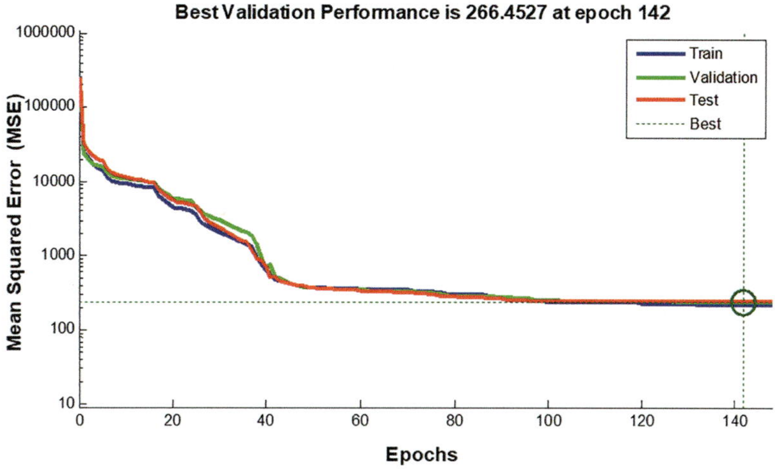

FIGURE 5.6 Validation performance (MSE) for the total number of active cases.

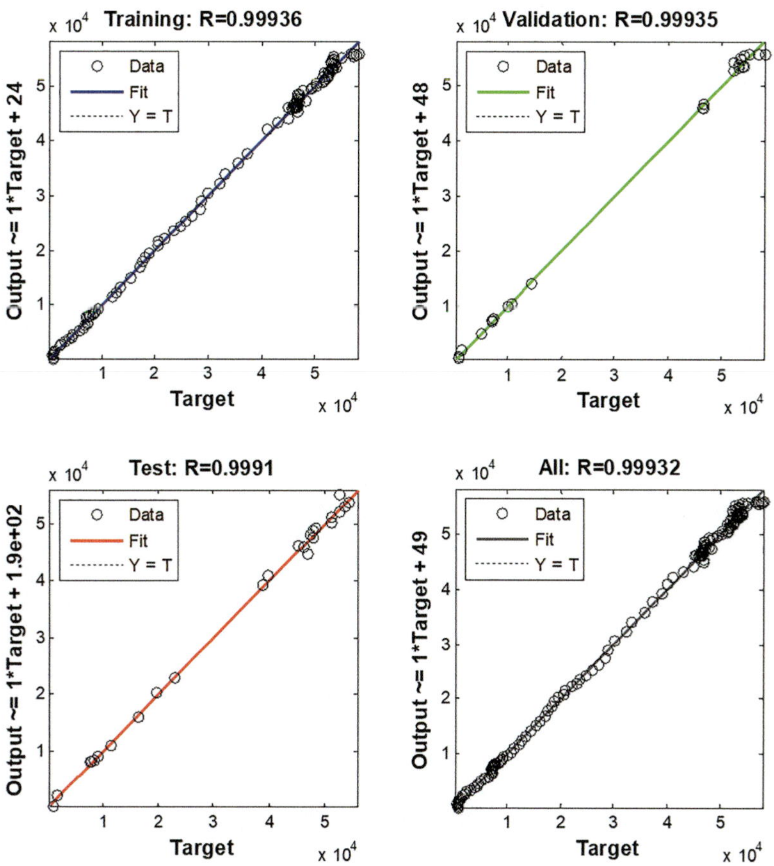

FIGURE 5.7 Regression map for total number of active cases.

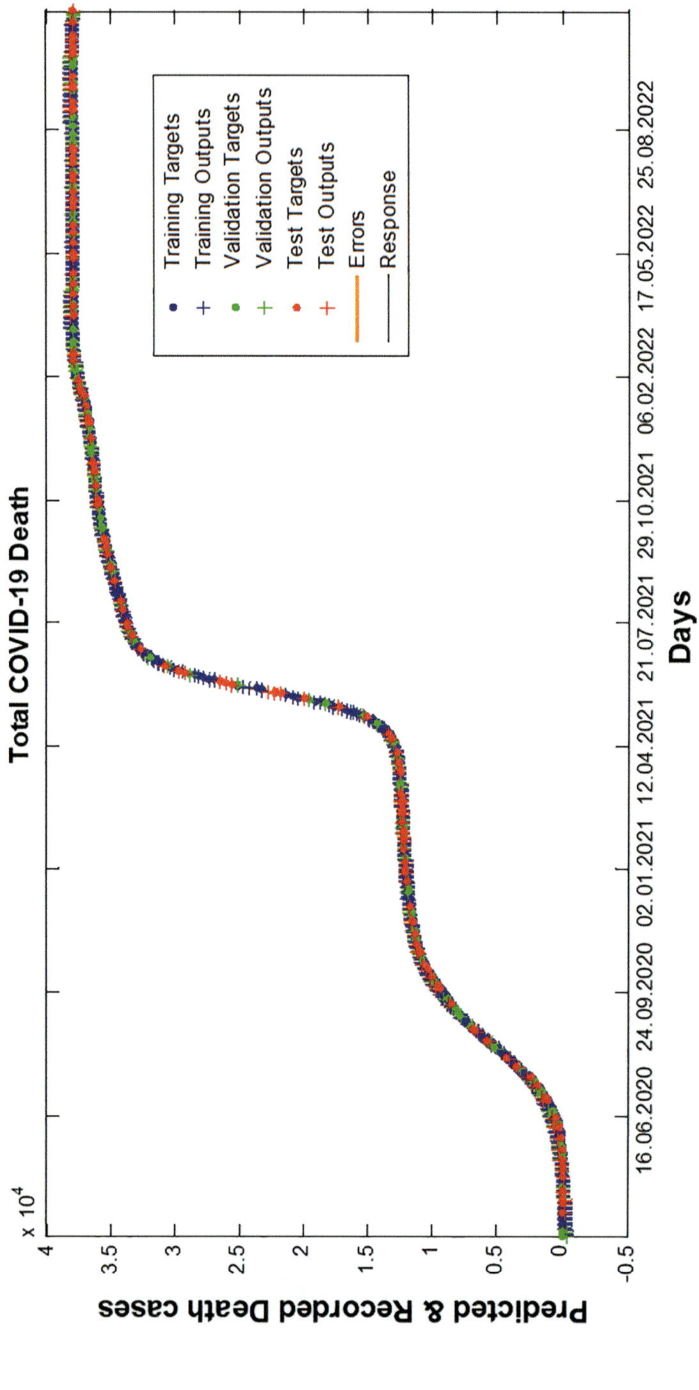

FIGURE 5.8 Response of the total number of deaths in Tamil Nadu state.

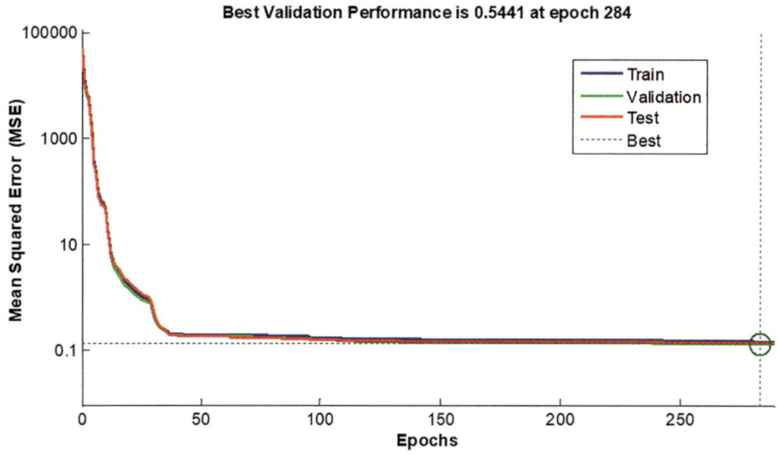

FIGURE 5.9 Validation performance (MSE) for total number of deaths.

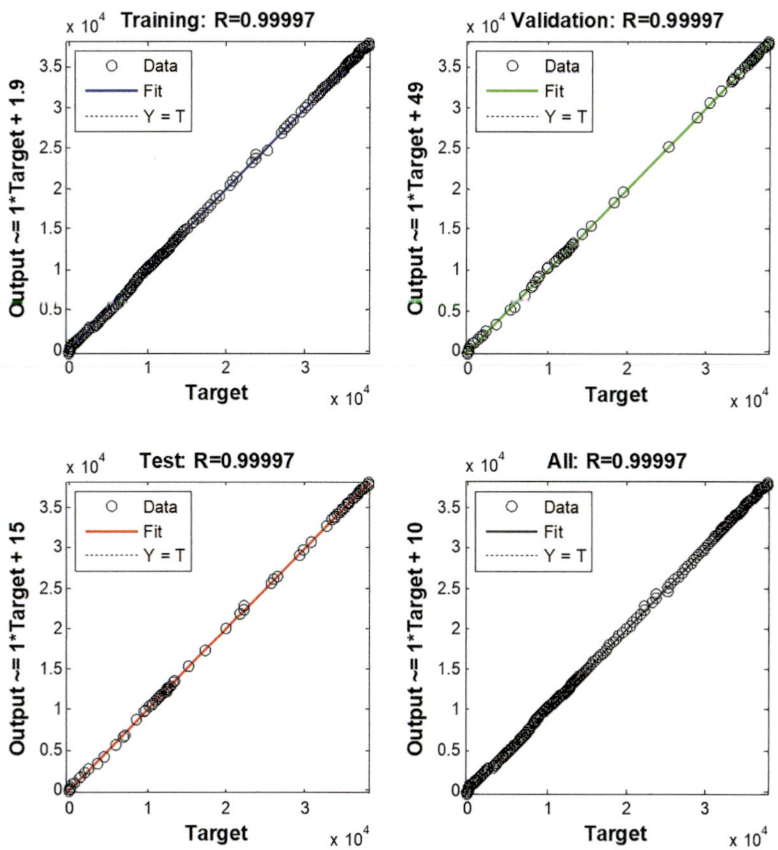

FIGURE 5.10 Regression map for total number of deaths.

TABLE 5.1
Performance Analysis in Terms of MSE and R^2 Value

DNN model	MSE	Maximum Epochs	R^2 scores
Total affected populations	0.26132	124	0.9959
Active cases	266.4527	142	0.99932
Deaths	0.5441	284	0.99997

TABLE 5.2
Prediction of Parameters Related to COVID-19 Spread for December 2022 and January 2023

Date	Total affected populations	Total active cases	Total deaths
20/12/2022	3594276	8	38049
05/01/2022	3594280	4	38049
20/01/2022	3594283	2	38049
05/02/2022	3594284	2	38049
20/02/2022	3594284	1	38049

scores that the predicted results obtained through DNN models are highly close to the reported data by the Tamil Nadu state government. Hence, the DNN can accurately model the transmission of the COVID-19 outbreak, which can be used as a decision-making tool for the government of Tamil Nadu, India.

5.6 FORECASTING ANALYSIS FOR THE EPIDEMIC CASE OF TAMIL NADU STATE

Through the use of DNN models, the transmission behaviour of COVID-19, such as the total affected population, mortalities, and the required number of beds in health centers, is estimated for the months of December 2022 to February 2023 in the state of Tamil Nadu, India, and the predicted data are recorded in Table 5.2. Figures 5.11 and 5.12 display the future predictions of the DNN epidemic models for all three attributes examined in the study. The future predictions of COVID-19 transmission characteristics are given below.

5.6.1 Epidemic Transmission

Figure 5.11 illustrates the DNN model-based analysis of future predictions for COVID-19-infected populations. As of December 3, 2022, 3,594,186 COVID-19 cases have been recorded in the state of Tamil Nadu. The results obtained indicate

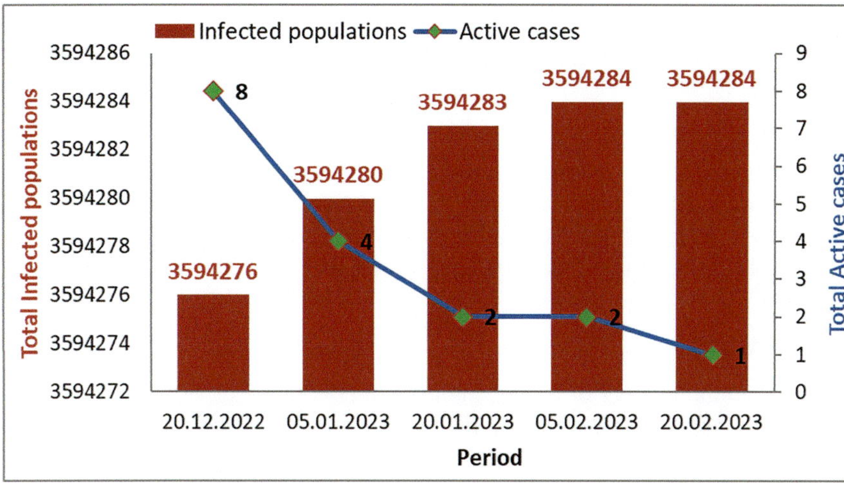

FIGURE 5.11 Future transmission trends of COVID-19 infected and active cases in Tamil Nadu.

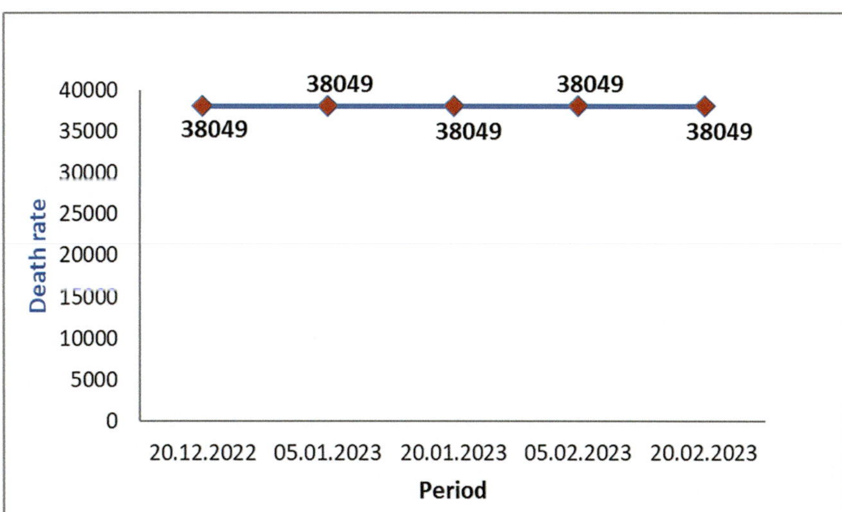

FIGURE 5.12 Future trends in the transmission of COVID-19 fatality rates in Tamil Nadu.

that the affected cases will decrease rapidly and are expected to reach 3,594,276 by the middle of December 2022 and 3,594,284 by the middle of February 2023.

5.6.2 Active Cases

According to the official report, the total number of cases admitted to the health center on December 3, 2022, is approximately 143. The forecast result (refer to Figure 5.11 and Table 5.2) indicates that the number of people to be hospitalized will be approximately 56,172 by the end of October 2020 and 63,983 by November 30, 2020.

5.6.3 Fatalities

Spotting the total number of deaths, the DNN model forecasts (refer to Figure 5.12 and Table 5.2) nearly 38,049 by the middle of December 2022 and 38,049 by February 20, 2023. Therefore, we recommend that severe restrictions be imposed on all affected areas, with strict contact tracing and continuous health monitoring of suspected cases, which in turn may effectively reduce the transmission of the epidemic.

It has been demonstrated that the DNN models reasonably predict the COVID-19 affected cases, which include several deaths and hospitalized people. These expected results demonstrate the superiority of the proposed DNN models in addressing the COVID-19 outbreak.

5.7 CONCLUSION

In this paper, we developed a DNN model with the ability to adapt to the characteristics of COVID-19. The work considered the total affected population, hospitalized cases, and deaths due to COVID-19 in Tamil Nadu. The veracity of the models developed for analysis has been verified using test inputs, and the numerical results align with the actual data, accurately reflecting reality in Tamil Nadu. In addition, the obtained results confirm the ground reality that DNN models can play a crucial role in predicting the trend in the transmission and impact of epidemics. The outcome of the analysis exactly predicts the future trend of the COVID-19 transmission in Tamil Nadu. Thus, the proposed models using the DNN approach may be a vital decision-supporting tool for estimating coronavirus transmission. For future work, we recommend exploring more advanced data-driven models that incorporate real-time data streams, additional epidemiological factors, and privacy-preserving techniques to enhance the accuracy and reliability of COVID-19 transmission predictions. Integrating these models with mobility, social behavior, and vaccination data could further improve prediction performance and provide more adaptive insights for public health interventions.

Data availability: The data supporting the findings of this study are available as open source (https://stopcorona.tn.gov.in/daily-bulletin/) by the Health and Family Welfare Department, Government of Tamil Nadu.

REFERENCES

[1] Roosa, K., Lee, Y., Luo, R., Kirpich, A., Rothenberg, R., Hyman, J. M., Yan, P., & Chowell, G. (2020). Short-term forecasts of the COVID-19 epidemic in Guangdong and Zhejiang, China: February 13–23, 2020. *Journal of Clinical Medicine*, 9(2), 596. https://doi.org/10.3390/jcm9020596

[2] Organization WH. (2020). Coronavirus disease (COVID-19) situation report-51. www.who.int/docs/default-source/coronaviruse/situation-reports/20200311-sitrep-51-covid-19.pdf?sfvrsn=1ba62e57_10 (accessed September 09, 2023).

[3] Organization WH. (2020). Coronavirus disease (COVID-19). www.who.int/emergencies/diseases/novel-coronavirus-2019 (accessed October 07, 2020).

[4] Organization WH. (2020). Global research on Coronavirus disease (COVID-19). www.who.int/emergencies/diseases/novel-coronavirus-2019/global-research-on-novel-coronavirus-2019-ncov (accessed August 07, 2023).

[5] Organization WH. (2020). Novel Coronavirus (2019-nCoV). India Situation Report-1. www.who.int/docs/default-source/wrindia/india-situation-report-1.pdf?sfvrsn=5ca2a672_0 (accessed October 07, 2020).

[6] Organization WH. (2020). An international randomised trial of candidate vaccines against COVID-19. www.who.int/publications/i/item/an-international-randomised-trial-of-candidate-vaccines-against-covid-19 (accessed May 20, 2023).

[7] India Ministry of Home Affairs. (2020). National executive committee guidelines – Order No. 40-3/2020-DM-I(A). www.mha.gov.in/sites/default/files/MHAorder%20copy.pdf (accessed June 24, 2020).

[8] Organization WH. (2020). Novel Coronavirus (2019-nCoV). India Situation Report-18. www.who.int/docs/default-source/wrindia/situation-report/india-situation-report-18.pdf?sfvrsn=7c00a3f_2 (accessed October 07, 2020).

[9] Government of India. (2020). COVID-19 daily updates. www.mygov.in/covid-19/ (accessed October 03, 2023).

[10] Health & Family Welfare Department, Government of Tamil Nadu. (2020). COVID-19 daily updates. https://stopcorona.tn.gov.in/wp-content/uploads/2020/07/Media-Bulletin-21.07.2020-26-Pages-English-469-KB.pdf (accessed October 03, 2023).

[11] Levenberg, K. (1944). A method for the solution of certain non-linear problems in least squares. *Quarterly of Applied Mathematics*, 2(2), 164–168.

[12] Wu, F., Liang, X., & Lei, J. (2023). Modelling COVID-19 epidemic with confirmed cases-driven contact tracing quarantine. *Infectious Disease Modelling*, 8(2), 415–426.

[13] Song, T. H., Clemente, L., Pan, X., Jang, J., Santillana, M., & Lee, K. (2025). Fine-grained forecasting of COVID-19 trends at the county level in the United States. *NPJ Digital Medicine*, 8(1), 204.

[14] Chakravarthy, S. P., Gunasundari, C., Bhuvaneswari, K. S., Sharma, B., & Chowdhury, S. (2022, December). Convolutional neural network (CNN) for image detection and recognition in medical diagnosis. In *The Institution of Engineering and Technology, 6th Smart Cities Symposium (SCS 2022)* (Vol. 2022, pp. 357–361). IET.

[15] Kuo, C. F. J., Tsai, W. L., Su, T. L., & Chen, J. L. (2011). Application of an LM-neural network for establishing a prediction system of quality characteristics for the LGP manufactured by CO2 laser. *Optics & Laser Technology*, 43(3), 529–536.

6 Federated Learning and Privacy-Preservation in Healthcare

Kamal Deep Garg, Karan Kalra, and Antra Soni

6.1 INTRODUCTION

Machine learning (ML) is expanding at an unprecedented rate and has become a vital technology in numerous sectors, including manufacturing, healthcare, and finance. As a result, the healthcare sector appears to be the most suitable area for the application of ML techniques, given the high volumes of data integrated in medical imaging studies and genomics studies. In addition to detecting illnesses and forecasting patient outcomes, machine learning (ML) models, particularly those based on intensive learning, have demonstrated outstanding potential in drug discovery and therapy customization. However, there are significant concerns regarding the use of ML in healthcare, particularly in terms of privacy and the security of sensitive data. Federated Learning (FL) is a cutting-edge method that offers an alternative by enabling decentralized model training. A shared model is trained across several decentralized devices or servers that have local data samples, without sharing these samples with a central server, using federated learning (FL), a state-of-the-art machine learning technique [1]. FL guarantees that data remains on the user's device, with only model changes (such as gradients or parameters) being shared with the central server. This contrasts with the traditional centralized "big data" strategy, which requires all data to be gathered in one place for model training. A global model is then improved by combining these updates, and it is then transmitted back to the local devices. Due to its inherent ability to enhance data confidentiality and privacy, FL is particularly well-suited for sensitive applications, such as healthcare. Since a large portion of the data handled is extremely sensitive, data privacy and security are crucial to the healthcare sector. Specifications that will determine how PETs will be acquired, stored, shared, and analyzed are provided under legalities such as the General Data Protection Regulation (GDPR) in Europe and the Health Insurance Portability and Accountability Act (HIPAA) in the United States.

The shift from centralized machine learning (ML) to federated learning (FL) is depicted in Figure 6.1. Healthcare organizations and providers must utilize innovative ML techniques to assist patients in this highly regulated environment while maintaining robust patient information protection. A potential remedy is FL, which permits cooperative model construction without requiring data centralization. Large

DOI: 10.1201/9781003561309-6

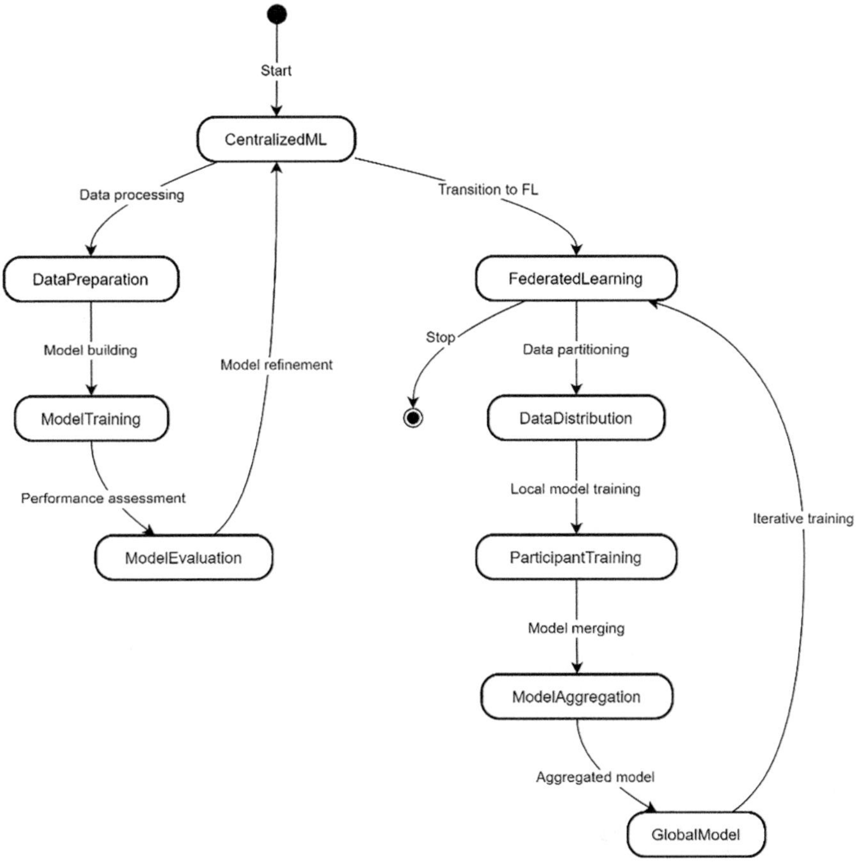

FIGURE 6.1 Transition from centralized learning to federated learning.

datasets collected from multiple sources and stored in a single database have historically been the foundation of machine learning (ML) in the healthcare industry. Models are trained on this aggregated data to account for patient, practice, and disease manifestation variability. Although this method has made it easier to develop strong models with excellent predictive accuracy, it also poses serious privacy hazards to individuals. Large volumes of data concentrated in one location raise the possibility of data breaches, making these repositories attractive targets for hackers. Financial fraud, identity theft, and the unapproved release of Protected Health Information (PHI) have all been outcomes of several instances of sophisticated assaults against healthcare institutions.

Additionally, data loss or corruption may occur during transit when moving data from local sources to a central server. By maintaining data decentralization, reducing the attack surface, and enhancing data security, FL mitigates these threats. FL does face particular difficulties in the healthcare sector, though. The heterogeneity of medical data and the unpredictability of data sources are among the primary challenges; they

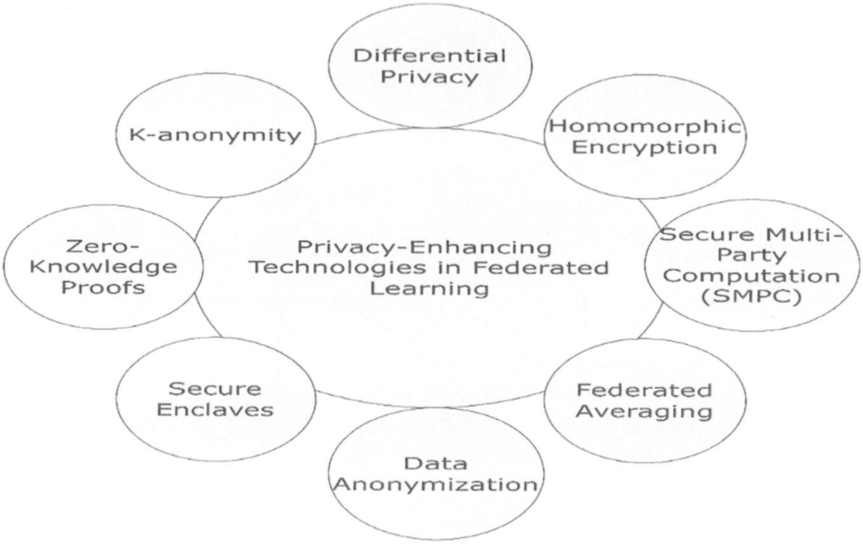

FIGURE 6.2 Technologies of privacy enhancing in federated learning.

may arise from variations in patient demographics, healthcare providers, illnesses, and data collection methods. For example, there may be substantial differences in diagnostic standards, treatment plans, and data collection procedures throughout institutions, which could result in inconsistent results. Furthermore, model training is made more difficult by the fact that healthcare data is frequently unbalanced, with some diseases being more prevalent than others.

6.1.1 Improving Confidentiality in Educated Learning

FL continues to raise privacy problems, especially concerning inference attacks. Even though FL eliminates the need for parties to disclose raw data, attackers may still use the model changes that are shared to deduce information about the underlying data. By reverse-engineering these updates, they can potentially reconstruct sensitive details from local datasets.

For instance, it can be used to reconstruct specific parts of local data, potentially identifying individual participants, particularly in cases where there are few participants. This concern underscores the importance of PETs in FL procedures to protect participant data. The technologies that improve privacy are shown in Figure 6.2. By hiding individual data contributions, techniques like Secure Multiparty Computation (SMPC), Homomorphic Encryption, and Differential Privacy (DP) help to improve FL security and reduce the possibility of inference attacks [2].

6.2 REVIEW OF LITERATURE

Various approaches have been proposed in the field of privacy-preserving AI, particularly in the context of federated learning (FL) in healthcare. These methods aim to strike a balance between performance and privacy, while addressing common challenges such as computational overhead and data security.

The authors of [3] proposed a blockchain-based Artificial Intelligence (AI) model for securing IoT data. Their approach enhanced security through a decentralized architecture, reducing vulnerabilities in data integrity and authentication. However, the model faced challenges related to scalability and lacked applications in healthcare. To address these limitations, future research aims to optimize blockchain-based AI for healthcare while enhancing scalability through the use of edge computing. The authors of [4] explored the use of FL in medical imaging to ensure privacy preservation in decentralized data sharing. Their model successfully maintained data security; however, it was limited to imaging datasets and required generalization to other medical applications. Future advancements will focus on expanding FL to electronic health records and improving model generalizability across different medical domains. Researchers [5] introduced a decentralized learning framework for multi-hospital data sharing, ensuring collaboration while preserving privacy. Although the approach strengthened data security across institutions, it had high computational costs and lacked lightweight implementations. Future studies aim to develop resource-efficient decentralized ML frameworks to optimize scalability and performance.

A study [6] proposed a privacy-preserving AI model that incorporates differential privacy (DP) and homomorphic encryption (HE). Their work highlighted the effectiveness of PETs in securing sensitive medical data. However, trade-offs in complexity and accuracy, along with challenges in clinical integration, remained significant drawbacks. Future research will focus on enhancing computational efficiency and integrating PETs into real-world clinical workflows. Researchers [7] implemented an agent-based model to address misleading data attacks, achieving an accuracy of 98.19%. Their study demonstrated the model's ability to maintain data integrity; however, the use of a small dataset limited its scalability and real-world applicability. Future efforts will focus on expanding dataset sizes and validating the model's performance in diverse environments. Researchers [8] developed an FDIA model to analyze the viability of false data injection attacks, achieving an accuracy of 80%. While the model effectively demonstrated the feasibility of the attack, it suffered from low detection accuracy. Future research will enhance model precision by utilizing advanced feature selection and deep learning techniques to improve cybersecurity measures further. The work in [9] proposed intrusion detection approaches for cybersecurity in cyber-physical systems (CPS), achieving an accuracy of 92%. Their framework effectively scanned vulnerabilities but was time-consuming, requiring extensive processing. Future improvements aim to automate and optimize detection processes with AI-driven solutions for real-time security monitoring. A study [10] introduced a theft detection model to identify advanced electricity theft attacks, achieving a 96% accuracy rate. While their approach proved effective, privacy and security concerns arose due to the sensitivity of meter data. Future research will focus on implementing privacy-preserving techniques and integrating AI with secure hardware solutions. Researchers [11] explored the integration of FL with HE and DP to enhance data security in multiple medical domains. Their approach provided strong privacy preservation but was computationally expensive and required significant infrastructure for secure model training. Future research will focus on optimizing FL frameworks for efficiency and developing hybrid encryption models. Table 6.1 summarizes the studies related to privacy preservation in FL.

TABLE 6.1
Summary of Studies Relating to Privacy-Preserving in Federated Learning

References/ Year	Model	Advantages	Limitations	Futuristic Approaches
[3] (2023)	Blockchain-based AI for IoT data	Enhanced security, decentralized architecture	Lacks healthcare applications, scalability issues	Implementing blockchain-based AI in healthcare, optimizing scalability with edge computing
[4] (2020)	FL in medical imaging	Privacy preservation in decentralized data	Limited to imaging data, needs generalization	Expanding FL applications to EHRs and other medical domains, improving model generalizability
[5] (2024)	Decentralized learning for multi-hospital data	Multi-hospital collaboration, privacy-preserving	High computational cost, lacks lightweight solutions	Developing lightweight decentralized ML frameworks, optimizing resource efficiency
[6] (2022)	Privacy-preserving AI (DP, HE)	Comprehensive PETs, robust privacy	Trade-offs in complexity and accuracy, clinical integration challenges	Enhancing computational efficiency, integrating PETs into real-world clinical workflows
[7] (2020)	Agent-based model	The integrity of misleading data attacks highlighted	Small dataset	Expanding dataset size, validating model performance in diverse environments
[8] (2022)	FDIA model	Demonstrates attack viability	Low accuracy	Improving model accuracy using advanced feature selection and deep learning techniques
[9] (2022)	Intrusion detection approaches	Effective vulnerability scanning for CPS	Time-consuming	Automating and optimizing detection processes with AI-driven solutions
[10] (2024)	Theft detection	Detects advanced electricity theft attacks	Privacy and security concerns	Implementing privacy-preserving techniques, integrating AI with secure hardware solutions
[11] (2023)	FL+ HE + DP	Strong privacy preservation, applicable to multiple medical domains, enhances data security.	Computationally expensive, requires significant infrastructure for secure model training	Optimizing FL frameworks for efficiency, developing hybrid encryption models

6.3 PRIVACY-PRESERVING MACHINE LEARNING: BACKGROUND AND TERMINOLOGY

Privacy-Preserving Machine Learning (PPML) is a relatively new field of study, largely emerging from the recognition of the importance of privacy in the context of ML applications. As ML systems are becoming more dependent on large sets of sensitive data, issues related to data privacy and security have become of utmost importance. The marriage of privacy and machine learning (ML) comprises several strategies designed to protect personal data while still enabling data collection for model building and usage. These strategies address the process of obtaining data for data preprocessing, model training, and utilization, as well as the specific methods for accessing or acquiring data. Healthcare information, by its nature, is always somewhat delicate, which makes data exchange problematic and frequently raises ethical and legal implications. The techniques of FL attempt to overcome these challenges by enabling collaborative training while avoiding the need for raw training data among participants. The server oversees the collective training process in the following manner: During the first stage, all entities send a copy of the model, and one round of local model updates using local training data is typically equivalent to one data pass. The parameters of the resultant model are then uploaded to the central server.

After that, the server computes the average of the model parameters' outcomes from all these entities and then sends the averaged model back to all the entities. Steps are repeated cyclically by interlinking until the enhanced performance level or a predetermined number of iterations is reached. The research shows that FL has relatively high efficiency in training models with high performance and accuracy, without the need for data sharing. Features of FL are shown in Figure 6.3.

Nevertheless, FL may be vulnerable to privacy threats such as reconstruction attacks; therefore, requirements for other privacy-preserving techniques are required to enhance privacy protection.

6.3.1 Encrypted Computation

Encrypted computing essentially means performing operations on data that stays encrypted at all times. The entire concept is relatively straightforward: while the data is first converted from plaintext into ciphertext, the operations performed on that ciphertext yield results precisely like those that were performed on the plaintext [12]. This way, sensitive data is protected during computation and the data remains encrypted. Probably the most well-known example of encrypted computation, Fully Homomorphic Encryption (FHE) allows the addition and multiplication of encrypted data [13]. FHE offers firm privacy guarantees, as computations can be performed without ever decrypting the data; however, its functionality is somewhat limited and requires a significant amount of processing power. Due to the numerous complex functions that require polynomial approximations, the Half-Wave Exponential Rectified Linear Unit (HE-RELU) is a homomorphic-based approximation of the Rectified Linear Unit (RELU) function. This approach introduces additional complications, thereby increasing the time required to execute, in contrast to operations on plaintext. Despite these challenges, encrypted computation remains a

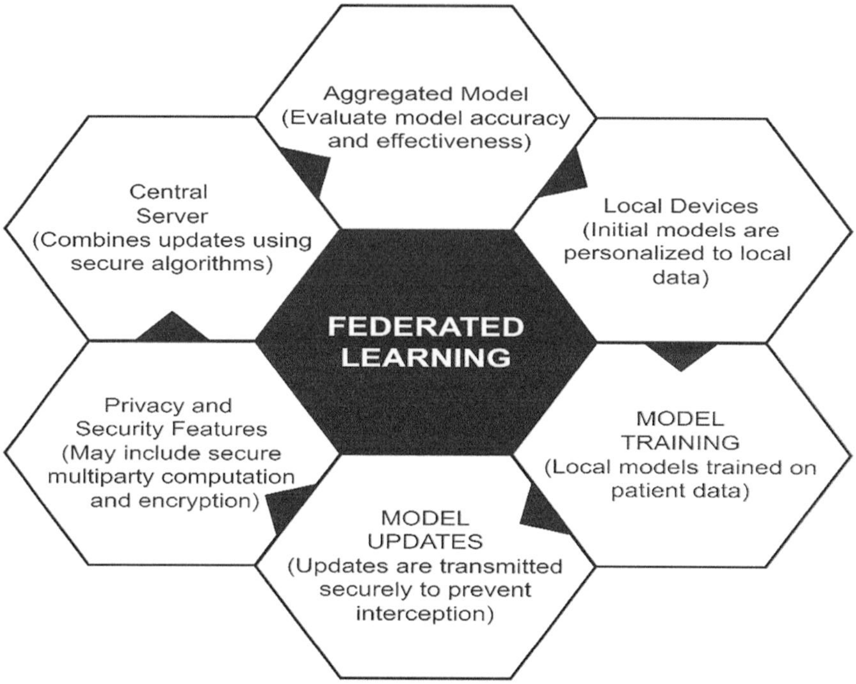

FIGURE 6.3 Features of federated learning.

successful technique for scenarios that require the critical protection of data privacy, particularly in secure data analytics and privacy-preserving machine learning. In general, this architecture is well-known as SMPC, which splits some secret input into several shares that are then distributed among the parties using some cryptographic technique such as Secret Sharing. SMPC stands as a closely related concept that frequently appears within Confidential Computing Systems (CCS). The encryption technique of SMPC distributes vital input information across multiple cryptographic parts that prevent any single user from holding complete master data access by applying Secret Sharing protocols, including Shamir's Secret Sharing. In additive Secret Sharing, the computation process becomes distributed among multiple secure parties. The distributed model training process of FL differs from SMPC because the latter relies on cryptographic encryption for security, albeit at the cost of high computational requirements. Since computation on these shares is performed in a way that reveals only the final output, no single party is capable of independently reproducing the original input [14]. Examples include Shamir's Secret Sharing and additive Secret Sharing; many such techniques have seen wide adoption in SMPC. Although CSC (Confidential Computing **Systems**) shares the same goal with FL, namely guaranteeing data privacy in the cooperation process, there is a key difference regarding the heavy reliance on cryptographic techniques. It makes the former suitable for both training and inference of ML models. Although CSC leaks some global data attributes in specific contexts, despite its strong privacy guarantee, it is computationally expensive. This highlights the need for ongoing research on these risks to potentially mitigate them.

6.4 FEDERATED LEARNING: A DISTRIBUTED COLLABORATIVE APPROACH

Due to challenges in adhering to strict legal norms regarding the collection and processing of personal data necessary for the extensive use of the cloud, it becomes highly or partially inappropriate to apply prior cloud-oriented machine learning (ML) techniques in numerous cases. The majority of personal data is generated at the edge by end-user devices, such as wearables, tablets, and smartphones, which are equipped with increasingly powerful computation capabilities and access to the Internet. Decentralized AI is therefore a trend that naturally emerges, given the widespread adoption of such personal devices and the corresponding rise in privacy concerns. In this regard, FL replaces cloud-centric ML methods, enabling multiple devices to jointly train an ML model while retaining the source personal data on the devices themselves, diminishing vulnerabilities associated with data privacy. With the help of this technique, cross-disciplinary topics such as machine learning, distributed computing, data privacy, and security can be addressed. It enables end users' devices to locally train a shared machine learning (ML) model using local data (also referred to as local nodes). Model aggregation and updates involve only the transfer of parameters related to the training process.

6.4.1 Model Training

FL is best suited for ML models whose objective functions are to estimate model parameters by minimizing some loss function over a particular training dataset [15].

On this count, gradient-based Optimization techniques assume centre stage. In this respect, let the optimization objective be cast as,

$$w \in \mathbb{R}^d f(w) = \left(\frac{1}{n}\right) \Sigma_{\{i=1\}}{}^{\{n\}f}_{i(w)} \tag{6.1}$$

The minimization objective can be formulated as follows:

Where the training dataset is in the form of a set of input-output pairs,

$$\left(x_i, y_i\right), x_i \in \mathbb{R}^d and\, y_i \in \mathbb{R}, \forall I \in \{1, 2, \ldots, n\} \tag{6.2}$$

where the training dataset consists of input-output pairs, with the parameter vector and loss function.

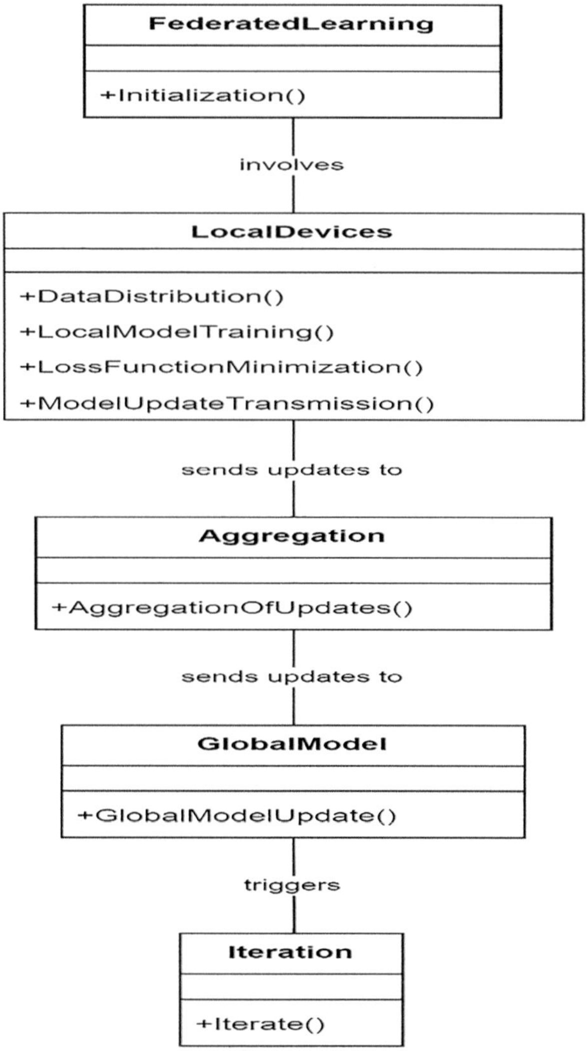

FIGURE 6.4 Process training of federated learning.

This formulation encapsulates a long list of models, including but not limited to linear and logistic regression, support vector machines, and even complex non-convex problems in Artificial Neural Networks (ANNs) and deep learning. The solution to this typically employs gradient descent algorithms, along with backpropagation, to minimize model parameters based on the overall loss. The process of training in FL is mentioned above in Figure 6.4, which is typically divided across centralized data servers that are usually interconnected by low-latency, high-throughput connections. However, in the context of FL, this site is significantly different: in FL, the data are usually unbalanced, Non-Independent and Identically Distributed (non-IID), and are distributed among millions of personal devices with higher latency and lower throughput compared to centralized servers. Moreover, data and computational resources on these devices are available intermittently. Therefore, FL requires optimization algorithms tailored to distributed environments, which necessitates the development of federated optimization techniques.

6.4.2 Optimized Federated Learning

FL is dependent on whether the optimization algorithms designed for federated settings, where training data is non-IID and distributed over a huge number of local nodes, are efficient or not. In the federated setting, fewer steps required by an optimization algorithm due to limited communication between local nodes and the central server are essential. To overcome these difficulties, a distributed version of gradient descent was developed, combining existing algorithms with FL techniques. It computes the gradients on local data, performs aggregation over weighted average parameters across all nodes, and issues updates each round based on them.

Local nodes are represented by K, which is the set of data samples stored in node k ∈ {1, 2, …, K}, and is the number of data samples stored in node k. Since personal data stored in each local node is not the same, we could consider that

$$P_k \cap P_l = \varnothing \, if \, k \neq l \, and \, \Sigma_{\{k=1\}_k^{\{K\}n}} = n \tag{6.3}$$

The distribution problem of the formulation for minimization is defined as follows: A key challenge in FL is that most conventional algorithms for distributed ML assume data independence across devices, which may not hold well in federated settings. Data across personal devices tends to be heterogeneous and non-IID, significantly reducing both model accuracy and convergence speed in federated settings [16]. To address these issues, efficient federated optimization techniques are being explored to reduce communication overhead between local nodes and the central server. Another variant of federated optimization, targeting the solution of non-IID data via a different framework is a promising approach. It improves model performance in a federated setting by leveraging shared features among models, thus guaranteeing better learning convergence.

FL consists of two types of architecture: centralized and decentralized. Distributed learning and FL systems can be designed with either a centralized or decentralized architecture. In centralized architecture, worker nodes perform the computation of gradients, which are then collected by a master node or parameter server and redistributed after updating the global parameters.

This concept has an extensive communication overhead even though it works well. Decentralized ring architecture, on the other hand, manages model parameter updates without the need for a central server. By using asynchronous update strategies to exchange information with neighbours, each node gathers updates and completes its local computation. The distinction between centralized and decentralized architecture is illustrated in Figure 6.5.

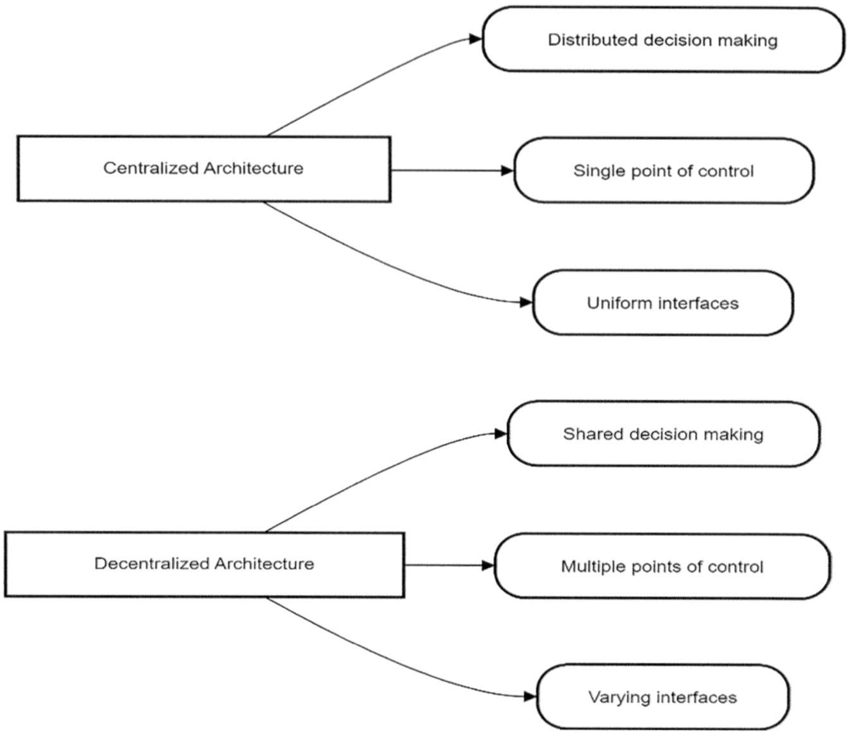

FIGURE 6.5 Features of centralized vs decentralized architecture.

In both centralized and decentralized architectures, model consistency is still essential. To ensure consistency across compute nodes, techniques such as Asynchronous Parallel, Bulk Synchronous Parallel, and Stale Synchronous Parallel are employed.

6.5 CENTRALIZED FEDERATED LEARNING FRAMEWORK: PRESERVING PRIVACY

Compared with screen standard approaches, ML approaches offer privacy-preserving advantages, as models can be collaboratively trained while keeping data and computations on-device.. Unfortunately, because some properties of the training data samples are inherent in such models, the personal data is still present in local ML model parameters even when the original data form is not uploaded to a coordinating server. As previously mentioned, a trained ML model inadvertently contains features that can be exploited to extract personal information. As a result, the local model parameters derived from a federated enhancing algorithm may be targeted by an adversary to infer personal data, especially when combined with supplementary details like model data structure. The extracted information could consist of the original training data samples, leading to what is called a reconstruction attack, or it could be used for membership inference. Interestingly, the ML attacking functions do not involve the actual participation of the attacker in the training process. For instance, it is possible to recover images of a specific man from a facial recognition model by estimating the weight-dependent probabilities of the feature vectors that define the man. Another privacy-hiding objective in centralized FL is to make it impossible for a coordinating server to gain access to the data for training at the local nodes. Nevertheless, this limitation compromises the openness of the training process [17]. Traditional model poisoning attacks mostly work by interrupting the training process by sending malicious local model updates to the coordination server. While in the case of data poisoning, the original training data is provided, model poisoning does not take place without the transmission of this data. This section primarily focuses on model poisoning attacks that exist in FL. In particular, model poisoning is performed on the client side, and the actual threat makes a subset of clients follow the same malicious scenario so that it controls the global model and guides it to a less optimal point; namely, the random type of attack.

6.5.1 Threat Model in a Centralized Framework

As the FL framework studied in this paper is centralized, it is susceptible to both interference and model poisoning attacks and thus requires careful design. Three categories are used to classify security and privacy threats. The three types of threats that exist within the implementation are: (1) threats from internal attackers to the coordinator server, (2) threats arising from outsiders to the communication channel, and (3) threats from dishonest participants. Speaking of possible threats from the position of an ill-intentioned coordination server and selected local nodes, this chapter describes threats to FL. This chapter explains how internal users can exploit parameter changes on local nodes containing data about the victim to perform passive inference attacks. In addition, these attackers may compel victims to participate in adversarial model training that is not an alternative. To enhance the privacy and data integrity of the current communication channels, Secure Sockets Layer/TLS (Transport Layer Security) is employed.

When there is a hacked local node that sends out wrong updates, Byzantine behaviour is likely to happen because it affects the overall model in some way [18]. Additionally, these attackers can strongly encourage victims to conduct adversarial model training. In that regard, the existing communication channels are protected by such protocols as SSL/TLS to enhance privacy and data integrity. The existence of compromised local nodes can bring about Byzantine behaviour in that they send wrong updates to distort the overall model. Figure 6.6 illustrates the centralized ML workflow, highlighting key considerations related to potential data breaches, including secure data handling, access controls, and risk mitigation strategies. This raises several open issues related to the quality of the models under consideration, as well as the safety of the data within the FL system.

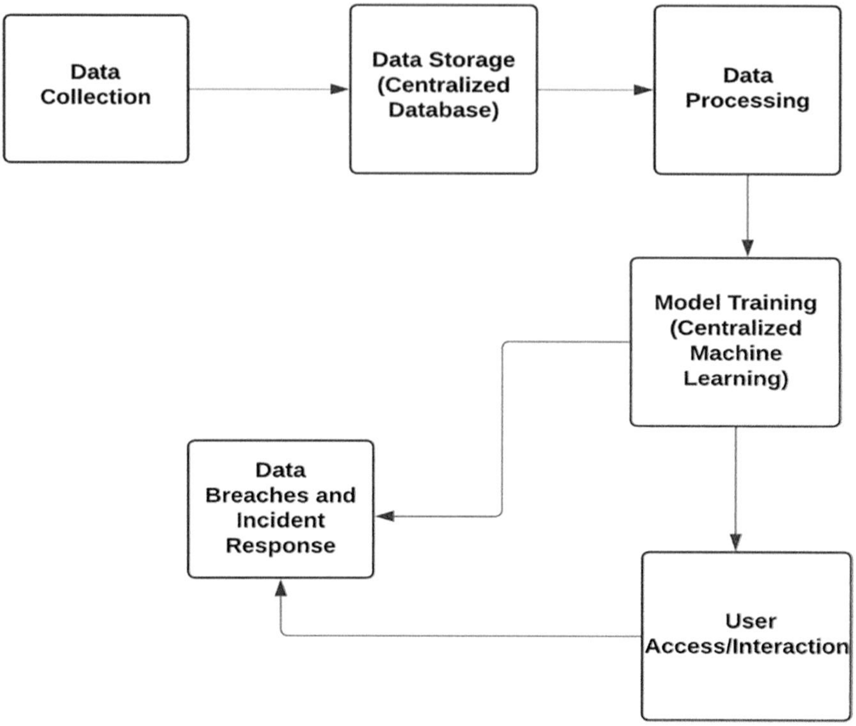

FIGURE 6.6 Centralized machine learning workflow with data breach considerations.

6.6 CENTRALIZED FEDERATED LEARNING AND GDPR COMPLIANCE

Based solely on data processing and storage (i.e., model training) at end-user devices (i.e., local nodes) and by aggregating the global ML model at a service provider's server (i.e., coordination server), federated learning (FL) offers a distinct approach to addressing the data privacy problem in ML applications. There is no denying FL's advantage in terms of privacy preservation over conventional centralized ML techniques: It enables the ML training model while keeping individual end-user training data gadgets. Locally trained model parameters, which have the necessary amount of data to be updated, are shared with a coordination server, which serves as the global model. This section carefully considers whether complying with the GDPR is necessary. There are three participant roles recognized by the GDPR: A data subject, a data controller, and a data processor, to which EU data protection law assigns related responsibilities. This is the legal requirement which is required of Data Controllers under the guise of the GDPR and is the same as the accountability that is required to explain the methods and purposes by which the data will be processed by the Data Processors, who are actively involved in making processing of the data on behalf of Data Controllers. The GDPR equally clearly outlines the rights of Data

Subjects. The subjects, which are the legal rights granted to data owners to exercise complete control over the data, include the right to correction and erasure, the right to restrict processing, the right to obtain from the controller information concerning processing activities, the right to be informed, and the right of access. However, where a service provider adopts an FL system, then the individual is both the Data Controller and the Data Processor. They inform the end-users, the Data Subjects, how to train an ML model with locally available training data and the locally constructed model. They also receive and handle the local model parameters that end users must input, and they aggregate and update the global model. Finally, they return to all end-users for the international models and ask them to update their models. Third, in centralized FL settings, a service provider never has access to other personal information, such as the original training data, as in traditional ML systems; the only information they can share with third parties is a global ML model, which can be deemed as least anonymous. The GDPR Article 5–11, which comprises six fundamental principles, offers service providers reasonable guidelines on how to manage personal data. These principles are similar to those outlined in the UK Data Protection Act of 1998 **United Kingdom**, in that they impose responsibility on Data Controllers to follow the principles and establish the required procedures to demonstrate compliance.

However, for service providers to expect end users to participate in FL training before using it to submit and process their data as a Data Controller, the company must provide its legal basis. As detailed in the GDPR, six legal bases must be met: It is possible to base the processing on the following grounds: (a) Consent; (b) Contract, (c) Legal obligation; (d) Vital interest; (e) Public task; and (f) Legitimate interest.

Healthcare, biomedical, and related fields, among the special category data, may require the above legitimate interests, alongside other legitimate interests beyond those mentioned. The appropriate one has to be chosen and used before the commencement of processing personal data; the choice made has to be documented, including the aims and context of processing. An FL system is designed to prevent the service provider, specifically the coordination server, from maintaining locally trained ML models on the end-user device and the original training data, thereby protecting users' anonymity. [19]. Instead, the end users will only provide feedback on all the findings to the coordination server in preparation for the participants of the FL system when they are ready.

The FL client-side application should provide a choice of actions to be taken by clients during the training process, as well as manage the transmission of, and reaction to, updates from and to the coordination server and the local training as a whole. Furthermore, FL systems transmit data—specifically the local ML model parameters—to other systems, while the system updates the global model and aggregates the results.Regarding the requirements for Fairness and Transparency, Deep learning and other AI and ML algorithms primarily work in a black-box setting without enough explanation of the treatment of data sample bias and the training process, or of how a particular decision is made. Figure 6.7 illustrates the principles of lawfulness, fairness, and transparency, highlighting their roles in ensuring ethical and accountable machine learning (ML) practices. In general, if the training set is inadequately gathered, purposefully biased, and put into an ML system that includes

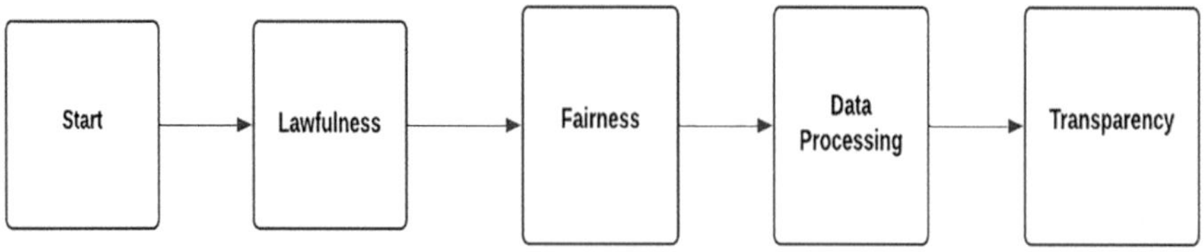

FIGURE 6.7 Lawfulness, fairness, and transparency.

an FL system, the outcome is biased. If this learned model is then used on a system that automatically comes to conclusions, then it can easily lead to discrimination and unfairness.

6.6.1 Rights of Data Subjects

The GDPR requires Data Controllers to provide to data subjects the following, if possible (The GDPR Articles 12–23). These are: (1) Right to information, (2) Right of subject access, (3) Right of rectification, (4) Right to be forgotten, (5) Right to processing, (6) Right to data portability, (7) Right to object, and (8) Rights concerning automated decision-making and profiling.

The challenge in enabling the right to information is that the GDPR requires the disclosing party to explain, in a brief and easily understandable way, the purpose of the local ML model constructed during the onset of FL training as well as the expected outcomes of the said system. As FL is a "black box" system in many nationwide ML methodologies, it is almost impossible to comprehend its working and future estimations. Since it is aware of this, the GDPR supervisory board has dispensed with the application of AI/ML techniques by allowing a general explanation to suffice as an affirmation of the types and objectives of processing personal data. Thus, for an FL system, the right to information is satisfied with privacy information that includes the purposes of processing local ML models, that is, to create a global. n addition, it is relatively straightforward to define elements such as retention periods—specifying how long data is kept after each training round—and to determine that the data will be shared only with the coordinating server. Such details can be set out in a Terms and Conditions statement when a client agrees to participate in an FL system. Rights related to computerized decision-making and profiling are mentioned in Articles 21–22 of the GDPR..

In this respect, under the GDPR, individuals have the right "not to be subjected to an automated processing of decision making which includes profiling." It means that an FL client, being a data subject, is used to receive information in an intelligible form that the program of the global ML model used in computerized decision-making may have legal effects on and/or be seriously adverse to them. Regrettably, like in any typical ML, as well as FL, there are "black-box" features inherent to the models being trained, and, as is expected, due to their lack of transparency, a product, such as the global ML model in FL, is usually created without a clear understanding of what causes given outcomes and what these outcomes might introduce. This makes it difficult to know whether the result of an ML model may impact the legal status or the right of the Data Subject or even harm his/her situation, action, or choices.

Because of this, FL systems do not, in general, fulfil the demands under the GDPR-related provisions of the Right of the Data Subject to be informed of automated decision-making. However, this duty may be waived where the controller has informed the data subject explicitly at the time when the request for consent is made that certain rights relating to automated individual decision-making and profiling do not apply. Some Other Rights are:

The decentralized nature of FL, which processes and stores data locally at the client side and only the aggregated models of ML, at the server side, reduces the number of Data Subject rights that can be exercised. These include: (1) a right of access to personal data, (2) right of rectification, (3) right to erasure, (4) right to restriction, (5) right to data portability, and (6) right to object. For instance, on "Right to erasure," if a user wishes to have their data deleted, it will only be possible to allow such a request if a new global model is trained anew without the data of the user in the round, and they contributed their local ML model parameters to the FL server [20]. This process is not feasible in FL settings because only the local ML model parameters, which can be sometimes augmented with private quality assurances such as DP, are reported back to the server in encrypted forms, using techniques such as Secure Aggregation and other cryptographic techniques. It has a small value to the Data Subject as control of their local ML model with three remaining strategies: (1) Privacy-preserving techniques to protect the model parameters against inference attacks; (2) the server cannot split gather data of any person from the blended models and delete individual model no longer when used to update fused model; and (3) the blended model itself is obscured and not possible to extract for use to derive personal information.

6.7 FINDINGS AND FUTURE WORK

The rapid advancements in AI have led to widespread digital transformations, resulting in fragmented and siloed data systems across enterprises. This lack of integration hinders seamless data sharing and collaboration, preventing businesses from fully leveraging their data's potential. To overcome these challenges, future innovations will focus on developing interconnected, AI-driven data ecosystems that enhance accessibility, security, and interoperability.

6.7.1 FINDINGS

AI technological advances have driven extensive digital transformations throughout industries, which has created spread-out data along with isolated data systems throughout businesses. Enterprises are unable to extract maximum value from their data because data sharing with collaboration has suffered major limitations. FL enables distributed ML operations while ensuring privacy protection and serves as a practical solution to resolve these problems [21]. FL meets extensive challenges, yet none of its solutions address every issue stopping its implementation from inference attacks. The adoption of PETs, including DP and HE, becomes vital.

The Research gives multiple Outputs:

1. **Data Security and Privacy Risks in Federated Learning**
   Privacy-Preserving Data Sharing FL protects against data centralization risks through efficient device-based training, which makes raw data transmission unnecessary. Data vulnerabilities persist in FL because hackers can break down updated model files to steal confidential information.
2. **Challenges in Encryption and Secure Communication**
   Security Challenges in FL implementations face major security threats because cyber-attacks such as Denial of Service (DOS) and Distributed Denial of Service (DDOS) attacks keep becoming more sophisticated. In FL systems, malicious clients can alter models during updates, thus damaging the overall model integrity. The current cryptographic methods might prove inadequate against escalating security threats, so engineers require more sophisticated encryption procedures.
3. **Scalability and Performance Bottlenecks**
   The increasing number of FL deployments reaching thousands of client nodes produces three main training efficiency problems: significant model convergence delays, massive communication requirements, and heterogeneity in device performance and bandwidth across the network.
4. **Advancements in Federated Learning Algorithms**
   Research is exploring FL as a solution that combines blockchain technology to build learning environments that both prevent tampering and maintain auditability. Equipment-based encryption methods combined with security techniques create improved protection mechanisms that produce lower computational burdens.

6.7.2 Future Work

The ongoing research requires improvement of security standards and scalability, and makes efficiency the main focus in FL systems. The upcoming research must concentrate on several main aspects that require attention.

1. **Strengthening Security Mechanisms in Federated Learning**
   Prospective research should create encryption methods that maintain data privacy together with reduced processing requirements. The research requires improvement of defense capabilities that identify and protect against model poisoning attacks and data inference attacks. The implementation of real-time systems that inspect model update behavior patterns for potential malicious activities should be introduced. The use of hardware-assisted encryption methods through secure enclaves provides better security protection for FL systems [22].
2. **Optimizing Communication Efficiency and Model Training**
   The system needs to enhance model training and communication performance to reach optimization goals. The development of model update compression

methods will help lower the communication efficiency costs. The concept of asynchronous FL algorithms requires examination to see if this approach permits clients to process model updates independently at different times for enhanced efficiency and reduced waiting periods. The approach should be enhanced for federated model aggregation to develop more secure global model convergence.

3. **Improving Trust and Accountability in Federated Learning Networks**
   FL networks require the implementation of strategies to enhance trust relationships and maintain network transparency. Trust evaluation methods must be created to determine the reliability of client contributions to the system. Through the deployment of SMPC and HE, users will obtain protection against unauthorized access to model updates. The development of decentralized reputation systems allows clients to obtain rankings by assessing their contribution quality and integrity.
4. **Addressing Bias and Fairness Issues in Federated Learning**
   Our focus is to develop approaches that combat biases together with unfairness requirements in FL systems. The development of fairness-aware FL algorithms enables the reduction of biases that occur due to non-IID distributed data. The system needs to develop approaches to modify client contribution weights because this will protect minority datasets from disappearing in the analysis.
5. **Scaling Federated Learning for Large-Scale Deployments**
   Extending FL operations to massive user bases in deployment environments. Research will focus on establishing hierarchical FL systems that arrange multiple client federations through layered networks to increase system capacity. The development of lightweight FL models requires attention to run efficiently on both IoT sensors and mobile phones, along with other low-power devices.
6. **Integrating Federated Learning with Emerging Technologies**
   Integrating FL with Emerging Technologies. The implementation of blockchain technology for Federated learning would establish safe protocols, leading to transparent model verification. Strategies to implement quantum-safe encryption methods will secure FL systems against future quantum attacks. New research should evaluate FL frameworks with automatic learning rate adjustments according to the present system conditions. In the future, a federated learning-based approach can be explored to enhance the privacy and scalability of the hatred and trolling detection transliteration framework. By training hierarchical LSTM models locally on user devices or distributed nodes without transferring raw code-mixed social media text to a central server, sensitive user data can be better protected [23].

6.8 CONCLUSION

Almost all industries have AI/ML-based applications and services a top priority in their agendas . However, there are significant and real concerns as to data protection due to the uncontrolled utilization or even unlawful utilization of individual data, which is growing at a rate. A large number of cases of serious data leakage and violation of personal confidentiality, such as the Cambridge Analytica case on Facebook, together with the urgent global need for mass applications for contact tracing and tracking movement during the Severe Acute Respiratory Syndrome Coronavirus 2 (SARS-CoV2) pandemic, pushed the problem of privacy into the public agenda around the world. Such problems entailed algorithm bias, ethical questions, the effects of political settings, and the question of legal accountability. This has resulted in a substantial need for good privacy-protection techniques, especially for the so-called "data-thirsty" AI/ML systems, for which FL is a possible approach. In the first instance, it should be noted that the introduction of ownership of personal data as well as the dispersion of storage and computation at user devices and integration of computing services at the server in FL, drastically diminishes the chances of an overall system data breach in a conventional centralized architecture. The data security platform FL shows great potential to safeguard privacy through distributed data management and computing, which prevents central data theft. FL differs from other ML approaches as it enables data to be installed on individual devices, which promotes both local control over information and adherence to laws like the Health Insurance Portability and Accountability Act (HIPAA) and GDPR. FL maintains numerous advantages, yet it faces several difficulties.

Moreover, since some of the existing privacy-preserving mechanisms like Specialty Medical Clinics (SMC) may introduce some deprecating performance costs, the proper application and use of more such methods for FL settings remains a challenge. Second, more research has to be conducted on algorithm biases, complexities, and explanations in FL systems. Despite great headway in studying these methods in centralized AI/ML settings, the applicability of such techniques in cases where training data are very non-IID, skewed, and distributed unevenly across sources, mostly in decentralized settings, is still an open question. More research is needed to examine the limitations of sampling concerning their effects and the possibility of minimizing bias in the global training model. More studies are required to understand how to deploy privacy-preserving mechanisms like SMC on FL applications since these have reasonable performance costs. Second, there should be more studies about the interpretability and fairness of algorithms used in FL systems. While there is a large body of work on centralized AI/ML scenarios, it is not clear if the developed techniques can be applied to decentralized scenarios where there is a significant amount of shift in the training data and high skewness. To understand the influence of the sample limitations as well as to realize measures for minimizing the bias effect of the global training model, it is necessary to explore the characteristics of the sample.

REFERENCES

[1] Alafif, Tarik, Abdul Muneeim Tehame, Saleh Bajaba, Ahmed Barnawi, and Saad Zia. 2021. "Machine and Deep Learning Towards Covid-19 Diagnosis and Treatment: Survey, Challenges, and Future Directions." *International Journal of Environmental Research and Public Health.* 16(9): 6092-6102. doi:10.3390/ijerph18031117.

[2] Arachchige, Pathum Chamikara Mahawaga, Peter Bertok, Ibrahim Khalil, Dongxi Liu, Seyit Camtepe, and Mohammed Atiquzzaman. 2020. "A Trustworthy Privacy-Preserving Framework for Machine Learning in Industrial IoT Systems." *IEEE Transactions on Industrial Informatics* 16 (9): 6092–102. doi:10.1109/TII.2020.2974555.

[3] Bansal, Himanshu, and Rizwan Khan. 2018. "A Review Paper on Human-Computer Interaction." *International Journal of Advanced Research in Computer Science and Software Engineering* 8 (4): 53. doi:10.23956/ijarcsse.v8i4.630.

[4] Fang, Congyu, Adam Dziedzic, Lin Zhang, Laura Oliva, Amol Verma, Fahad Razak, Nicolas Papernot, and Bo Wang. 2024. "Decentralised, Collaborative, and Privacy-Preserving Machine Learning for Multi-Hospital Data." *EBioMedicine* 101, 105006. (March). doi:10.1016/j.ebiom.2024.105006.

[5] Gandhi, Neel, Shakti Mishra, Santosh Kumar Bharti, and Kaushal Bhagat. 2021. "Leveraging towards Privacy-Preserving Using Federated Machine Learning for Healthcare Systems." In *Proceedings of CONNECT 2021: 7th IEEE International Conference on Electronics, Computing and Communication Technologies*. Institute of Electrical and Electronics Engineers Inc. doi:10.1109/CONECCT52877.2021.9622730.

[6] Grama, Matei, Maria Musat, Luis Muñoz-González, Jonathan Passerat-Palmbach, Daniel Rueckert, and Amir Alansary. 2020. "Robust Aggregation for Adaptive Privacy Preserving Federated Learning in Healthcare." September. http://arxiv.org/abs/2009.08294.

[7] Guerra-Manzanares, Alejandro, L. Julian Lechuga Lopez, Michail Maniatakos, and Farah E. Shamout. n.d. 2023. "preserving Machine Learning for Healthcare: Open Challenges and Future Perspectives." *Trustworthy Machine Learning for Healthcare*, 25-40, Springer.

[8] Jamil, Danish, Sellappan Palaniappan, Asiah Lokman, Muhammad Naseem, and Syed Saood Zia. 2021. "Diagnosis of Gastric Cancer Using Machine Learning Techniques in Healthcare Sector: A Survey." *Informatica (Slovenia)*. 45(7): 147-166. doi:10.31449/inf.v45i7.3633.

[9] Kaissis, Georgios A., Marcus R. Makowski, Daniel Rückert, and Rickmer F. Braren. 2020. "Secure, Privacy-Preserving and Federated Machine Learning in Medical Imaging." *Nature Machine Intelligence* 2 (6): 305–11. doi:10.1038/s42256-020-0186-1.

[10] Li, Jiachun, Yan Meng, Lichuan Ma, Suguo Du, Haojin Zhu, Qingqi Pei, and Xuemin Shen. 2022. "A Federated Learning Based Privacy-Preserving Smart Healthcare System." *IEEE Transactions on Industrial Informatics* 18 (3): 2021–31. doi:10.1109/TII.2021.3098010.

[11] Mercier, Dominique, Adriano Lucieri, Mohsin Munir, Andreas Dengel, and Sheraz Ahmed. 2022. "Evaluating Privacy-Preserving Machine Learning in Critical Infrastructures: A Case Study on Time-Series Classification." *IEEE Transactions on Industrial Informatics* 18 (11): 7834–42. doi:10.1109/TII.2021.3124476.

[12] Mestari, Soumia Zohra El, Gabriele Lenzini, and Huseyin Demirci. 2024. "Preserving Data Privacy in Machine Learning Systems." *Computers and Security* 137(C): 103605, (February). doi:10.1016/j.cose.2023.103605.

[13] Rajput, Amit, and Suraksha Tiwari. 2023. "A Review on Privacy Preserving Using Machine Learning and Deep Learning Techniques." *International Journal for Research in Applied Science and Engineering Technology* 11 (3): 1785–90. doi:10.22214/ijraset.2023.49781.

[14] Gupta, Manik, Rakesh Kumar, Shashi Shekhar, Bhisham Sharma, Ram Bahadur Patel, Shaily Jain, Imed Ben Dhaou, and Celestine Iwendi. 2022. "Game Theory-Based Authentication Framework to Secure Internet of Vehicles with Blockchain." *Sensors* 22 (14): 5119.

[15] Reddy, Vonteru Srikanth, and Kumar Debasis. 2023. "DLSDHMS: Design of a Deep Learning-Based Analysis Model for Secure and Distributed Hospital Management Using Context-Aware Sidechains." *Heliyon* 9 (11). doi:10.1016/j.heliyon.2023.e22283.

[16] Aadiwal, Vikrant, Bhisham Sharma, and D. P. Yadav. 2024, September. "Enhancing Breast Cancer Detection with Neural Networks: A Machine Learning Approach for Improved Diagnostic Accuracy." In *2024 3rd International Conference for Advancement in Technology (ICONAT)* (e22283). IEEE.

[17] Rigaki, Maria, and Sebastian Garcia. 2023. "A Survey of Privacy Attacks in Machine Learning." *ACM Computing Surveys* 56 (4): 1-34. doi:10.1145/3624010.

[18] Sinaci, A. Anil, Mert Gencturk, Celia Alvarez-Romero, Gokce Banu Laleci Erturkmen, Alicia Martinez-Garcia, María José Escalona-Cuaresma, and Carlos Luis Parra-Calderon. 2024. "Privacy-Preserving Federated Machine Learning on FAIR Health Data: A Real-World Application." *Computational and Structural Biotechnology Journal* 24 (December): 136–45. doi:10.1016/j.csbj.2024.02.014.

[19] So, Jinhyun, Basak Guler, and Salman Avestimehr. 2020. "A Scalable Approach for Privacy-Preserving Collaborative Machine Learning." *Advances in Neural Information Processing Systems* 33: 8054–66.

[20] Torkzadehmahani, Reihaneh, Reza Nasirigerdeh, David B. Blumenthal, Tim Kacprowski, Markus List, Julian Matschinske, Julian Spaeth, Nina Kerstin Wenke, and Jan Baumbach. 2022. "Privacy-Preserving Artificial Intelligence Techniques in Biomedicine." *Methods of Information in Medicine 61* (June): E12–27. doi:10.1055/s-0041-1740630.

[21] Wang, Lianhai, Lingyun Meng, Fengkai Liu, Wei Shao, Kunlun Fu, Shujiang Xu, and Shuhui Zhang. 2022. "A User-Centered Medical Data Sharing Scheme for Privacy-Preserving Machine Learning." *Security and Communication Networks* 2022. doi:10.1155/2022/3670107.

[22] Zerka, Fadila, Samir Barakat, Sean Walsh, Marta Bogowicz, Ralph, T H Leijenaar, Arthur Jochems, Benjamin Miraglio, David, and Philippe Lambin. 2020. "Systematic Review of Privacy-Preserving Distributed Machine Learning From Federated Databases in Health Care." *JCO Clinical Cancer Informations* 4: 184-200.

[23] Shekhar, Shashi, Hitendra Garg, Rohit Agrawal, Shivendra Shivani, and Bhisham Sharma. 2023. "Hatred and Trolling Detection Transliteration Framework using Hierarchical LSTM in Code-Mixed Social Media Text." *Complex & Intelligent Systems 9* (3): 2813–26.

7 Revolutionizing Patient Care with Biomedical Robotics in Modern Healthcare

Moniga K and Premkumar M

7.1 INTRODUCTION

The cutting-edge discipline of biomedical robotics combines the knowledge of biology, medicine, and robotics to develop systems that enhance medical operations, improve patient care, and facilitate research. One area of study in this discipline is the development of surgical robots, such as the da Vinci Surgical System, which enables surgeons to perform intricate procedures with greater flexibility and accuracy. Furthermore, biomedical robotics is essential to treatment, as patients recovering from surgery or accidents use robotic exoskeletons to regain physical function. Another area where biomedical robots have made significant progress is in advanced prosthetics, which are driven by neural signals and enable artificial limbs to mimic natural movement. Medical diagnostics are more accurate and efficient when diagnostic robots help with imaging, testing, and data processing. Additionally, the discipline is exploring the potential of medical nanorobots that could revolutionize disease treatment by delivering medications directly to target cells in the body. Biomedical robotics is revolutionizing healthcare by enhancing the safety, effectiveness, and minimally invasive nature of healthcare procedures.

Biomedical robots require precise control, biocompatible materials, and sterile environments to operate effectively in healthcare applications, such as surgical procedures, diagnostics, and patient care. On the other hand, generic robots are employed in a wide range of fields, including manufacturing, supply chain management, and services. Due to their proximity to the human body, biomedical robots are subject to stringent safety and regulatory requirements, whereas conventional robots are subject to less stringent norms. The goal, architecture, working conditions, and human-robot interaction set biomedical robots apart from their more widely used general counterparts.

Artificial intelligence (AI) applications in medicine primarily rely on machine learning. This technique involves creating classifiers and methods [1] to develop models that can predict new data by learning from existing sources [2]. As shown in Figure 7.1, AI in medicine enhances patient experiences and outcomes by leveraging machine learning to analyze and evaluate vast amounts of medical data [3].

DOI: 10.1201/9781003561309-7

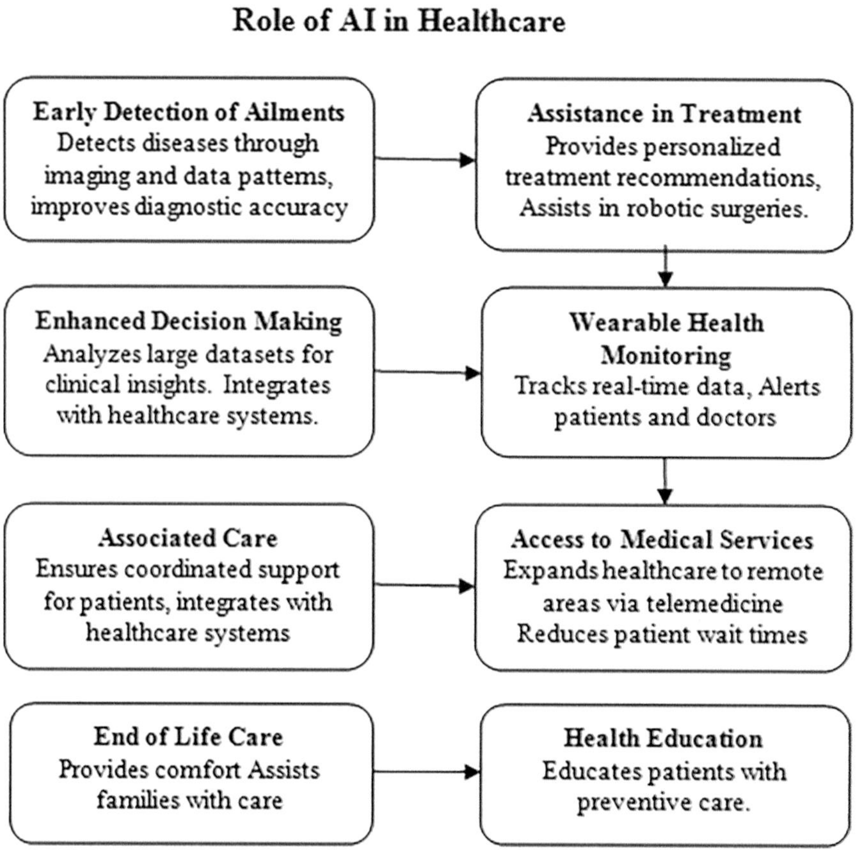

FIGURE 7.1 Biomedical robots applications

Artificial intelligence (AI) is becoming increasingly important in advancing clinical studies, reducing healthcare costs, and enhancing the quality of life. This is due to advancements in processing power, machine learning algorithms, and the increasing access to vast amounts of data through smartphones, wearable devices, and electronic medical records.

7.2 IMPORTANCE OF MODERN HEALTHCARE

By increasing surgical precision, supporting rehabilitation, and automating repetitive chores, robotics dramatically improves patient care. Robotic technologies in surgery enable more precise, minimally invasive procedures, resulting in faster healing and fewer complications. Through individualized therapy, robotic devices help patients regain their movement during rehabilitation. Furthermore, robots perform repetitive tasks such as patient monitoring and medication distribution, freeing up healthcare workers to focus on delivering essential care. In general, robotics enhances patient outcomes by increasing the accuracy, effectiveness, and personalization of therapy [4].

With the worldwide surgical robot market expected to expand from $5.5 billion in 2020 to $16.7 billion by 2026, biomedical robotics has had a tremendous impact on healthcare. Compared to traditional surgery, robotic-assisted treatments result in 20–30% fewer issues and a 15–20% reduction in hospital stays. In 2020, over 1.2 million procedures are expected to be conducted worldwide. By 2027, the global demand for robotic devices in rehabilitation is projected to reach $6.4 billion, with robotic exoskeletons expected to reduce recovery times for stroke patients by 30–50%. In addition, the functional skills of amputees have been improved by 60–80% thanks to robotic prosthetics, with over 70% of users reporting notable improvements in their quality of life and everyday activities [5].

Machine learning aids doctors in various clinical settings, including identifying high-risk ICU patients, detecting respiratory disorders in X-rays, and analyzing claims related to health insurance by analyzing vast quantities of data from electronic health records (EHRs). Yet, implementing these strategies can be challenging because it requires time- and labor-intensive collaboration [6].

By identifying potential failure areas that traditional methods, such as models and psychological studies, overlook, this methodology ultimately supports the development of trustworthy and efficient human-machine interfaces. As shown in Figure 7.2, by offering immersive and creative solutions for enhanced patient and provider interactions, the developing metaverse—powered by technologies like block chain technology, quantum computation, AI, virtual reality, augmented reality, and the Internet of Medical Things (IoMT) [7]—holds promise for revolutionizing the healthcare industry.

This chapter will examine how improved surgical precision and shortened recovery times resulting from minimally invasive treatments utilizing biomedical robotics are transforming patient care. The future of minimally invasive medicine will be explored through existing applications, technical advancements, and emerging developments in biomedical robotics.

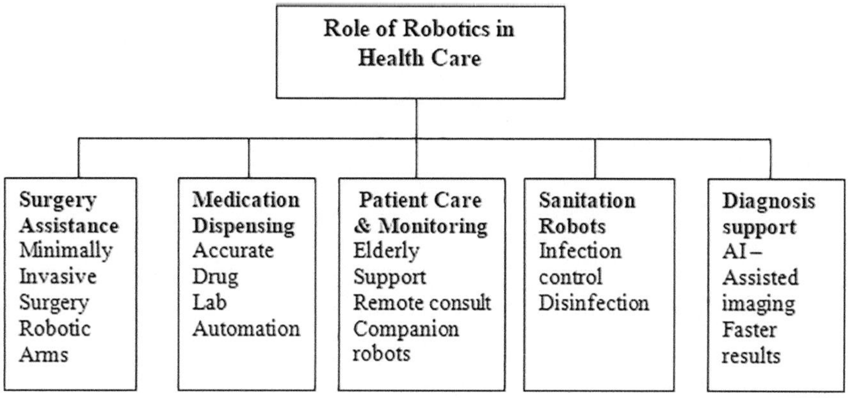

FIGURE 7.2 Role of robotics in health care

7.3 ORIGINS AND EARLY DEVELOPMENTS OF BIOMEDICAL ROBOTICS

The route of revolutionary developments in medical technology can be traced through the evolution of biomedical robots over time. Robotics has introduced new levels of precision to surgical procedures since its introduction in the 1980s, with devices such as the PUMA 560. The applications of biomedical robotics have evolved, enhancing surgical outcomes and rehabilitation through advancements such as exoskeletons and AI-driven surgical robots [8]. This development is a result of the continuous improvement of medical procedures and patient care through the use of modern innovations in healthcare.

7.3.1 Early Innovations

Table 7.1 illustrates the evolution of surgical robotics across various stages of development. Medical robotics began to take shape in the mid-20th century, when the concept of utilizing machines to assist with medical procedures emerged. Advances in robotics and computer technology propelled early innovations; the release of the "PUMA 560" robot in 1985 marked a significant turning point in history. At Memorial Sloan-Kettering Cancer Center, this robot was utilized for a neurosurgical biopsy, demonstrating how robotics can improve surgical precision [9].

The launch of the da Vinci Surgical System in 1999, which revolutionized minimally invasive surgery, marked a breakthrough in the 1990s. The da Vinci system's success sparked broad adoption, leading to further innovations that resulted in advancements in telemedicine and robotic rehabilitation equipment [10]. This chapter examines the development of medical robotics and its early achievements, laying the groundwork for an understanding of its present and potential effects on healthcare.

7.3.2 Milestones and Advancements in Biomedical Robots

Several groundbreaking efforts have revolutionized the field of medical robotics, representing significant achievements in the discipline. A breakthrough in surgical

TABLE 7.1
Early Stages of Surgical Robotics

Year - Stages of Surgical Robots
1970 - NASA explores telesurgery
1983 - Introduction of surgical robotics for orthopedic procedures
1985 - PUMA 560 used to obtain brain biopsy
1990 - ROBODOC performed total hip arthroplasty
1997 - First laparoscopy performed
2000 - Da Vinci – the first robotic system for general and laparoscopic surgery
2001 - Cyberknife does procedures automatically
2019 - Over 5000 Da Vinci surgical systems installed globally

robotics was achieved with the introduction of the "PUMA 560" robot in 1985, specifically for use in neurosurgery, which exhibited improved control and precision [11]. The da Vinci Surgical System, developed in 1999, revolutionized minimally invasive surgery with its precise robotic arms and high-definition 3D imaging, enabling more dexterity and improved patient outcomes.

Robotic devices for telemedicine and remote surgery represent a breakthrough in medical robotics. With the advent of telesurgery, exemplified by the Raven II surgical robot, surgeons can now perform procedures remotely, expanding access to specialized treatment and overcoming geographic constraints in the healthcare system.

7.3.3 AI AND ML IN MEDICINE

Recent developments have led to AI quickly becoming a crucial component of contemporary healthcare, as illustrated in Figure 7.3. Planning an appropriate course of therapy and ensuring patients' well-being depend heavily on accurate diagnosis of the illness. Diagnostics are less precise due to human error, as analyzing medical information is a challenging and cognitive process. AI has the potential to improve diagnosis efficiency and accuracy.

Machine learning algorithms, for example, can identify skin lesions in skin images, predict the likelihood of a heart attack using cardiac magnetic resonance imaging (MRI), or detect lung cancer through computed tomography (CT) scans. These algorithms can also identify psychological symptoms, such as depression, thanks to the abundance of data they process, which makes their decisions informed

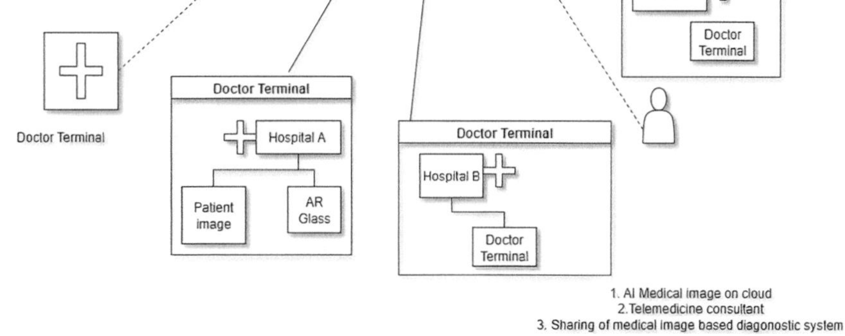

FIGURE 7.3 Virtual and real worlds

Source: **Reprint from [12]**

and efficient. As a subclass of machine learning, deep learning is particularly significant, especially in the areas of identification and detection.

Multiple clinical applications of machine learning (ML) have been successfully implemented. In robotic surgery, where the AI system assists surgeons in treating patients more precisely and with less discomfort, while also minimizing surgeon variance that may impede patient recovery, AI-based solutions are anticipated to have a significant impact. AI is also being used in pathology, nephrology, endocrinology, and medical imaging [12].

7.3.4 Technical Advancement in Biomedical Robotics

The quick development of technology and its application to healthcare is reflected in the growth of healthcare robotics over the years. Early research and development in the 1980s and 1990s focused on simple robotic systems, such as the PUMA 560, which pioneered the concept of robotic assistance in surgery, enhancing control and precision. A significant breakthrough occurred in 1999 with the release of the da Vinci Surgical System, which revolutionized minimally invasive treatments with its advanced robotic arms and high-definition 3D vision. During this time, robotic prosthetics and rehabilitation devices were also developed, illustrating the potential of robotics for uses beyond surgery.

As cutting-edge technologies such as artificial intelligence, machine learning, and new materials have been integrated, the field of biomedical robotics has advanced significantly in the 2000s and beyond. Advances in processing power, sensor technology, and data analysis have led to the development of innovations such as automated surgical robots and robotic exoskeletons for rehabilitation [13]. The application of AI has expanded the capabilities and efficacy of medical robotics by enabling robots to assist with intricate tasks, such as remotely performing surgeries and creating customized treatment plans. This constant growth underscores the dynamic character of biomedical robotics and its growing influence in reshaping healthcare through ongoing improvements in patient care and the expansion of medical professionals' skills.

7.4 TYPES OF BIOMEDICAL ROBOTS IN HEALTHCARE WITH THEIR APPLICATIONS

7.4.1 Surgical Precision and Assistance

Surgical techniques that utilize robotic assistance are referred to as robotic-assisted techniques. The primary objective of integrating robotics into surgery is to overcome the limitations of conventional methods, including open surgery and minimally invasive surgery, by enabling medical professionals to navigate the complexities of the human body more effectively. In robotic surgery, a tiny incision is made, and a robotic arm with visual 3D imaging and surgical instruments is inserted through it [14]. Through the use of an interface that telemanipulates the robotic arm's movements, the surgeon can perform precise and regulated procedures. Robotic surgery combines sophisticated control systems with real-time visual feedback to enhance surgeons' skills and simplify complex surgical procedures.

Despite early triumphs, ambiguities and worries about robot safety hampered the acceptance of robotic surgery in several nations. But the release of the revolutionary

Da Vinci robot in 2000 completely changed the industry, was an enormous success, and is now the most widely used surgical robot in the world. A turning point was reached with the deployment of the Da Vinci robot, which rekindled interest in robotic surgery and spurred the creation of numerous more robotic surgical systems.

Numerous surgical robots have been used worldwide, but as time has progressed, these robots have undergone improvements, and the upgraded versions are currently in use. Figure 7.4 illustrates the various types of surgical robot systems.

Increasingly, surgical robots are being utilized to reduce operating times, minimize the risk of infection, and expedite recovery. Surgeons have also profited from robotic surgery in addition to patients. Surgeons can operate on complex areas of the human body more skillfully by using robotic assistance to enhance their physical and mental abilities during surgeries. By improving control and precision, surgical robotics has significantly revolutionized surgery, making complex procedures more precise and accurate. Minimally invasive procedures, which involve tiny incisions, result in fewer complications, less tissue damage, and a quicker recovery, thanks to these devices [15]. Robotic systems, equipped with sophisticated imaging and high-definition cameras, offer a comprehensive view of the surgical field, thereby enhancing target recognition. Robotic arms' dexterity imitates precise hand movements, offering stability and making complex moves easier. Additionally, ergonomic forms reduce physical strain on surgeons, and they can benefit from training simulation tools. Robotic surgery enhances clinical outcomes by reducing the risk of infection, minimizing complications, and facilitating a faster recovery. Here is a comparative table highlighting the Features and Capabilities of various surgical robotic systems in Table 7.2.

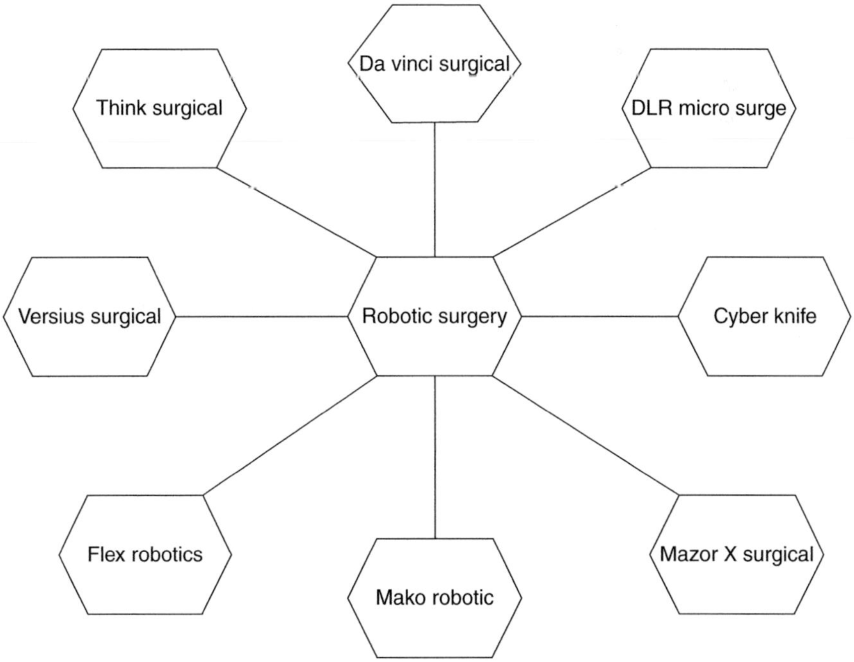

FIGURE 7.4 Types of surgical robots

TABLE 7.2
Features and Capabilities of Surgical Robots

Feature/ Capability	Primary Use	Precision	Visuali-zation	Control System	Types of Procedures	Robotic Arms	Unique Features
Da Vinci Surgical System [15]	Minimally invasive surgery	3D visualizati-on with high precision	3D vision	Controllby hand	Urology, cardiac, gynecology	4 robotic arms	Most widely used
Cyber Knife System [17]	Stereo-tactic Radio surgery	Targeting tumors with high accuracy	Real-time image (X-ray)	Image-guided robotic system	Non-invasive tumor treatment	Robotic arm with multiple angles	Non-invasive surgery
Mako Robotic-Arm Assisted Surgery [16]	Ortho-pedic surgery	Real-time haptic feedback with high precision	CT-real-time Image	Assist by robots	Knee and hip replacement	1 robotic arm	Real-time tactile feedback
Versius Surgical Robotic System [13]	Laparoscopic surgery	Flexible modular arms (high accuracy)	3D vision	Surgeon console, open design	General surgery (hernia repair)	3-4 modular arms	Modular design

7.4.2 Rehabilitation Robots

Robotic rehabilitation is a significant development in physical therapy and rehabilitation, offering patients new ways to treat chronic illnesses or heal from traumas. These robots, which are frequently used in hospitals, rehabilitation facilities, and home care settings, are designed to assist with therapeutic activities and movement training. Rehabilitation robots can be customized to meet the unique requirements of each patient by providing accurate, repeatable movements and varying resistance levels. This personalization enhances the effectiveness of rehabilitation programs, resulting in a quicker and more comprehensive recovery. Robotic arms that assist with repetitive motion workouts and exoskeletons equipped with robotic components that support and enhance limb mobility are two notable examples. These devices aid patients in regaining their strength, balance, and mobility, which is especially advantageous for individuals recuperating from spinal cord injuries and strokes [16].

Figure 7.5 shows various rehabilitation robots, including those for the upper and lower limb, exoskeletons, hand rehabilitation, robotic treadmills, ankle rehabilitation robots, balance training robots, and complete–body rehabilitation robots. Examples with specific applications and their primary functions are given in Table 7.3.

Regaining strength and mobility is made possible by the precise, repeated motion therapy that these robots offer, especially in situations such as stroke recovery or post-orthopedic surgery rehabilitation. These systems may monitor patient development and modify therapy in real time, assuring efficient treatment and better results, by utilizing sophisticated sensors and control algorithms [17].

Innovative prosthetic limbs and wearable robots that combine biomechanical design and state-of-the-art robotics are revolutionizing mobility support. These tools are designed to enhance the mobility of individuals who have lost limbs or experience mobility issues. Examples of these tools are prosthetic limbs and robotic limbs. With the help of sensors, actuators, and control systems, robotic prosthetic limbs can move in a way that is intuitive and natural, much like biological limbs. Exoskeletons and other wearable robots help enhance the wearer's natural abilities, allowing for improved walking, balance, and even the capacity to perform challenging activities. These devices not only help people regain lost function but also enhance their quality of life by promoting independence and reducing physical strain from daily tasks [18].

7.4.3 Assistive Robots

The development and use of assistive robots, which provide solutions that increase independence and raise the standard of care, is growing. Such robots are used to monitor patients and assist the elderly.

These robots enable seniors to enjoy a greater degree of autonomy while reducing the strain on caregivers by assisting with everyday tasks, including mobility, medication schedules, and social interactions. AI and sophisticated sensors are combined to create assistive robots that can adapt to the unique needs of each user, offering personalized care that evolves, as illustrated in Figure 7.6. This flexibility is particularly crucial for meeting the diverse and constantly changing demands of the growing elderly population. Assistive robots not only help with everyday tasks but are also

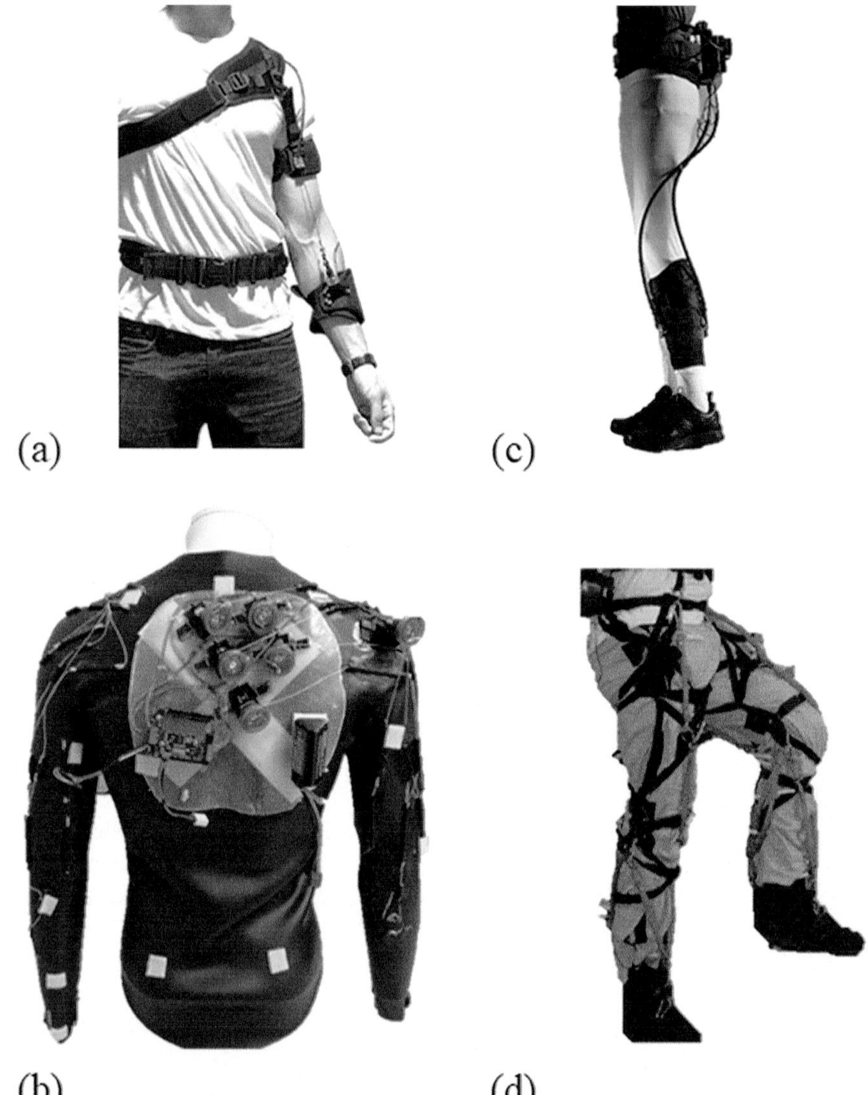

FIGURE 7.5 Examples of soft exoskeleton

Source: **Reprint from https://doi.org/10.1017/wtc.2021.13**

essential for monitoring patients. Robots like these have sensors and communication systems that enable them to recognize falls, continuously track energy levels, and monitor medical conditions in real-time. By detecting health problems early, continuous monitoring reduces the likelihood of severe consequences and enables prompt action. Moreover, the information gathered by these robotic devices can be examined to reveal long-term health patterns, improving patient management and

TABLE 7.3
Rehabilitation Robotic Types

Rehabilitation Robot Type	Examples	Specific Applications
Exoskeletons [18]	ReWalk	Assisting walking and mobility in people with paraplegia, stroke
Robotic Gait Trainers [19]	Lokomat	Improving gait in neurological impairments
Upper Limb Rehabilitation Robots [17]	ArmeoSpring	Arm and hand movement recovery post-stroke
Ankle-Foot Orthoses (AFOs) [18]	WalkAide	Supporting ankle and foot movement
Hand Rehabilitation Robots [13]	Amadeo	Enhancing hand strength and dexterity
Therapeutic Robots [15]	MIT-Manus	Repetitive therapy for motor skill recovery
Robotic Physiotherapy Assistants [19]	Robot-Assisted Therapy (RAT)	Assisting with repetitive tasks, assessments
Balance Rehabilitation Robots [16]	Biodex Balance System SD	Improving balance and coordination

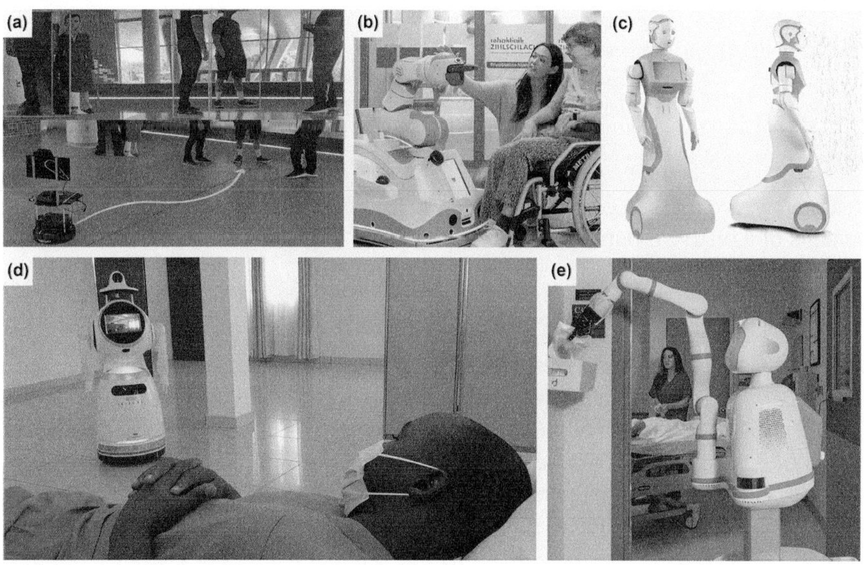

FIGURE 7.6 Elderly care and patient monitoring

Source: **Reprint from https://10.1109/ACCESS.2020.3045792**

TABLE 7.4
Types of Assistive Robots

Assistive Robot	Function	Benefits	Example Applications
PARO Therapeutic Robot [15]	Provides emotional support and companionship	Reduces stress and anxiety, improves mood in elderly patients	Nursing homes, hospitals, mental health therapy
Jibo Social Robot [18]	Social interaction, daily assistance	Enhances social engagement, supports independent living	Home care for elderly, social companionship
ROBEAR [18]	Assists in lifting and transferring patients	Reduces physical strain on caregivers, improves patient mobility	Elderly care facilities, hospitals
ASIBOT [17]	Assists with daily activities for disabled individuals	Supports self-care tasks like feeding and grooming, enhances autonomy	Homes of disabled individuals
Buddy Companion Robot [16]	Provides reminders, security, and social interaction	Improves daily task management, enhances safety and social connection	Smart homes, elder care, daily assistance
ReWalk Exoskeleton [18]	Provides mobility assistance to paraplegics	Enables walking, improves physical health, increases independence	Rehabilitation centers, personal mobility
Care-O-bot [13]	Domestic assistance, elderly care	Supports daily living activities, improves quality of life for elderly	Assisted living, private homes

treatment approaches in general. Table 7.4 highlights and compares the functions and benefits of assistive robots, with their applications detailed.

7.4.4 Diagnostic Robotics

Medical procedures and analyses are being carried out in a completely new way thanks to robots, which are dramatically improving precision as well as effectiveness in diagnosis and laboratory automation. Robotic systems can precisely handle huge amounts of samples in diagnostic applications, lowering the possibility of human mistakes and guaranteeing consistent results. These systems might streamline repetitive activities like pipetting procedures, sample sorting, and preparation, which makes them very useful in high-throughput situations like clinical laboratories. Robots optimize overall lab efficiency by streamlining these operations, which not only speeds up diagnosis but also frees up human technicians to work on more difficult duties [19].

Robotic technologies are increasing diagnostic procedure accuracy while simultaneously increasing the efficiency of common laboratory activities. To help with the

TABLE 7.5
Types of Diagnostic Robots

Robot Type	Primary Function	Examples
Imaging Robots [22]	Enhanced diagnostic imaging	Firefly (Fluorescence Imaging), Viking 3DHD (3D Imaging)
Biopsy Robots [18]	Precision tissue sampling	NeuroMate (Brain), Ion (Lung)
Endoscopic Robots [30]	Minimally invasive internal exams	Flex Robotic System (Gastrointestinal)
Ultrasound Robots [21]	Automated ultrasound scanning	SonoSiteiViz (Portable), InTouch Health (Remote)
Robotic Scanners [17]	Improved scanning and image quality	CyberKnife (Radiosurgery), ARTAS iX (Hair Imaging)
Blood Analysis Robots [24]	Automated blood sample processing	ClearPath Robotics, Abbott Diagnostics
Micro/ Nano robots for Diagnostics [27]	Cellular-level disease detection	Magnetically Guided Nanobots (Cancer Detection)
AI-Powered Diagnostic Robots [26]	AI-based medical data analysis	IBM Watson Health, Zebra Medical Vision

interpretation of medical photos, for example, robots outfitted with AI algorithms and cutting-edge imaging technology can detect abnormalities more accurately than with conventional techniques. In domains such as radiology and pathology, where timely and precise illness identification can greatly influence patient outcomes, this cap acity is essential. Furthermore, real-time analysis made possible by the integration of lab automation robots with data management platforms facilitates smooth data flow, improves making decisions, and expedites the diagnostics procedure [20]. Table 7.5 highlights the functions and applications of diagnostic robots.

7.4.5 Nano and Micro Robots

7.4.5.1 Targeted Drug Delivery

By facilitating exact and focused medication delivery, especially in the treatment of cancer, through which they can recognize and destroy tumor cells while preserving healthy tissue, nanorobots are radically changing the medical industry and decreasing side effects. Furthermore, these nanorobots can move within the human body utilizing external inputs like magnetic fields, which makes them more successful in addressing deeply rooted malignancies [21]. Moreover, multipurpose nanorobots that integrate medication and scanning are being developed. This enables real-time diagnosis and modification, which enhances the outcome of patients. Additionally, they are being developed to overcome biological obstacles such as the blood-brain barrier, opening

TABLE 7.6
Applications and Benefits of Nano Robotics

Application	Medical Procedure	Benefits
Targeted Drug Delivery	Delivering chemotherapy directly to tumors	Precision in drug delivery, fewer side effects
Minimally Invasive Surgery	Navigating and performing surgery through small incisions	Faster recovery, less pain, lower infection risk
Precision Diagnostics	Detecting early-stage cancer cells	Early detection, accurate diagnosis
Tissue Repair	Delivering stem cells or growth factors to damaged tissues	Accelerated healing, effective tissue regeneration
Blood Clot Removal	Breaking down clots in blood vessels	Stroke/heart attack prevention, minimally invasive
Intracellular Surgery	Repairing or modifying cells at the molecular level	Precise cell-level interventions, potential genetic repair

up new avenues for the treatment of neurological conditions that were previously challenging to manage with conventional techniques.

7.4.5.2 Minimally Invasive Surgery (MIS)

The safety and accuracy in surgery have been greatly improved by robots created for minimally invasive surgery (MIS) [22]. Compared to open procedures, these surgical robots can carry out intricate tasks with tiny incisions, minimizing recuperation times, minimizing damage to the patient, and minimizing the risk of infection. The creation of robots with improved delicacy and control has enabled surgeons to do more precise operations in tight areas like the brain or heart. The accuracy of these procedures is further enhanced by the incorporation of robotic equipment and real-time imaging, which allows surgeons to explore and manipulate tissues with minimal interruption. This technique offers patients less intrusive options with better results, which is a significant advancement in surgical care. The applications and benefits of nano and micro robots are shown in Table 7.6.

7.5 IMPACT ON PATIENT CARE AND OUTCOMES

By giving surgeons instruments that are more precise, stable, and controlled than those used in manually operated surgery, robotics dramatically reduces human error and improves surgical outcomes. The chance of unintentional harm to tissue is decreased by these robotic systems' superior imaging and motion-scaling technologies, which convert the surgeon's movements into accurate motions on a smaller

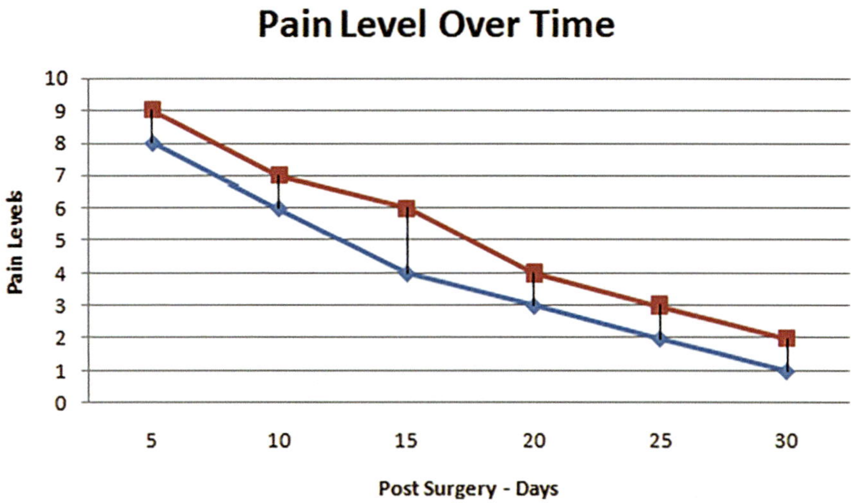

FIGURE 7.7 Pain Levels over time by robotic surgery

scale. Furthermore, tremor filtration—a function that further reduces the influence of spontaneous hand tremors—is frequently seen on robotic platforms. This contributes to improved accuracy and reliability of surgical procedures [23]. Because of this, incorporating robots into surgery merely lowers the possibility of difficulties but also enhances patient outcomes overall, resulting in quicker recovery periods and better postoperative outcomes.

In Figure 7.7, a graph that shows the important parameters for each method can be created in order to evaluate robotic surgery and normal human-performed surgery in terms of speedy healing times and post-operative results. The structure of this comparison graph can be as follows.

Figure 7.8 compares the post-operative results and recuperation time between robotic and conventional human-performed surgery, highlighting pain levels over time and complication rates. In terms of pain management, robotic surgery demonstrates a quicker recovery than traditional surgery. Additionally, in categories such as infection, hemorrhage, and reoperation, robotic surgery shows a reduced rate of complications.

7.5.1 Enhanced Recovery and Rehabilitation

By reducing surgical interference and increasing precision, robotically assisted surgeries help patients recuperate from their treatments more quickly and effectively. These robotic technologies minimize harm to tissues and postoperative suffering by employing smaller incisions than open surgery, which results in faster recovery periods and less damage [24]. Furthermore, surgical problems are less common thanks to robotic systems' improved precision and control, which can speed up recovery and reduce time in the hospital.

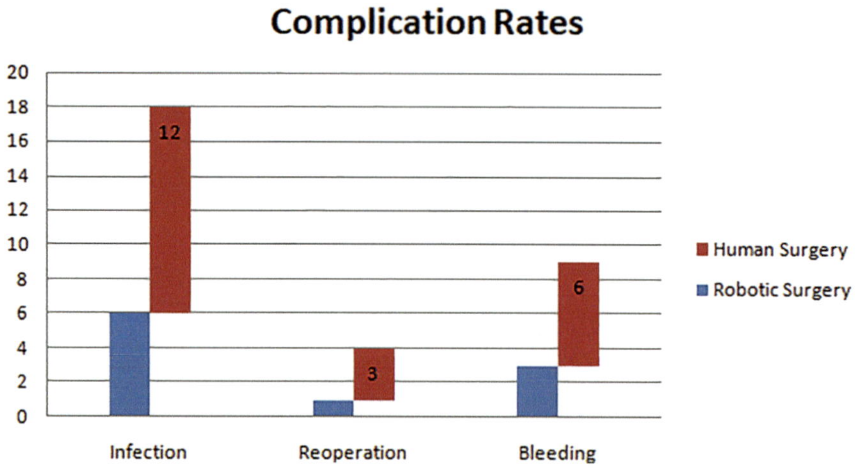

FIGURE 7.8 Complication rates of human surgery

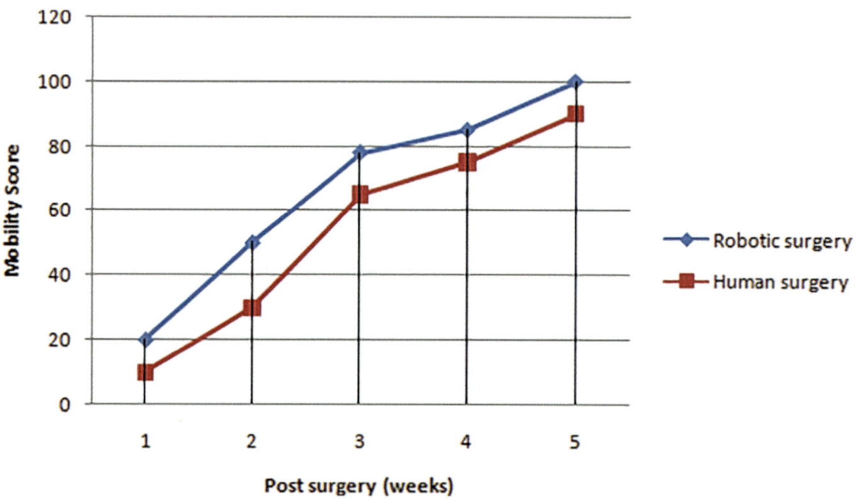

FIGURE 7.9 Mobility improvements over time

Figure 7.9 compares the post-operative results and hospital stay duration between robotic and human-performed surgery. Mobility improvement over time is evident, with patients regaining movement more quickly following robotic surgery. Additionally, reduced hospital stays are typical for patients who undergo robotic surgery.

7.5.2 Increased Accessibility to Quality Care

Through telecommuting and robotic-assisted treatments, biomedical robots are serving a critical role in enabling access to advanced medical treatments in rural or disadvantaged places. Through remote communication, these robots allow highly qualified surgeons to perform complicated operations from a distance, bridging the medical knowledge gap between rural and urban areas. This technology improves overall healthcare equality by decreasing the need for patients to travel great distances for specialized treatment and increasing access to superior medical care in underprivileged areas.

7.5.3 Patient Satisfaction and Quality of Life

By providing more accurate, minimally invasive, and tightly regulated surgical treatments, these robots greatly enhance patient satisfaction and provide long-term health advantages. By lowering intra operative trauma, these robots improve the overall surgical experience and facilitate faster rehabilitation to regular activities and less discomfort following surgery. Furthermore, the precision of robotically assisted surgeries lowers the risk of difficulties, which can improve long-term health outcomes by, among other things, lowering the need for repeat surgery and guaranteeing a more functional recovery. Shorter hospital stays and better cosmetic results have been demonstrated to increase patient satisfaction with biomedical robots in surgery, which over time improves quality of life.

7.5.4 Cost Effectiveness and Efficiency

Healthcare expenses are directly reduced by the use of robotics in operations and other applications in medicine, which result in a lower risk of problems and post-operative treatment, which saves money for patients as well as healthcare providers. Robotic systems facilitate the optimal deployment of medical personnel and facilities by streamlining processes and enhancing operating room efficiency [24]. This results in increased productivity and more efficient utilization of healthcare assets. Table 7.7 highlights various metrics of robotic surgery and human surgery.

TABLE 7.7
Traditional Care and Robotic Care Metrics Comparison

Metric	Traditional Care	Robotic-Assisted Care
Precision	Moderate, variable	High, consistent
Invasiveness	Larger incisions, more invasive	Minimally invasive
Recovery Time	Longer due to larger incisions	Shorter due to minimally invasive procedures
Cost	Lower initial cost, higher long-term costs	Higher initial cost, potential for lower long-term costs
Treatment Duration	Longer, manual techniques	Shorter, efficient procedures
Consistency	Variable, dependent on skill	High, automated precision
Patient Comfort	More pain, larger incisions	Enhanced comfort, smaller incisions
Risk of Complications	Higher risk of infections and errors	Lower risk due to precision and minimal invasiveness
Skill Requirements	High skill and experience	Specialized training for robotic systems

robotic technology greatly shortens the healing period for patients, lowers the risk of complications from surgery. Another such is the Cyber Knife technology, which is utilized in radiotherapy to precisely treat cancers. Oncology patient satisfaction has improved as a result of the system's continual imaging and adaptive therapy capabilities, which have improved cancer treatment while sparing normal tissue [34].

7.8.2 Understanding Challenges

Although there have been a lot of achievements in healthcare robotics, there have also been some significant disappointments and setbacks that offer important lessons for the future. One noteworthy instance is the early difficulties encountered in the application of robotic systems in orthopedic surgery, where a lack of strong clinical procedures and inadequate instruction led to higher-than-expected rates of complications in certain early implementation [35]. An additional instance underscored the important role of thorough testing and validation before clinical implementation; wherein specific robotic surgical instruments were recalled because of software glitches that resulted in harming patients. These failures highlight the necessity of extensive testing, continuous monitoring, and extensive education to guarantee the security and efficacy of robotic systems in therapeutic settings. These incidents additionally demonstrate the significance of open communication and evaluation. Table 7.9 shows the Summary of Case Studies in Biomedical Robotics.

7.9 CONCLUSION

The main developments, uses, and difficulties of biomedical robotics were covered in this chapter. It discussed the effective application of technological innovations such as the Cyber Knife system, which has transformed radiation therapy with its accurate tumor targeting, and the Da Vinci Surgical System, which is renowned for its ability to shorten recuperation times and improve surgical precision. We also discussed the combination of AI with customized healthcare, which enables more individualized and efficient care. A number of difficulties were also looked at, including the costly nature of robotic systems, the requirement for specific education, and the difficulties in winning over patients. Additionally, we emphasized the significance of drawing lessons from previous mistakes and the necessity of thorough testing, extensive training, and continuous supervision for the secure and effective utilization of these technologies.

Biomedical robots have the capability to revolutionize healthcare in the future. Significantly bettering outcomes for therapy, these devices provide unmatched precision and may be customized to meet the demands of specific patients. These robots' use of AI and machine learning is especially promising since it allows for continuous acquisition of knowledge and decision-making in real time, both of which increase the robots' efficacy. Furthermore, telemedicine and robotic systems have the opportunity to improve availability of high-quality medical care in underprivileged and rural places, which is a major step towards lowering inequality in health care. These advancements are poised to become an essential component of contemporary medicine

TABLE 7.9
Summary of Case Studies in Biomedical Robotics

Case Study	Robot Type	Application	Key Outcomes	Challenges	Lessons Learned
1. Robotic-Assisted Heart Surgery [19]	Surgical Robot	Minimally Invasive Cardiac Surgery	- 30% faster recovery - 25% fewer complications	- High cost - Surgeon training required	- Cost-effective models needed - Training is crucial
2. Stroke Rehabilitation Robotics [24]	Rehab Robot	Upper Limb Rehab	- 50% better limb function - 40% faster recovery	- Customization challenges - Tech malfunctions	- User-friendly design - Regular maintenance
3. Elderly Care in Assisted Living [25]	Assistive Robot	Elderly Monitoring & Assistance	- 60% fewer falls - 35% better med adherence	- Resistance from elderly - Privacy issues	- Gradual tech introduction - Privacy safeguards
4. Nanorobots for Cancer Treatment [21]	Micro/Nano Robot	Targeted Drug Delivery	- 80% tumor size reduction - Minimal side effects	- High cost - Regulatory hurdles	- Cost reduction strategies - Clear regulations needed
5. Robotic-Assisted Spinal Surgery [24]	Surgical Robot	Spinal Fusion Surgery	- 35% shorter surgery - 40% less pain	- High system cost - Extensive planning	- Pre-op planning crucial - Imaging integration
6. Tele presence in Remote Monitoring [20]	Tele presence Robot	Remote Consultation	- 50% more consultations - 30% fewer readmissions	- Connectivity issues - Elderly tech adaptation	- Improve rural tech - Patient tech education
7. Exo-skeletons for Paraplegic Patients [33]	Rehab Robot	Mobility Assistance	- 70% mobility improvement - Psych benefits	- High cost - Adaptation period	- Affordable models - Psychological support
8. Automated Pharmacy Dispensing	Assistive Robot	Medication Dispensing	- 60% fewer errors - 30% more efficient	- High setup costs - System integration	- Seamless IT integration - Regular updates

as they develop further, accelerating the transition to more effective, individualized, and widely available healthcare.

It is essential to keep developing science and technology while tackling the moral, authorized, and safety concerns that come with these advancements if biomedical robotics is to reach its maximum potential. This entails encouraging interdisciplinary cooperation, making sure that emerging technologies are thoroughly tested and validated, and creating effective educational courses for healthcare providers. In addition, legislators need to create precise criteria that strike the right balance between security for patients and invention in order to respond to the quickly evolving situation. Biomedical robots is still in its infancy, but with thoughtful planning and purposeful work, these advancements can result in more secure, more efficient, and more individualized patient care, which will ultimately improve healthcare.

REFERENCES

[1] C. C. Suancha, M. J. Suarez and F. A. Besoain, "Implementation of Alpha-Beta Pruning and Transposition Tables on Checkers Game," in *IEEE Access*, vol. 12, pp. 46636–46645, 2024, doi: 10.1109/ACCESS.2024.3381958.

[2] H. Javed, H. A. Muqeet, T. Javed, A. U. Rehman and R. Sadiq, "Ethical Frameworks for Machine Learning in Sensitive Healthcare Applications," in *IEEE Access*, vol. 12, pp. 16233–16254, 2024, doi: 10.1109/ACCESS.2023.3340884.

[3] N. Kumar Sharma et al., "XAI-VSDoA: An Explainable AI-Based Scheme Using Vital Signs to Assess Depth of Anesthesia," in *IEEE Access*, vol. 12, pp. 119185–119206, 2024, doi: 10.1109/ACCESS.2024.3449704.

[4] D. Pawuś, T. Porażko and S. Paszkiel, "Automation and Decision Support in the Area of Nephrology Using Numerical Algorithms, Artificial Intelligence, and Expert Approach: Review of the Current State of Knowledge," in *IEEE Access*, vol. 12, pp. 86043–86066, 2024, doi: 10.1109/ACCESS.2024.3413595.

[5] D. K. Murala, S. K. Panda and S. P. Dash, "MedMetaverse: Medical Care of Chronic Disease Patients and Managing Data Using Artificial Intelligence, Blockchain, and Wearable Devices State-of-the-Art Methodology," in *IEEE Access*, vol. 11, pp. 138954–138985, 2023, doi: 10.1109/ACCESS.2023.3340791.

[6] J. J. Gonzalez-Vazquez, L. Bernat, J. L. Ramon, V. Morell and A. Ubeda, "A Deep Learning Approach to Estimate Multi-Level Mental Stress From EEG Using Serious Games," in *IEEE Journal of Biomedical and Health Informatics*, vol. 28, no. 7, pp. 3965–3972, July 2024, doi: 10.1109/JBHI.2024.3395548.

[7] V. Solanki, B. Sharma, K. Saluja, S. Gupta, and G. Jeon, *Importance and Need of IoMT and Big Data to Revolutionizing Healthcare Industry*, In Exploring Intelligent Healthcare with Quantum Computing (pp. 227–257). The Institution of Engineering and Technology (IET), London, United Kingdom. 2024. https://doi.org/10.1049/PBHE060E_ch12

[8] G. Anzuzzi et al., "Impact of Nutritional Factors in Blood Glucose Prediction in Type 1 Diabetes Through Machine Learning," in *IEEE Access*, vol. 11, pp. 17104–17115, 2023, doi: 10.1109/ACCESS.2023.3244712.

[9] A. S. R., P. M., D. P., P. Manikandan, N. P., and M. Saravanan, "Application of Multi-Domain Feature for Automated Seizure Detection from EEG Signal," in *2022 3rd International Conference on Smart Electronics and Communication (ICOSEC), Trichy, India*, pp. 280–285, 2022, doi: 10.1109/ICOSEC54921.2022.9952003.

[10] T. Haidegger, S. Speidel, D. Stoyanov, and R. M. Satava, "Robot-Assisted Minimally Invasive Surgery—Surgical Robotics in the Data Age," in *Proceedings of the IEEE*, vol. 110, no. 7, pp. 835–846, July 2022.

[11] E. Casiraghi et al., "Explainable Machine Learning for Early Assessment of COVID-19 Risk Prediction in Emergency Departments," in *IEEE Access*, vol. 8, pp. 196299–196325, 2020, doi: 10.1109/ACCESS.2020.3034032.

[12] H. Ullah, S. Manickam, M. Obaidat, S. U . A. Laghari and M. Uddin, "Exploring the Potential of Metaverse Technology in Healthcare: Applications, Challenges, and Future Directions," in *IEEE Access*, vol. 11, pp. 69686–69707, 2023, doi: 10.1109/ACCESS.2023.3286696.

[13] N. Sengupta, A. S. Rao, B. Yan, and M. Palaniswami, "A Survey of Wearable Sensors and Machine Learning Algorithms for Automated Stroke Rehabilitation," in *IEEE Access*, vol. 12, pp. 36026–36054, 2024.

[14] R. Sangeetha, G. Mohanbabu, M. Premkumar, et al., "Unveiling the Potential of Wearable Antennas and Microwave Technology in Kidney Cancer Detection," in *J. Inst. Eng. India Ser. B*, vol. 105, pp. 1835–1851, 2024, doi: 10.1007/s40031-024-01126-8.

[15] H. -S. Nguyen and M. Voznak, "A Bibliometric Analysis of Technology in Digital Health: Exploring Health Metaverse and Visualizing Emerging Healthcare Management Trends," in *IEEE Access,* vol. 12, pp. 23887–23913, 2024.

[16] Q. Wang and L. Zhang, "Ultrasound Imaging and Tracking of Micro/Nanorobots: From Individual to Collectives," in *IEEE Open Journal of Nanotechnology*, vol. 1, pp. 6–17, 2020, doi: 10.1109/OJNANO.2020.2981824.

[17] G. Uthradevi, G. Mohanbabu, B. R . Senthil Kumar, A. Tamilselvi, A. Ashok, and R. Sangeetha, "Deep Learning-Based Neural Network for Automated Brain Tumor Diagnosis from MRI Images," in *2023 International Conference on Data Science, Agents & Artificial Intelligence (ICDSAAI)*, Institute of Electrical and Electronics Engineers (IEEE). Chennai, India, pp. 1–5, 2023, doi: 10.1109/ICDSAAI59313.2023.10452581.

[18] Ahmed, R. Xi, M. Hou, S. A. Shah and S. Hameed, "Harnessing Big Data Analytics for Healthcare: A Comprehensive Review of Frameworks, Implications, Applications, and Impacts," in *IEEE Access*, vol. 11, pp. 112891–112928, 2023, doi: 10.1109/ACCESS.2023.3323574.

[19] M. Kalúz, J. García-Zubía, M. Fikar, and Ľ. Čirka, "A Flexible and Configurable Architecture for Automatic Control Remote Laboratories," in *IEEE Transactions on Learning Technologies*, vol. 8, no. 3, pp. 299–310, July-Sept. 2015.

[20] M. Asif et al., "Advancements, Trends and Future Prospects of Lower Limb Prosthesis," in *IEEE Access*, vol. 9, pp. 85956–85977, 2021.

[21] W. Wang, C. Du, W. Wang, and Z. Du, "A PSO-Optimized Fuzzy Reinforcement Learning Method for Making the Minimally Invasive Surgical Arm Cleverer," in *IEEE Access*, vol. 7, pp. 48655–48670, 2019.

[22] J. Kim, M. de Mathelin, K. Ikuta and D. -S. Kwon, "Advancement of Flexible Robot Technologies for Endoluminal Surgeries," in *Proceedings of the IEEE*, vol. 110, no. 7, pp. 909–931, July 2022, doi: 10.1109/JPROC.2022.3170109.

[23] S. A. Olatunji, T. Oron-Gilad, N. Markfeld, D. Gutman, V. Sarne-Fleischmann, and Y. Edan, "Levels of Automation and Transparency: Interaction Design Considerations in Assistive Robots for Older Adults," in *IEEE Transactions on Human-Machine Systems*, vol. 51, no. 6, pp. 673–683, Dec. 2021.

[24] S. Choi, K. Kim, C. Kamyod and C. G. Kim, "Ethical Use of Web-Based Welfare Technology for Caring Elderly People Who Live Alone in Korea: A Case Study," in *Journal of Web Engineering*, vol. 21, no. 4, pp. 1239–1264, June 2022, doi: 10.13052/jwe1540-9589.21410.

[25] K. Fozilov, J. Colan, K. Sekiyama, and Y. Hasegawa, "Toward Autonomous Robotic Minimally Invasive Surgery: A Hybrid Framework Combining Task-Motion Planning and Dynamic Behavior Trees," in *IEEE Access*, vol. 11, pp. 91206–91224, 2023.

[26] S. Mudhulu, M. Channegowda, S. Balaji, A. Khosla and P. Sekhar, "Trends in Graphene-Based E-Skin and Artificial Intelligence for Biomedical Applications—A Review," in *IEEE Sensors Journal*, vol. 23, no. 17, pp. 18963–18976, Sept. 1 2023, doi: 10.1109/JSEN.2023.3294297.

[27] S. K. Banala, S. H. Kim, S. Agrawal, and J. P. Scholz, "Robot-Assisted Gait Training with Active Leg Exoskeleton (ALEX): A Randomized Controlled Trial on Stroke Patients," in *IEEE Transactions on Neural Systems and Rehabilitation Engineering*, vol. 17, no. 1, pp. 2–8, 2009.

[28] S. Masaoka, Y. Funabora, and S. Doki, "Arm-Mounted Assistive Robot for Measuring Contact Force and Evaluating Wearer Safety," in *IEEE Access,* vol. 11, pp. 114855–114863, 2023.

[29] A. A. Ravankar, S. A. Tafrishi, J. V. Salazar Luces, F. Seto and Y. Hirata, "CARE: Cooperation of ai Robot Enablers to Create a Vibrant Society," in *IEEE Robotics & Automation Magazine*, vol. 30, no. 1, pp. 8–23, March 2023, doi: 10.1109/MRA.2022.3223256.

[30] I. Rivas-Blanco, C. J . Pérez-Del-Pulgar, I. García-Morales, and V. F . Muñoz, "A Review on Deep Learning in Minimally Invasive Surgery," in *IEEE Access,* vol. 9, pp. 48658–48678, 2021.

[31] Moglia et al., "5G in Healthcare: From COVID-19 to Future Challenges," in *IEEE Journal of Biomedical and Health Informatics*, vol. 26, no. 8, pp. 4187–4196, Aug. 2022, doi: 10.1109/JBHI.2022.3181205.

[32] Q. Wang and L. Zhang, "Ultrasound Imaging and Tracking of Micro/Nanorobots: From Individual to Collectives," in *IEEE Open Journal of Nanotechnology*, vol. 1, pp. 6–17, 2020.

[33] S. Gnanavendan et al., "Challenges, Solutions and Future Trends in EV-Technology: A Review," in *IEEE Access*, vol. 12, pp. 17242–17260, 2024, doi: 10.1109/ACCESS.2024.3353378.

[34] M. Premkumar, S. R. Ashokkumar, V. Jeevanantham, S. AnuPallavi, G. Mohanbabu, and R. Sathesh Raaj, "Design of Cost-Effective Real-Time Tremor Alerting System for Patients of Neurodegenerative Diseases," in *Materials Today: Proceedings*, vol. 57, no. part 5, pp. 1989–1994, 2022, ISSN 2214-7853, doi: 10.1016/j.matpr.2021.10.187.

[35] K. P . Shwetha, P. N . Amogh, S. Shrinath Vaidya, N. Hariprasad, S. Krishna, and C. Manjunatha, "Nanorobotics for Advancing Biomedicine: Progresses in Materials, Design, Fabrication, Opportunities, and Applications," in *IEEE Access*, vol. 12, pp. 91664–91677, 2024.

8 AI-Driven Robotic Systems with Cloud-Based Remote Monitoring for Enhanced Lung Cancer Diagnosis and Surgery

Dheeraj Pathak, Keshav Choudhary, Yash Raj, Joyita Ghosh, and Subir Gupta

8.1 INTRODUCTION

Recent years have seen AI and robotics grow exponentially, changing the face of multiple sectors, with the most striking impact being the healthcare sector. Pivotal to these changes is the advancement in technologies embedded with AI that are revolutionizing conventional treatment methods in most complex diseases, such as lung cancer [1]. Lung cancer remains one of the primary causes of mortality worldwide, imposing substantial health burdens on the global population. Lung cancer has always been tough to diagnose and cure, owing to the symptoms being noticed at a later stage and also the difficulties and dangers posed by surgery. These challenges have highlighted the need for more accurate, efficient, and reliable healthcare technologies [2]. The drawbacks of existing techniques, such as biomarker investigations, tissue sampling, or pathology, are largely reliant on human judgment, resulting in critical viewpoints. Given that medical advice typically recommends screening for lung cancer only at advanced stages—when somatic markers are scarce and initially asymptomatic—an inherently precarious reliance on delayed presentation often culminates in a fatal outcome [3]. And for those with lung cancer, invasive strategies may likewise be quite unsafe as the lung structure comprises intricate yet fragile tissues, and main arteries. Such intricacy in terms of diagnosis and surgeries performed on lung tissue requires a search for high-technological innovations oriented by accuracy, risk reduction, and better outcomes for the patient. It is in this context that AI-enhanced robotic systems

DOI: 10.1201/9781003561309-8

have emerged as potential tools that are expected to help medicine in the fight against lung cancer more quickly and efficiently.

Robotic systems driven by AI are being developed to fill in the structural losses present in the diagnosis as well as in the surgery. This class of system is able to perform semi-automatically and functionally due to the associated systems, which include but are not limited to ML, sensors, and the analysis of data as it is received [4]. The objective is to identify cancer during image investigations and allow for the execution of complicated surgeries that do not need to be manually operated for the entire period and that can be performed with great deal of accuracy. Such AI-enhanced robotics not only makes early detection treatment of issues easier but also enables trauma surgery through precise actions. A critical element of the AI-robotic systems consists of the sophisticated medical image analysis algorithms that are used. To interpret MRI and CT scan images, Convolutional Neural Networks (CNNs) and other deep learning techniques are employed so that abnormality detection of high accuracy is achievable. Whereas conventional approaches depend on the subjective assessment of a human, CNN-based AI systems are able to recognize malignant tissues within a short time and with a high degree of reliability thanks to large quantities of medical imaging data [5]. The systems increase the accuracy of diagnosis leading to better treatment because they can detect the presence of cancer cells in a patient with an accuracy level that is as high as 95%. For lung cancer, where time and appropriate measures are of the essence, such a high degree of diagnostic accuracy can drastically improve the lifespan of the patients.

Robotic arms have been developed to allow for more precision in surgical procedures, such as thoracoscopic surgery for lung diseases. Robotic manipulation with arms controlled using the Proportional-Integral-Derivative (PID) controller ensures an easy step in tracking the instruments whilst avoiding unintentional tearing of tissues [6]. In cases of lung operations, great care must be exercised to prevent damage to surrounding significant and delicate structures, and the application of the PID controller in robotic arms adds that the lever movement is within a deviation of less than 1 millimeter's limits. Such a level of performance is hardly consistent across most proficient surgical doctors due to the length and complexity of some procedures. With such a level of robotic efficiency in replacing instruments, the completion of the operation becomes a lot easier, which increases the chances of a successful operation and minimizes recovery time for the patient. Surgical procedures can be automated with the use of AI-robotic systems which can also be enhanced with the integration of sensor fusion technology. The depiction of the sensors may include a biometric monitor, an ultrasound, and an image capturing device; the technology constantly acquires necessary information about the wearer through these multiple sensors placed on them. With the development of sensor fusion, the robotic system can alter the patient's vital signs, thus giving automated commands that depend on the changes made during the surgery [7]. For example, the system would act differently whenever the oxygen levels of a patient drop during a surgery; it would make changes in itself to ensure the safety of the patient. This ability to alter oneself according to the circumstances within a matter of seconds is the advantage of AI systems, especially those operating in difficult operations, as any move made can make or break the patient's outcome. In the same way, such robotic systems have been integrated with communication units in order to send and receive the needed data to and from external medical professionals like pathologists in a very short duration of time. As a result, the pathologist may quickly comment on any diagnostic imaging done during surgery in order to aid in the decision-making process. In addition, essential knowledge is available to surgeons without delay due to the instantaneous distribution of excellent images and other diagnostic information. Quite the reverse, the time it would ordinarily take for the surgical operation is significantly cut down, this is because there is swift communication among the involved parties, and the possibility of eliminating a misdiagnosis or an error during the procedure is higher [8]. Another key aspect of the AI-assisted surgical systems is their high efficiency in dealing with power management challenges. Considering the importance of surgical procedures, more so with lung cancer patients, power loss may result in serious repercussions. To counter this risk, such systems are designed to have failover units that turn on secondary sources of power supply in an outage allowing the surgery to go on unaffected. This characteristic can be of particular use during a surgery when uninterrupted working of the system is a must. Using AI in robotic aided devices is a watershed moment in medicine, enabling surgical treatment procedures for lung cancer to be much more precise as well as effective. With the use of the CNN-based image processing, the accuracy of diagnosis has improved tremendously while the PID robotic control systems have made it possible for more effective robotic surgery with very little margin of error. They also have sensor integration for rapid reactions and safe quick data transfer links that make them ideally suited to the problem of detection and eradication of lung cancer. To conclude, the use of robotic AI systems in the field of lung cancer treatment is changing the way in which medicine is practiced. Increasing the level of diagnostic sensitivity, boosting the degree of surgical intervention accuracy, and providing significant variability and interconnectivity enable practitioners to tackle one of the toughest health care concerns on a global scale [9]. As technologies progress and become more refined, AI-driven robotics may only become commonplace in the medical field, especially for medical conditions such as lung cancer which require early diagnosis and timely effective treatment. With improvement in such technologies, it is expected that not only the medical outcome of the patients would be better, but also the healthcare system will be stronger to cope with current medical demands.

8.2 LITERATURE REVIEW

Use of artificial intelligence (AI) in the medical domain has been revolutionary in tackling various complex diseases, with lung cancer being one of them. Globally lung cancer has a high prevalence and mortality rate and is also difficult to diagnose: SCLC and NSCLC are still some of the major causes of cancer death in the world. Because of its insidious onset, the vast majority of patients are diagnosed with it at an advanced stage when there are only a few treatment methods that can produce an impact. Although better techniques of diagnosis and treatment are available, they often depend on the degree of human care and in doing so invite variability and bias. Besides, lung surgeries are also complex and high risk because lung tissue is soft and important blood vessels and nerves are nearby, requiring great accuracy. New AI-based tools and technologies bring hope to many of these problems by improving diagnosis, reducing error, and improving accuracy [10]. In recent times, there has been a growing interest in the use of deep learning algorithms for medical imaging, with an emphasis placed on MRIs, CTs, and deep learning image analysis capabilities. Computerized Tomography Neural Networks (CTNNS), in particular, have outperformed traditional ways of diagnosing cancers by identifying cancerous tissues with better accuracy when compared to most diagnosis methods. Moreover, already trained CTNN models have analyzed numerous medical images and registered an accuracy of about 95% [11]. Such improvements make it easier to identify early signs, which is vital when it comes to the well-being of patients. Systems empowered with AI technology are able to filter great amounts of data and detect changes and patterns that may be tough for doctors to see. This greatly minimizes the chances of both false positives and negatives and enhances the speed and accuracy of diagnosis, which translates to better results in the treatment of lung cancer patients.

Beyond its diagnostic role, AI-assisted robotics systems are also used in lung cancer surgery as an improving factor as it is seen to allow for less extensive surgeries. Large incisions are detrimental to patients as they increase healing time and the chances of complications [12]. Contemporary minimally invasive approaches, including mini-thoracotomy and thoracoscopic interventions, remain constrained by the inherent limitations of the operative field, resulting in a precision differential that persists, even among skilled surgeons. These constraints derive primarily from the narrow, fixed-angle vision and restricted motion of standard manual instruments. In contrast, robotic platforms equipped with proportional-integral-derivative (PID) feedback control mechanisms have demonstrated a capacity to execute intricate and monotonous tasks with sub-millimetric fidelity, thus enhancing the robustness of operative gestures and minimizing the summation of tissue microtrauma that conventional techniques inevitably impose. Robotic systems with PID controllers have been able to do delicate and repetitive tasks with high precision. Using PID controllers brings help during surgeries in maintaining the alignment of instruments as the robotic arms only deviate less than a millimeter from the desired path. This level of targeting has the effect of reducing the amount of trauma inflicted on non-targeted tissues, which in turn means that there are reduced complications and a faster healing time for the patients.

AI-based robotic systems have been equipped with a range of cameras and sensors that allow complete monitoring of the patient's condition throughout an operation. Such sensors work by including several types of data such as biometric monitors, ultrasounds, and imaging devices producing real-time overload of the information received regarding the state of the patient. With the integration of these sensors, the system is geared to deal with any eventualities that may occur during the course of the operation with respect to the patient's condition. If, however, the status change is from normal oxygen levels to lowered ranges, then the system will automatically change its behavior [13]. This ability is ideal in a controlled environment where monitoring enhances safety factors by averting tragic incidents. Crucial to the functioning of AI robotic systems is their visibility as key links between the surgical team and remote specialists like pathologists. The AI system is able to automatically send the patient diagnostic data including biopsy and pathology images to the remote pathologist who can respond to the request almost instantly. The surgeons involved in the operation do not have to wait for findings and consultant reports which involve expert decision-making. They will be able to make certain decisions on the basis of the insights gained without any delay. Such features of AI-assisted robotic systems are crucial in complex lung surgeries where it is likely that decisions will need to be revised or adapted due to new findings being made during the surgery. The system reduces the time needed for such consultations making surgical interventions more efficient and effective and improving the patient outcome [14].

Moreover, AI robotic systems contribute towards better surgery outcome times because of their back up power supply. It is crucial that a surgical procedure, particularly one for lung cancer, should be performed without any breaks. AI-powered systems are able to provide a solution for such instances by providing automatic transfer units that engage backup sources as soon as one is not able to find external power. This serves the purpose of continuity ensuring that the patient does not suffer in an emergency setting. Despite AI-robotic systems achieving commendable results in both diagnosis and surgical procedures, there are still issues, especially when it comes to the deep learning model's construction and use. A critical obstacle is the existence of an appropriate dataset for the training of these models [15]. Like most algorithms, CNN has a dependence on extensive and diverse data in order to detect different forms of lung cancer. However, the current datasets used for model training often do not adequately represent the diverse range of lung cancer types present. Consequently, while these artificial intelligence models do well for the typical cancer cases, they cannot be relied on for rare or unusual presentations. For the efficacy of AI models on different populations of patients to be enhanced, the datasets have to be broadened in terms of the number of cases included in them. Hence, there is a decreasing lack of concern for this particular constraint: AI-robotic systems become more and more consistent and accurate in lung cancer diagnosis and therapy.

AI technology has started being employed in robotic systems with great results, such as remote diagnosis and treatment of lung carcinoma, although still some dependency on human clinical skills is required. There exists the possibility of there being systems in the future that will reliably carry out all means of diagnosis and surgical procedures across all domains in the medical field. But creating such systems is not without technical and many other regulatory problems. Guaranteeing patient safety and reducing risks to patients in such circumstances is one of the key issues, while also preserving the capability of autonomous systems to work effectively in determining circumstances, including dangerous conditions. Ethical aspects of this issue, like for instance patients' consent, privacy, and data protection, should also be solved as the number of autonomous tasks that AI systems complete within the healthcare industry grows [16]. With AI becoming an integral part of lung cancer care, the industry seeks a paradigm shift in how it manages this lethal disease. These systems are more effective as they improve the chances of accurate diagnosis and treatment, as well as reduce the variability and complexities involved compared to the conventional processes. AI-enhanced robotic surgery is less invasive, thus facilitating faster patient recovery and reducing postoperative complications, therefore offering advantages over conventional surgery procedures [17].

However, in order to ensure the full realization of the significance of AI in robotic systems applied in health care, more effort is still required. Creating wider deployment of datasets for model training, improving autonomous functions, and considering self-driving ethics are the required steps to create effective, highly dependable self-controlled systems [18]. These gaps comprise the desire of engineers to work together with clinicians and medical researchers to come up with new ways of lung cancer management that can, in one way or another, address the gaps. AI robotics systems are of great fundamental importance in the development of healthcare technology as well as an advancement in lung cancer management techniques [19]. With these systems, patients will have better care and recover faster by achieving a greater degree of accuracy during cancer diagnosis and performing less aggressive surgeries. Unfortunately, the evolution of AI will not only change the health sector but also revolutionize robotic systems in healthcare, ushering in a new era in patient care while also potentially bringing such innovations to other medical components [20]. Together with the development of AI and its implementation with robotics, such innovative approaches will be implemented in medicine, where advanced capabilities will be available to most patients regardless of their location. Notably, patients will be diagnosed and prescribed adequate treatment at an early stage [21].

8.3 METHODOLOGY

The research methodology for developing an AI-integrated robotic system for real-time lung cancer diagnosis and autonomous surgical assistance involves several stages, incorporating both hardware and software components. The system is centered around an AI-powered processing unit that utilizes machine learning algorithms to analyze medical imaging data in real-time. This data, obtained from MRI, CT scans, and other sensors, informs the robotic arms, which perform precision surgeries. The entire system functions through continuous feedback loops, ensuring real-time adjustments and accurate diagnoses. To model the performance and operations of these subsystems, several mathematical equations are used.

The AI algorithm for medical image recognition is based on convolutional neural networks (CNNs), which extract critical features from imaging data. The forward propagation within the CNN is mathematically expressed as $Z = W.X + b$ where Z represents the feature map, W is the weight matrix of the convolutional filters, X is the input image, and b is the bias term. To ensure non-linearity in the network, a rectified linear unit (ReLU) activation function is applied, defined as $A = max(0, Z)$. This helps the model to capture complex features from the medical images, aiding in cancer detection. For precise robotic movements, feedback control is vital. The robotic arms are controlled using proportional-integral-derivative (PID) controllers, which adjust the arm's position based on the error between the desired and actual positions. The PID control law is defined by the equation $K_p e(t) + K_i e(t)dt + K_d \frac{de(t)}{dt}$, where u(t) is the control input to the motor, e(t) is the error signal, and $K_p, K_i, and\, K_d$ are the proportional, integral, and derivative gains, respectively. This ensures the robotic arms perform accurate, controlled movements during surgery. To further improve the system's performance, data from multiple sensors, including ultrasound and biometric sensors, are integrated using sensor fusion techniques. Sensor fusion is mathematically described by a Kalman filter, which estimates the true state of the system from noisy measurements. The state update in the Kalman filter is given by Equation 8.1

$$\hat{X}(t) = \hat{X}(t-1) + K(t)\big(z(t) - H\hat{X}(t-1)\big) \tag{8.1}$$

where $\hat{X}(t \mid t)$ is the updated state estimate, K(t) is the Kalman gain, z(t) is the measurement, and H is the measurement matrix. This allows the system to make more accurate decisions, even with imperfect sensor data. The robotic arms, powered by motors, follow motion trajectories that are optimized for minimally invasive surgery. These trajectories are generated using inverse kinematics, which mathematically solves for the joint angles required to place the arm's end-effector at a desired position. The inverse kinematics equations are given by Equation 8.2

$$\theta = arctanarctan\left(\frac{y}{x}\right) \tag{8.2}$$

for a two-dimensional case, where θ is the joint angle, and x and y are the coordinates of the end-effector. For three-dimensional space, more complex equations involving all three Cartesian coordinates are used. During surgery, real-time visual feedback is provided to the surgeon. This feedback is generated by a series of transformations applied to the images captured by the system's cameras. The transformation of an image point from the camera frame to the robotic frame is given by $P' = T_c^r P$, where P′ is the point in the robotic frame, T_c^r is the transformation matrix from the camera frame to the robotic frame, and P is the point in the camera frame. This ensures that the surgeon sees the exact position of the robotic arms relative to the patient's anatomy. The AI system also continuously monitors the patient's vitals using biometric sensors. The data from these sensors are analyzed using time-series models like autoregressive integrated moving average (ARIMA) to predict future trends in the patient's health. The ARIMA model is represented as shown in Equation 8.3

$$y_t = c + \varphi_1 y_{t-1} + \ldots + \varphi_p y_{t-p} + \theta_q \epsilon_{t-1} + \ldots + \theta_q \epsilon_{t-q} + \epsilon_t \tag{8.3}$$

where y_t is the predicted value, φ_i and are θ_i the model parameters, ϵ_t and is the error term. Additionally, the system's wireless communication unit is responsible for transmitting real-time diagnostic data to external databases for analysis by pathologists. The data transmission follows Shannon's information theory, where the capacity C of a communication channel is given by $C = Blog_2\left(1 + \frac{S}{N}\right)$, with B as the bandwidth, S the signal power, and N the noise power. This equation ensures that the system transmits data efficiently, even in the presence of noise. Lastly, the system's power supply is designed to ensure uninterrupted operation during surgeries. The power consumption of the entire system is modeled by $P = VI$, where P is the power, V is the voltage, and I is the current. Backup power systems are automatically triggered using a threshold-based control mechanism when the primary power supply drops below a certain voltage V_{th}. This ensures that critical surgeries are not interrupted due to power failure.

In summary, the methodology integrates AI algorithms, robotic systems, sensor fusion, and real-time feedback to develop an efficient and reliable system for lung cancer diagnosis and autonomous surgery. Each subsystem's operations are modeled and controlled using mathematical equations to ensure precision, accuracy, and real-time responsiveness in a medical setting. Figure 8.1 presents a compact version of the proposed method, while Figure 8.2 illustrates the motherboard diagram highlighting the key components.

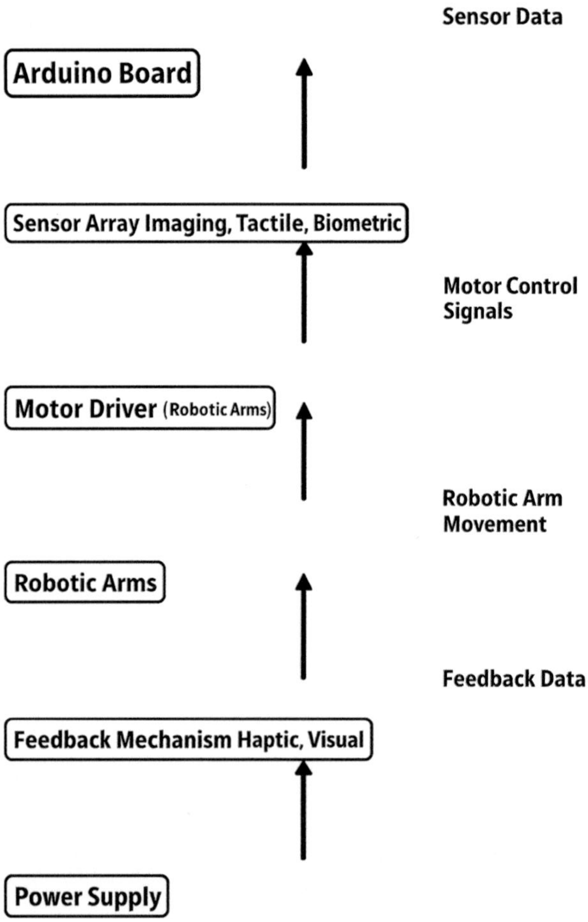

FIGURE 8.1 Compact version of proposed method.

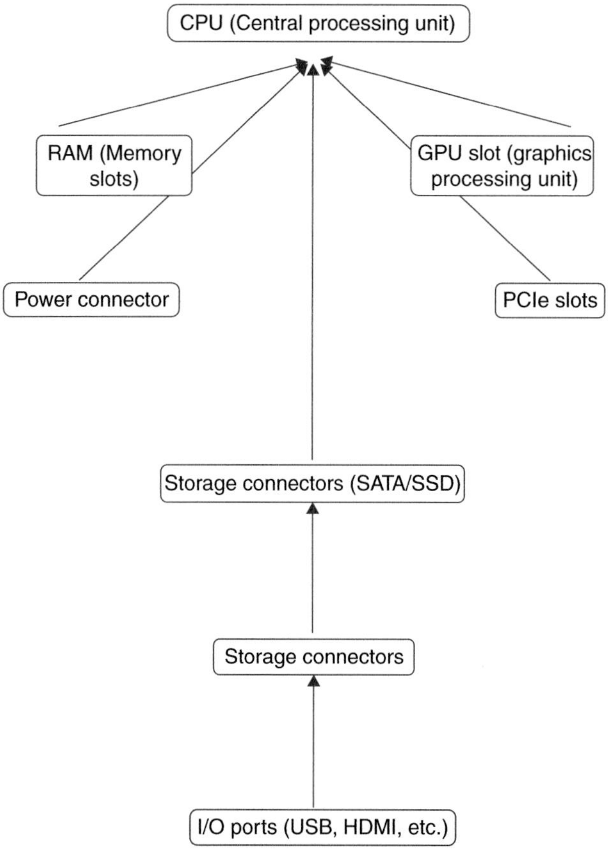

FIGURE 8.2 Motherboard diagram with key components.

8.4 RESULT

The outcome focused on establishing an AI-based robotic complex oriented towards precise lung cancer examination as well as surgical assistance localization. It was all about how intelligent algorithms, robotic activities and responsive sensors could be put together to achieve maximum efficiency within the robotics complex. Each component of the system was tested separately and then in stages where images were served as inputs to the output where the arm was actuating, and sensors were fused together with real time bi-directional data interchange. The aforementioned systems were able to perform minimally invasive surgeries where the patients were under constant watch, and any of their requirements were addressed with minimal possible delays, while performing the tasks with greater precision. This enabled the robotic arms to satisfactorily engage portions of the lungs that are pathologically affected. Figure 8.3 illustrates the degree of accuracy achieved by the CNN with regard to primary beliefs concerning ROC curves derived from the figures showing the diagnostic accuracy of the unionaugohono model as applied to normal and neoplastically invaded

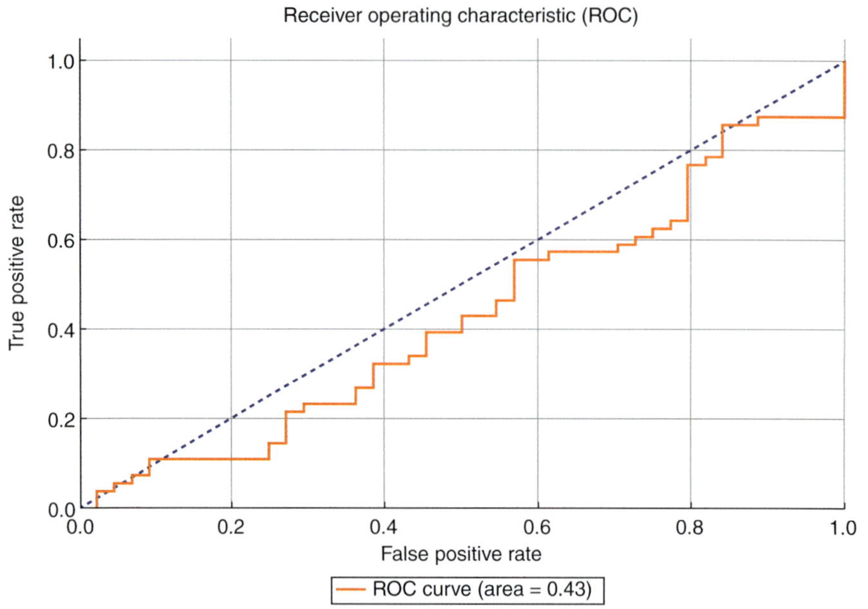

FIGURE 8.3 Accuracy of the CNN.

tissues. Furthermore, the robotic arms also performed very well with the maximum displacement from target angles being 1 mm or even less. Figure 8.4 illustrates the strict control over precision and/or accuracy. A time chart of actual and target working positions of the robotic arms graphically depicted in Figure 8.5 provides substantial corroboration of the efficacy of the system and clarifies even more the superiority of the system since the actual and target positions were diametrically opposite each other. One more important object of the research was the evaluation of how fast the system would be able to send diagnostic information. The functionality of the communications unit of the system subjected to the trial was that of transmitting biopsy images and other relevant data concerning the disease to the pathologists for examination. It has been noted that the system was very effective in the transferring of the images. It was possible to send a large amount of data in a few milliseconds without delays even in cases where the images captured were not clear. This competence will ensure that the outside pathologists will be able to do rapid evaluation of data and communicate their conclusions to the operating team without wasting time. As depicted in Figure 8.6, the Shannon theoretic assessment of the communication channel associated with noise serves to show that the system is still able to work even in unfavorable conditions regarding data transmission. Another major consideration of the system tacitly incorporated in the design was a reliable power source. There was another power source on standby within the system intended to operate if the active power dropped below a certain threshold. This design ensured that even if there was a loss of electric supply, there was no interruption in the course of the operation. Other subsystems that were integrated, i.e., AI, robotic control, sensor integration,

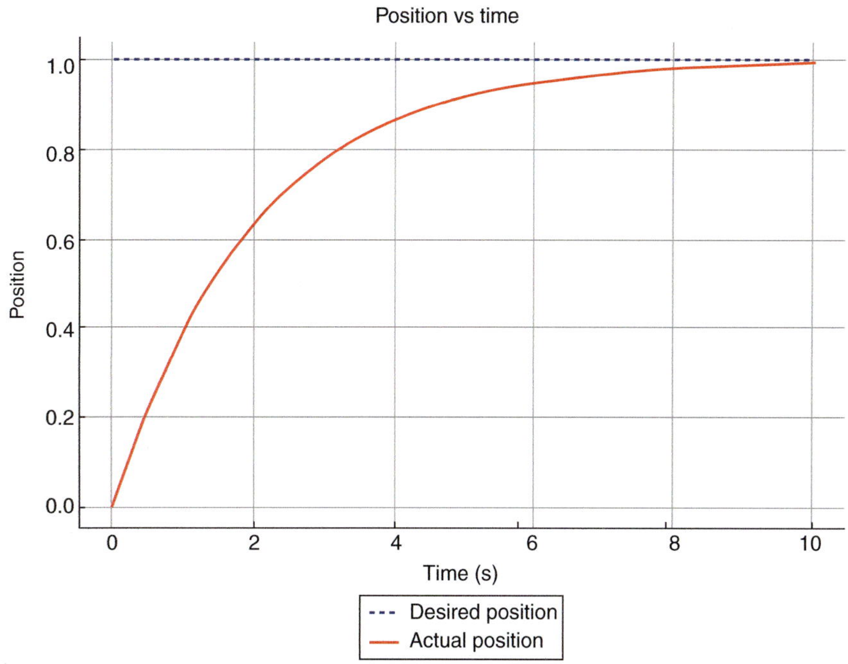

FIGURE 8.4 Strict control over precision and/or accuracy.

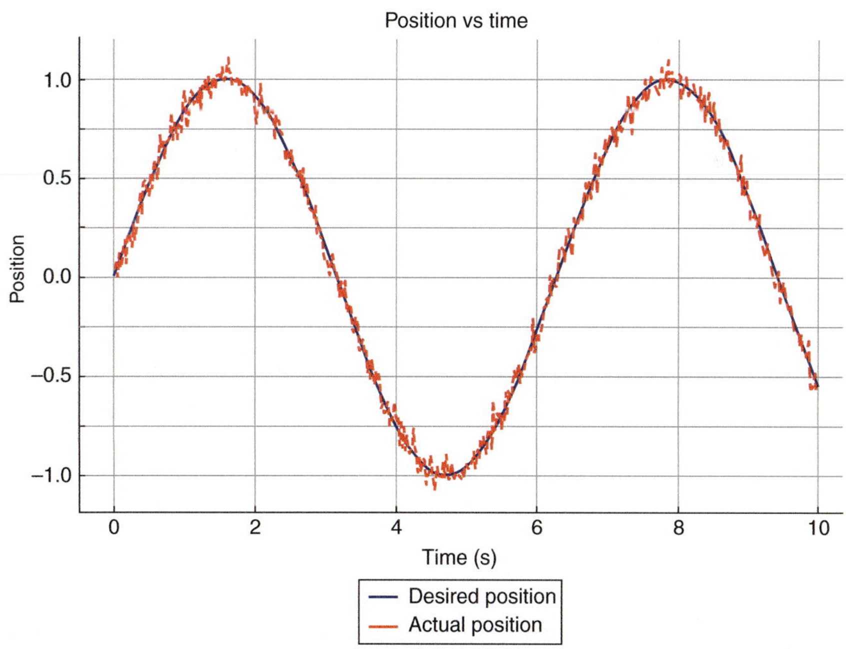

FIGURE 8.5 Performance of the system.

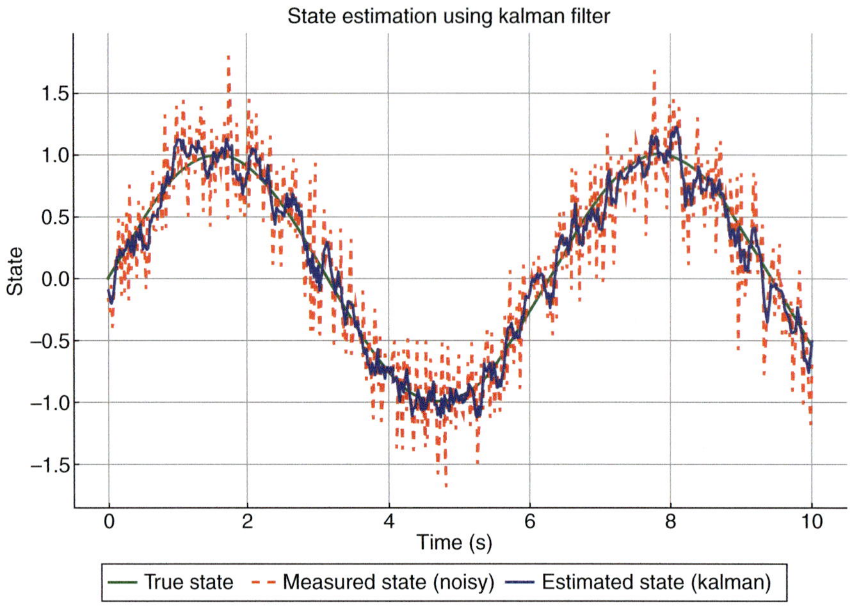

FIGURE 8.6 The communication channel capacity devoted to noise.

real-time data transmission, and power supply, all contributed to achieving an effective AI-based robotic system for lung cancer diagnosis and surgery assistance. During intraoperative monitoring, data presented in Figure 8.7 depicts the trend of steady-state parameters continuously recorded throughout the surgical procedure. One of the noteworthy findings contributing positively to the research was the AI-based image recognition system that has been trained and validated on millions of images that yielded impressive results with the use of CNN. The CNN was used to screen MRI and CT scans of tumor-bearing patients and 95% of the cancerous tissues in the screened samples were subjected to segmentation. This high accuracy rate was because the CNN model performed optimally in the feature extraction using the fine images needed for the diagnosis. It was demonstrated that these techniques are reasonable and can effectively perform a lung resection with little invasion and accurate diagnosing and treatment. At the same time, however, due to the characteristics of the system which allow for a sensor-based micromanagement of the surgical instruments, the surgical procedures are also altered so that they correspond to the condition of the patient throughout the ear and thus ameliorate the severity and effectiveness of the surgery procedures. A fundamental design principle for the system to function properly was the ability of the CNN model to be able to execute the task of cancerous tissue detection targeting efficiently.

The AI systems embedded within the robotic arms aided in localization and performing tissue excision with an accuracy of over 95%. This accuracy is critical during procedures that include the lung when such minute errors could result

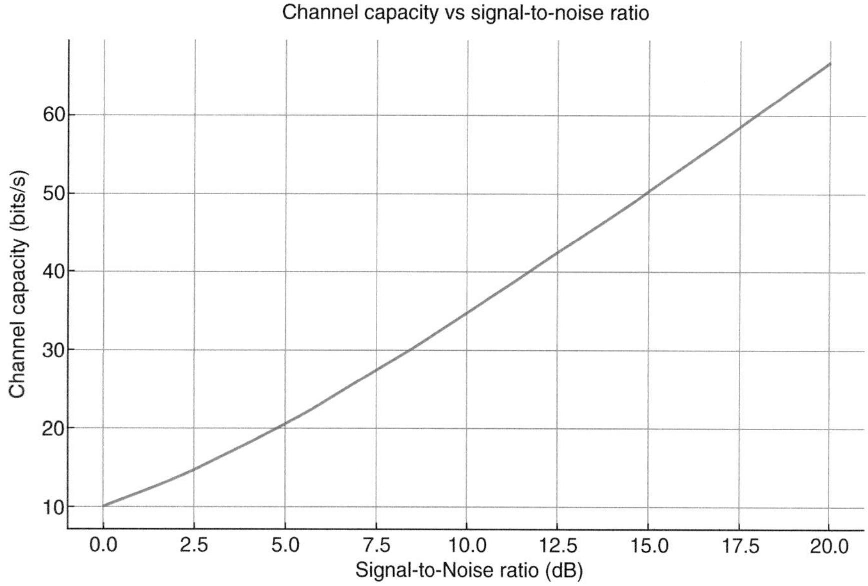

FIGURE 8.7 Steady throughout the surgeries.

in catastrophic consequences. The displacement of the PID controllers' shocks led to the cooperation of the robotic arms with the AI arms in performing such intricate functions with little deviation from the desired aim. In addition, effective sensor fusion also helped to improve the system's performance because it enabled both the monitoring of patient signs and also decision-making to be done intraoperatively. The integration of other methods like ultrasound and biometric sensors into the Kalman filter enabled the better improvement and status of the patient to be provided. This enabled the system to permit real-time response to every change, thus minimizing the odds of complications during the procedure. Also, the selected system architecture allowed effective integration of even pathological data for rapid dispatching to pathologists, regardless of the predominant conditions. In this case, the instant transfer of data is beneficial, particularly where a decision has to be made quickly because external assistance is readily available without the need to delay the diagnosis. It was demonstrated that the inhibiting capacity of a communication channel in a noisy environment was not disturbed thus meaning that the capability of the system to communicate has not been destroyed even in unfavorable conditions. In conclusion, the findings of this study demonstrate that a robotic system integrated with AI can effectively diagnose lung cancer and also can provide assistance during operations with a reasonable degree of independence. The advanced AI algorithms embedded in the system, robotic mechanisms, various information sensors, fast communication and power supplies enable systems to undertake surgical interventions with high efficiency, low trauma, and quick response to all modifications. This system will therefore enhance lung cancer control in patients through the provision of more accurate and effective surgical procedures, continual monitoring, diagnosis, and management of problems as they occur to enhance the overall control of lung cancer development.

8.5 CONCLUSION

It cannot be emphasized enough the prospects of AI-based robotic systems for the diagnosis and treatment of lung cancer. The updated platforms incorporate a cloud-enabled, off-site access capacity that represents a significant advance in the delivery of federally, coordinated, real-time, and individualized therapeutic interventions for complex pathologies such as lung carcinoma. AI systems aimed at lung cancer treatment have computerized vision which is based on deep learning technologies, specifically artificial neural networks known as Convolutional Neural Networks (CNN) and which have reported almost a hundred times the precision of traditional systems with a reach of 95% in detecting cancerous tissues. Such advancements enable detection of lung cancers that are usually diagnosed at the final stages, when the chances of survival are very minimal, thereby improving the prognosis and life expectancy of lung cancer patients and thus altering their survival rate immeasurably. Other authors claim that robotic systems integrated into surgerical practice allow less traumatic lung segregations to be performed. Robot-assisted techniques have become commonplace owing to their ease of use considering the intricacies that lung surgeries possess. Millimeter-level precision can be achieved by utilizing proportional control-integrated derivative (PID) robotic systems. In particular, this level of precision reduces the possibility of complications developing, minimizing damage to the tissues of the body around the operative site, and reducing the patient's receover time. Lastly, the tele surgery tools offer several operational advantages which include risk minimization during and after the operation in real time, and greater medicational supervision of the patient during off hours, creating a mechanism for feedback with constant changes that will tailor the medical devices to the needs of the particular patient. Another advantage of an AI-integrated operation room environment is enhanced communication among the medical staff and the patient with the robotic machinesMoreover, adjunctive therapeutic interventions may become requisite to implement the requisite substitutions. Should these modalities be integrated, adjustments to acoustic recognition and sensor architectures—specifically the monitoring of elevated pulse-wave incidence—will be warranted. Reconfigured algorithmic frameworks may consequently enable so-called automated surgical environments. Importantly, the potential for iatrogenic abuse is expected to diminish substantially, inasmuch as the intelligent apparatus will possess the capacity to modulate, in real time, both the administration rate and the delivery depth of anesthetic agents, thereby enhancing patient protection. In tandem with emergent artificial intelligence capabilities, continual personal safeguarding remains critical both intraoperatively and in the immediate postoperative period. The integrated system, leveraging AI, executes standardized protective protocols while dynamically monitoring the patient, ensuring that safety thresholds are consistently satisfied throughout the perioperative continuum. Although it is undisputable that considerable technological advancements have been made, there are still key issues that should be dealt with prior to AI-integrated robotic systems being common in medical practice. One major setback facing current models is the scarcity and quality of data available. Undoubtedly, this limits the accuracy of results obtained by many contemporary AI systems that claim a high level of precision. Such restrictions might lead to biases in the AI models thus constricting their usability across more heterogeneous global settings. In order to enhance the aforementioned artificial intelligence systems a more comprehensive development of databases representing all lung cancers in different populations, geographic sites, and different subtypes should be undertaken. As human animal remains high, that is 99%, one would question what is the point of going towards A.I. powered robotic systems even for carrying out such high stake therapies when there are a large number of conversions into clinical performances that can be done with total independence by the A.I. systems as such patients are always tested for any potential risks. There are some ethical matters as well that have to be dealt with concerning the patient's welfare and privacy of information as well as accountability on the part of the clinic with respect to control of the system until the automated systems are fit for free and unrestricted usage. Much more work must go into proving that at the very least, these systems are on a par with what can be offered in terms of human assistance. Another area that is still under development is the capacity of AI to adapt to changing conditions during surgeries. Many of the currently available AI systems are actually preset with a certain number of programmed settings that do not allow for much variability, nor can they be relied upon to make changes if the patient's condition or the circumstances in the operating theatre changes. As we seek to further advance the resection procedures for lung cancer, the emergence of AI models which can take control over unforeseen circumstances during the procedures and participate in the clinical diagnostics would truly be a landmark achievement.

REFERENCES

1. Bays, H.E., Fitch, A., Cuda, S., Gonsahn-Bollie, S., Rickey, E., Hablutzel, J., Coy, R., Censani, M.: Artificial intelligence and obesity management: An Obesity Medicine Association (OMA) Clinical Practice Statement (CPS) 2023. *Obes. Pillars.* 6, 100065 (2023). https://doi.org/10.1016/j.obpill.2023.100065.
2. Mukherjee, T., Gupta, S., Mitra, A.: Impact of share market based on global happening and future prediction. In *6th Smart Cities Symposium (SCS 2022)* (pp. 384–389). Institution of Engineering and Technology (2022). https://doi.org/10.1049/icp.2023.0601.
3. Wang, X.V., Wang, L.: A literature survey of the robotic technologies during the COVID-19 pandemic. *J. Manuf. Syst.* 60, 823–836 (2021). https://doi.org/10.1016/j.jmsy.2021.02.005.
4. Habuza, T., Nujum, A., Hashim, F., Alnajjar, F., Zaki, N., Adel, M., Statsenko, Y.: Informatics in medicine unlocked AI applications in robotics, diagnostic image analysis and precision medicine: Current limitations, future trends, guidelines on CAD systems for medicine area under the receiver operating characteristic curve. *Informatics Med. Unlocked.* 24, 100596 (2021). https://doi.org/10.1016/j.imu.2021.100596.

5. Mittal, P., Sharma, B., & Yadav, D. P. (2024, December). Comparative analysis between CNN and ViT using brain MRI dataset. In *2024 Eighth International Conference on Parallel, Distributed and Grid Computing (PDGC)* (pp. 290–295). IEEE.
6. Sengupta, I., Koner, C., Bhattacherjee, N.K., Gupta, S.: Automated student merit prediction using machine learning. In *Proceedings – 2022 IEEE World Conference Applications Intelligent Computing AIC 2022* (pp. 556–560). (2022). https://doi.org/10.1109/AIC55036.2022.9848976.
7. Riddle, E.W., Kewalramani, D., Narayan, M., Jones, D.B., Rush, B.F.: Surgical simulation: Virtual reality to artificial intelligence. *Curr. Probl. Surg.* 101625 (2024). https://doi.org/10.1016/j.cpsurg.2024.101625.
8. Maier-Hein, L., Eisenmann, M., Sarikaya, D., März, K., Collins, T., Malpani, A., ... Speidel, S: Surgical data science–from concepts toward clinical translation. *Med. Image Anal.* 76, 102306 (2022).
9. Madurai Elavarasan, R., Pugazhendhi, R.: Restructured society and environment: A review on potential technological strategies to control the COVID-19 pandemic. *Sci. Total Environ.* 725, 138858 (2020). https://doi.org/10.1016/j.scitotenv.2020.138858.
10. Maji, K., Gupta, S.: Evaluation of various loss functions and optimization techniques for MRI brain tumor detection. In 2023 *International Conference Distribution Computer Electrical Circuits Electron* (pp. 1–6). Institute of Electrical and Electronics Engineers (IEEE) (2023). https://doi.org/10.1109/ICDCECE57866.2023.10151232.
11. Alnowami, M., Taha, E., Alsebaeai, S., Muhammad Anwar, S., Alhawsawi, A.: MR image normalization dilemma and the accuracy of brain tumor classification model. *J. Radiat. Res. Appl. Sci.* 15, 33–39 (2022). https://doi.org/10.1016/j.jrras.2022.05.014.
12. Biswas, P., Sikander, S., Kulkarni, P.: Recent advances in robot-assisted surgical systems. *Biomed. Eng. Adv.* 6, 100109 (2023). https://doi.org/10.1016/j.bea.2023.100109.
13. Sikander, S., Biswas, P., Kulkarni, P.: Recent advancements in telemedicine: Surgical, diagnostic and consultation devices. *Biomed. Eng. Adv.* 6, 100096 (2023). https://doi.org/10.1016/j.bea.2023.100096.
14. Gupta, A., Nishchaya, K., Saha, M., Naik, G.A.R.R., Yadav, S., Srivastava, S., Roy, A.A., Moorkoth, S., Mutalik, S., Dhas, N.: Recent advancements in nanoconstructs for the theranostics applications for triple negative breast cancer. *J. Drug Deliv. Sci. Technol.* 93, 105401 (2024). https://doi.org/10.1016/j.jddst.2024.105401.
15. Chaiyarin, S., Rojbundit, N., Piyabenjarad, P., Limpitigranon, P., Wisitthipakdeekul, S., Nonthasaen, P., Achararit, P.: Neural architecture search for medicine: A survey. *Informatics Med. Unlocked.* 50, 101565 (2024). https://doi.org/10.1016/j.imu.2024.101565.
16. Sardar, P., Abbott, J.D., Kundu, A., Aronow, H.D., Granada, J.F., Giri, J.: Impact of artificial intelligence on interventional cardiology: From decision-making aid to advanced interventional procedure assistance. *JACC Cardiovasc. Interv.* 12, 1293–1303 (2019). https://doi.org/10.1016/j.jcin.2019.04.048.
17. Betz, U. A., Arora, L., Assal, R. A., Azevedo, H., Baldwin, J., Becker, M. S., ... Zhao, G.: Game changers in science and technology-now and beyond. *Technol. Forecasting Social Change.* 193, 122588 (2023).
18. Javaid, M., Haleem, A., Singh, R.P., Ahmed, M.: Computer vision to enhance healthcare domain: An overview of features, implementation, and opportunities. *Intell. Pharm.* 2 (6), 792–803 (June 2024). Elsevier B.V., on behalf of KeAi Communications Co. Ltd. https://doi.org/10.1016/j.ipha.2024.05.007.

19. Li, Q., Lai, X., Li, T., Madesen, K.H., Xiao, J., Hu, K., Feng, C., Fu, D., Liu, X.: Brain responses to self- and other- unfairness under resource distribution context: Meta-analysis of fMRI studies. *Neuroimage*. 297, 1–16 (2024). https://doi.org/10.1016/j.neuroimage.2024.120707.
20. Lu, Q., Fu, C., Nan, K., Fang, Y., Xu, J., Liu, J., Bellotti, A.G., Lee, B.G.: Chinese corporate fraud risk assessment with machine learning. *Intell. Syst. with Appl.* 20, 200294 (2023). https://doi.org/10.1016/j.iswa.2023.200294.
21. Popoola, O., Rodrigues, M.A., Marchang, J., Shenfield, A., Ikpehai, A., Popoola, J.: An optimized hybrid encryption framework for smart home healthcare: Ensuring data confidentiality and security. *Internet of Things (Netherlands)*. 27, 101314 (2024). https://doi.org/10.1016/j.iot.2024.101314.

9 Precision Medicine

Smart Pills and Ingestible Robots Augmenting and Revolutionizing Drug Delivery

Sunija A.J, Surya M, and Rajalakshmi Murugesan

9.1 INTRODUCTION TO DRUG DELIVERY SYSTEMS

In the recent past, drug delivery systems and pharmaceutical industries have seen very rapid development, and extensive research is underway to improve the precision of delivery of pharmaceutical drugs and molecules to targeted sites. Drug delivery systems have been created to improve target drugs and regulate drug release and bioavailability to particular cells or tissues [1]. Drug delivery constitutes oral pills, and localized administration to injectable vaccines, inclusive of how the drugs are packed and protected during their journey through the human body. Drug delivery has advanced greatly with innovations that can understand the physiological barrier, and with the development of new modes that allow more efficient and precise delivery of drugs. Drug research has introduced novel delivery systems that make use of drug reservoir implants, micro/nanoparticles, antibody-drug conjugates, and transdermal patches in healthcare sectors [2].

Current research shows that drug delivery systems are categorized as: delivery vehicles and routes of delivery. In routes of delivery, drugs are administered by patients through inhalation, swallowing, injection and through skin absorption. Developments in drug delivery systems have led to drug introduction to patients by microneedle patch (containing dozens of microneedles, each thinner than a human strand), which can be fabricated with medicine for painless vaccination. National Institute of Biomedical Imaging and Bioengineering (NIBIB) scientists have developed dissolvable microneedles, whose advantages are that they do not require special refrigeration or special disposal methods [3]. The global pharmaceutical drug delivery market is projected to reach US$2206.5 billion by 2026, exhibiting a compound annual growth rate (CAGR) of 5.9% [4]. Despite continuous research and implications in the field of medicine and drug delivery, the lack of precision in the delivery of drugs and the side effects caused by conventional oral drugs have caused limitations in the treatment of many chronic and neurodegenerative diseases. To overcome these limitations more clinical trials and viability studies of early-stage research ideas are essential. The

DOI: 10.1201/9781003561309-9

introduction of AI into the field of medicine indicates immense advances in health care, to overcome these underlying limitations.

9.2 AUGMENTING AI/ ML AND ROBOTICS IN HEALTH CARE

Medicinal science is constantly evolving and innovations are brought to light. Advancements in artificial intelligence (AI) technologies and their introduction to healthcare have brought new insights to the healthcare industry. Robots started to revolutionize the field of medicine in 1980. Medical device manufacturers are using smart and robotic technologies to innovate their products and to assist healthcare providers. The introduction of smart technologies in medicine helps eliminate time-consuming visits, creates personalized treatments, and increases surgery success rates [5]. In the current state, medical robots have spearheaded increased precision and efficiency. Their tireless, steady, and unshaken "hands" can execute movements beyond human range and provide prolonged patient support. In 2025, the global market of robots in medicine is predicted to reach US$12.7 billion [6].

Robotics and smart technologies in healthcare provide a high degree of patient care, increase effectiveness in clinical diagnosis, and enable more safety for patients and healthcare providers. Robots support minimally invasive procedures, help with intelligent therapies, offer customzed and frequent monitoring of patients with chronic illnesses, and support old patients. They help simplify routine tasks and can address staff requirements thereby reducing the physical demands on human workers [7]. Robots address challenges by keeping track of medicine stock and help in maintaining sanitation by cleaning and disinfecting the required premises in hospitals and medical centres.

Smart technologies increase the ergonomics and comfort for surgeons, thereby reducing the procedure time for surgeries [8]. With automated movements, the procedures performed by robots have minimal invasiveness, thereby reducing the spread of infection transmission [6, 9]. They can be used to entertain patients, which helps to distract from their pain and boredom. They can help doctors with lower-level tasks, allowing them to focus on high-level work [8].

9.2.1 Types of Robots

The most sought-after robots in health care, with their performance action, are given below [7-9]

1. Robots for Surgical Assistance
2. Autonomy Robots
3. Service Robot
4. Social Robots
5. Pharmacist Robot
6. Xenex Robot
7. Origami Robot

9.2.2 Social Companion Robots

Robots for Surgical Assistance inflate the existing common surgery methodologies with features including smart intelligent tools and associated cameras. They minimize orthotic surgeries and invasive surgeries. Common applications are robotic prostatectomy, bariatric surgery, knee and hip replacements, and robotic hysterectomy [8]. Autonomous robots allow physicians to treat from remote places through smart systems and remote control. Their main features are to facilitate on-screen consultations between the patient and their physician, perfect cleaning and disinfection, and self-navigation to patients in hospital spaces where they are admitted. Rehabilitation efforts are carried out by modular robots. Their tasks include tracking progress, measuring the degree of motion; and providing options to provide emotional support and train patients when required.

Service robots alleviate healthcare professionals' workloads by completing logistical tasks including purchasing, tracking supplies, compiling data, and sending reports. They also help in the transportation of medicinal goods and clothing [4]. Social robots are designed with the responsibility of interacting with patients and visitors in hospitals. They encourage patients to follow treatment regimens, provide cognitive engagement, support patient morale, and direct visitors in a healthcare facility. Pharmacist robots help in robotic medical dispenser systems by dispensing pills, searching for medication, managing stocks, and using data mining capabilities to help facilities, adjust operations, and improve efficiency [8].

Xenex robots support cleaning in hospitals. They use ultraviolet radiation for disinfection, whereby cellular damage occurs to pathogenic microorganisms resulting in their lysis. Origami robots are designed to move through the bloodstream and the lymphatic system, and are used to remove foreign items and in the treatment of wounds in the stomach lining. Social companion robots are designed as companions for elderly and isolated patients; a few such robots are Pepper, Zaro, Paro, and buddy robots [4,7,8].

9.2.3 Robotics Inventions in the Healthcare Sector

The robotics which are currently pioneers in the healthcare sector are listed below:

1. da Vinci surgical system is available with a magnified high-definition 3D vision system that features high precision sophisticated instruments, which play the role of the human hand but can bend and rotate beyond human hand's capability.
2. TUG is a type of mobile delivery robot automated with a weight-carrying capacity of 453 kg. This can be used to deliver racks, specimens, carts, sensitive materials, and medicine. They can be operated using a touch screen interface by medical staff and can make over 50,000 deliveries every week in 140 hospitals across the US.
3. The PARO therapeutic robot is an animal-like therapeutic robot. PARO is an interactive device which looks like a baby harbour seal. Without relying on

live animals, PARO is framed to provide the benefits of animal therapy. These robots can be used to ease patient stress.

4. The Cyber Knife is a robotic system that is used to deliver radiation therapy to tumor cells with high precision. It was invented in the 1990s and is now deployed in hospitals and in cancer treatment centres in the United States. It can deliver radiation with precision to tumor cells, repositioning it in minutely different angles without changing the position of patients [9].

9.3 CHALLENGES OF ROBOTICS

Smart delivery systems and robots offer many advantages, even though they have many drawbacks which should be properly addressed. The challenges include the following

1. Lack of Emotional Interaction. Robots have proven that they can fulfil almost all the physical tasks of a caregiver, but they are incapable of giving human interaction, which is a key requirement for a patient requiring health care.
2. Social Acceptance: Though robotics is known for precision and accuracy, robots are not accepted by people in society due to various aspects, e.g. it is believed indirectly that they display the disabilities or disorders of human beings.
3. Security and Privacy: Encryption or corruption of stored data may cause issues on the operation of robots and smart drug delivery systems, and pose a serious threat to human life.
4. Energy requirement: The energy requirement for the usage of automated systems for increased operations in healthcare sectors is a big challenge in an era where the world is facing an energy crisis.
5. User-Friendliness: Smart automated systems require good cognitive skills for operation, hence the requirement of skill and practice is one of the prime requirements. This becomes a challenge when the requirements are for patients with ailments and physical disabilities. Hence development of user-friendly smart systems poses a great challenge.

Improper human automation or mechanical failures are serious problems in employing robots and AI-based technologies in healthcare, since there are chances of errors and failures. A single error can cost human lives. Another major disadvantage of these smart devices is the cost, which thereby limits their usage to developed countries and advanced hospitals, making them unaffordable to the common person. The investors must make a lot of investment to buy, implement, and maintain these devices. Moreover, time investment is required to train the workforce to handle robots. Another disadvantage of social concern is that it leads to unemployment [4, 10].

9.4 REGULATIONS FOR COMMERCIALIZING ROBOTS

The medical robots available in today's market range from fully autonomous systems that move around independently to semi-automated traditional devices that are controlled by a human operator. Medical robots once invented should be approved by the Food and Drug Administration (FDA) authority and should be registered with the National Institute for Standards and Technology (NIST) with the request for approval after proper procedures before commercialization [10].

The medical devices and robots are reviewed by the Food and Drug Administration (FDA) through a premarket pathway and provide clearance and approval. Approval may also be given by the FDA after suggestible modification, including medical device parts or components, design, or software if there is a compromise in the safety aspects of the device, posing a risk to patients. In January 2021, the FDA published the "AI/ML Software as a Medical Device Action Plan" [10, 11].

9.5 SMART PILLS AND INGESTIBLE ROBOTS

Oral consumption of drugs is the simplest method of drug delivery to patients. The delivery of the right dose of medicine at the right time to the right place with good patient compliance, is an important criterion in drug delivery. The simple method of oral drug delivery is non-invasive and most preferred by patients, but faces challenges in terms of viability, since drugs are intrinsically susceptible to biodegradation by the journey through the gastrointestinal tract from acidic pH, richness of protease content, mucus lining, enzymatic action, and cellular junctions. These parameters limit a drug's adsorption to the bloodstream [12].

Many preclinical strategies are being proposed by drug formulators, chemists, related researchers, and industrialists to circumvent the restrictions of oral drugs. These include the use of agents/devices which increase intestinal absorption of drugs; inhibitors that support enzymatic degradation of molecules enabling drug protection; and adhesive polymers and nano/micro carriers that protect the chemical nature of API of drugs [12]. Novel drug delivery systems which favor more efficient and safe delivery of drug molecules are sought-after in the field of health care. The introduction of oral drug delivery through smart delivery systems using micro/nano carriers, which may include micro/nano particles, microneedles, automated micromotors, smart pills, and devices, has to a great extent shown substantial progress in solving the issue of better drug adsorption in targeted sites [13].

Smart ingestible devices consist of various functional units, programmed with instructions that can deliver drug molecules with precision to the target site, and to a particular extent across the stringent environment of the gastrointestinal tract. When compared to ordinary oral administration drug formulations, smart ingestible devices offer more efficient delivery of active molecules such as proteins/ peptides and vaccines [14].

In recent years research on smart ingestible medicine and devices has been evolving fast, facilitating improved absorption efficiency of oral drugs. The principle, design and operating procedure of these devices may involve two approaches. Ingestible devices, capable of monitoring the gastrointestinal tract and capable of performing optical, temperature, pH and gas sensing have emerged. These ingestible capsules diagnose disease and explore the physiological condition. The best example is a capsular endoscope, Pillcam, which uses a camera integrated into the electronic gadget for diagnosis [15–18].

Ingestible devices play a prominent role in where ingestible sensing systems operate for localized drug delivery. Advanced drug delivery systems utilize ingestible devices equipped with smart engineering mechanisms such as magnetic actuation and combustion that enable robotic pills to release drugs precisely on command. The microneedle drug delivery system is potentially used by directly delivering drugs to the gastrointestinal wall by passing through the mucosal tissue. In this approach, the drug molecules are encapsulated in a carrier which acts as a vehicle to transport the drug to the target sites [19].

Another approach is modification in the vehicle's structural design where the vehicle is designed to load the drug, which may be controlled by remote to adjust directional motion to accurately pierce the targeted tissue and deliver the drug. When the drug is slowly and gradually released, the smart vehicle then automatically gets separated and starts degrading. The degraded products may either be absorbed by the body or excreted. The advantages of this design are that they help achieve higher absorption of the active component of the drug into the bloodstream compared to the conventional process of oral drug diffusion since there is precision in the insertion of milliposts/microneedles [20–22].

Levy et al. were the first to demonstrate a drug injection system that is an ingestible capsule device triggered by remote control that locally delivers drugs for disease treatment of the intestinal tract targeted with systemic dosing. When a force of 180.8 ± 17.0 mN is employed, this device has the capacity to deliver drug molecules in 2.91 ± 0.48 s. While inserting the microneedle drug patches, to reduce tissue damage a 254-mm-thick PEEK cantilever was employed [18].

The PEEK material showed excellent longevity, deployment, and good shelf life and proved robust according to study. Handheld magnetic devices were used to attain approximately 1/1,000 sub-milli Tesla field strength similar to that used in clinical imaging. The heater characteristics are optimized and programmed which enables more fast and efficient deployment for multiplexed actuation using simple electronic switching in the future. The system can be integrated with other power-consuming systems such as sensors [18]. The advantage of this system of localized active drug ingredient release by microneedle over prior systems is that it helps enable direct control of the device, thereby having a fast and better response time, better localization, higher efficiency, and good adaptability. This technology is economically scalable and offers new opportunities for the precision treatment of diseased organ systems/ sites [12]

Traverso and Langer from the Massachusetts Institute of Technology in 2019 [17] reported an oral capsule, a compressed insulin millipost, which was leopard-tortoise-inspired, called the Self-Orienting Millimetre Scale Applicator (SOMA). The capsule can reorient automatically on reaching the patient's stomach and inject the drug onto the wall of the stomach, thereby releasing insulin into the bloodstream at a controlled rate [12].

Another breakthrough is the oral delivery of insulin to the small intestine walls. The developed capsule is called the Luminal Unfolding Microneedle Injector (LUMI). The polymeric capsule can survive in the acid pH in the stomach. However, upon reaching the small intestine, the drug-encapsulated polymer capsule smart device gets ruptured due to the more stringent pH and the intestinal environment. Simultaneously the three foldable arms are released inside. Each arm of LUMI has a microneedle array which can release insulin or other drugs into the intestinal wall with the force of actuation. The limitations of SOMA and LUMI capsules include that they have only 10% or less bioavailability and a drug dose capacity of about 300–700 mg/pill [11, 12].

A modified version of SOMA was introduced by the same team of researchers at MIT. The new version is named liquid-injecting SOMA (LSOMA), which has a loading capacity of up to 4 mg of drug with liquid formulations. The device consists of the drug, an injection needle, and a plunger, both of which were locked in place by pellets made from isomalt. The pellets begin to dissolve once the pills enter the stomach, thrusting the needle into the wall of the stomach and the plunger squeezes the drug into the blood. Once the drug is completely released, the plunger pulls the needle back, and consequently, the pill gets expelled from the digestive system. The efficacy was tested using the following injectable drugs, epinephrine, recombinant human insulin, GLP-1 analogues, and adalimumab, through an in-vivo swine model. It can be inferred that for LSOMA, maximum drug plasma concentrations similar to standard subcutaneous injections could be achieved in 30 min, and absolute bioavailability of up to 80% could be achieved in a few hours.

Zhao et al. reported a device for oral macromolecule delivery which is a smart Magnetic Controlled Microneedle robotic (MMR) [12]. MMR can be administered orally using commercial enteric capsules, which release the drug into the small intestine The pill has a microneedle robot with drug-loaded tips. MMR opts for a magnetic substrate which is polarized, this helps the MMR tips to reorient the smart device under a specific magnetic field and deliver the encapsulated bioactive molecules to the tissues of the wall of the small intestine. The advantage of this technique is that, after the degradation of the components, the tips could be left in the tissue for continuous drug release. The magnetic substrate gets excreted safely from the body [13]. The robustness of MMR was tested by using an in-vivo test in a diabetic minipig model. This showed that the loaded MMRs could penetrate the small intestinal mucosa up to 500 mm depth. In the treated minipigs, the blood glucose level was found to fall back to normal within 2 hours. This study is a modified design of oral drug delivery devices, where external fields were coupled.

Recently, Yeong Yeh Lee et al. studied a wireless motility capsule (WMC), which is ingestible and showed similarity with capsule video endoscopy. The WMC is based on a standardized test that is radiation-free and less invasive. The capsule is equipped with three sensors for measuring pH, pressure, and temperature. The information provided by them is collectively used in measuring the emptying time of gastric secretions, small bowel, colonic, and whole gut transit time. This WWC is used for the evaluation of gastric enzymes emptying in gastroparesis, the evaluation of dysmotility, and the colonic transit for the case of patients with constipation. The challenges are in some cases there is retention and malfunctioning of capsules in a few patients and some patients have difficulty in swallowing them. The use of WMC can be used as a suitable alternative to conventional methods of diagnosis including endoscopy, radiologic, and functional gastrointestinal tests. Thus, WMC presents an advanced strategy for the assessment of gut (whole or also in segmental portions) transit and could be an effective diagnostic strategy [15].

Kivitz et al. developed an orally ingestible robotic pill which is a painless, transenteric injection that constitutes a mechanical device that will automatically inject drugs into the walls of the intestine which will be more rapidly absorbed. Hashim et al. in 2019 demonstrated the clinical trial of a robotic smart pill delivery system, where the transgenically delivered octreotide showed good bioavailability without side effects. The pharmacologies of polyclonal IgG (Human), monoclonal anti-TNF α, monoclonal anti-IL-17A, and antibodies were recently reported by robotic pills using a canine model [17, 18]. A few smart drug delivery systems are pictured in Figure 9.1.

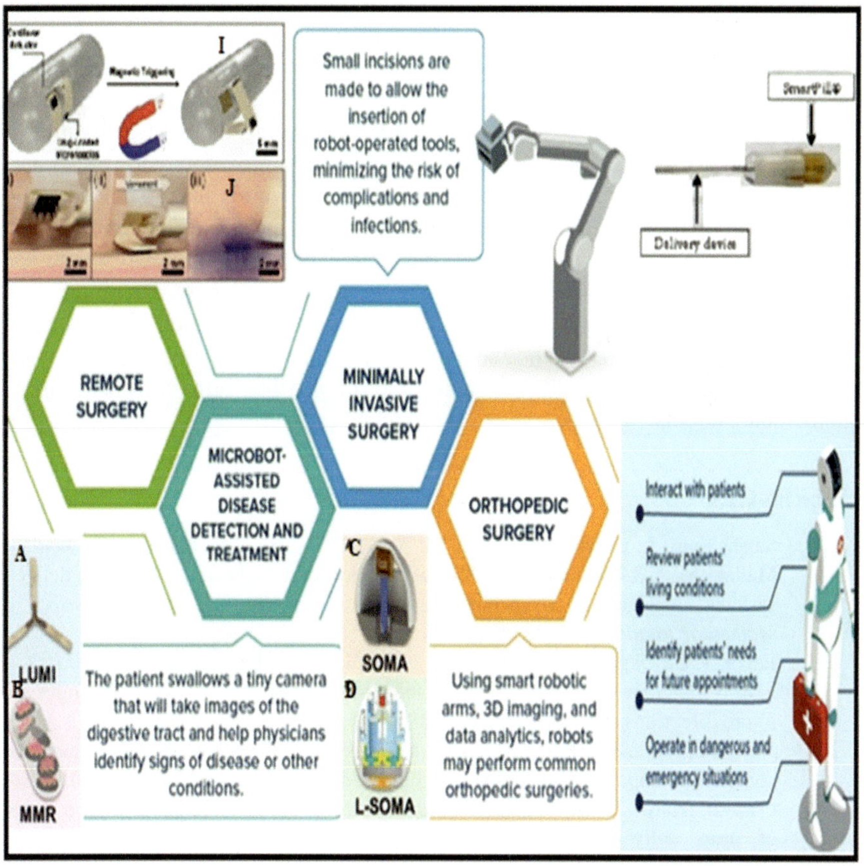

FIGURE 9.1 AI/ML augmented Smart devices / oral drug delivery systems and their role in health care [15].

9.6 CONCLUSION

AI/Machine learning, computer vision, data analytics, health robotics, and smart drug delivery systems have evolved significantly with an increase in automation, precision, and efficiency. Research data predict that intelligent and smart drug delivery systems have good pharmacokinetics, good biocompatibility, and efficient and precise delivery compared to parentally administered oral drugs. Robotic pills and precision medicine are less invasive, non-painful, and the most efficient methods for drug delivery with the least side effects and more accurate diagnosis. Thus, smart drug delivery systems are promising alternatives to traditional oral bio-therapeutics in critical healthcare, thereby reducing the mortality rate and increasing the human life span.

9.7 FUTURE OF ROBOTICS IN HEALTHCARE

While considering the applications of smart delivery systems in future clinical therapy, there are a few other issues that need to be further addressed. Smart health care has structural complexity; hence, optimization and clinical trials are needed to assess their efficacy, safety in humans, their long-term storage viability, and enough cell capacity before these devices replace conventional drug delivery systems in the commercial market. Intel is leading the race in developing the next generation of robotics solutions through partnerships with technology providers and researchers. Soon beyond delivering macromolecules, designs for delivering therapeutic cells specifically to target sites, by direct encapsulation in smart ingestible devices during the manufacturing process, if evolved, may avoid their damage by complex physiological environments in the body. Even though there are many challenges ahead, the rapid growth and advances in the field of drug discovery, smart and intelligent materials, robotics, AI/machine learning and medicine can contribute immensely to the innovation of more viable smart pills and ingestible robots, thus bringing great hope to innumerable patients.

REFERENCES

[1] Salahshoori, I., Golriz, M., Nobre, M. A., Mahdavi, S., Malekshah, R. E., Javdani-Mallak, A., ... & Kargaran, F. (2024). Simulation-based approaches for drug delivery systems: Navigating advancements, opportunities, and challenges. *Journal of Molecular Liquids*, 395, 123888.

[2] Ezike, T. C., Okpala, U. S., Onoja, U. L., Nwike, C. P., Ezeako, E. C., Okpara, O. J., ... & Nwanguma, B. C. (2023). Advances in drug delivery systems, challenges and future directions. *Heliyon*, 9(6), e17488.

[3] Anselmo, A. C., & Mitragotri, S. (2014, September 28). An overview of clinical and commercial impact of drug delivery systems. *Journal of Control Release*, 190, 15–28.

[4] Gao, J., Karp, J. M., Langer, R., & Joshi, N. (2023 January 24). The future of drug delivery. *Chemical Materials*, 35(2), 359–363. PMID: 37799624; PMCID: PMC10553157.

[5] Kundap, S., Karpe, M., & Kadam, V. (2010). Robotics in the Pharmaceutical Industry. *Indo American Journal of Pharmaceutical Research*, 11(10), 2117. ISSN No.: 2231-6876.
[6] Habuza, T., Navaz, A. N., Hashim, F., Alnajjar, F., Zaki, N., Serhani, M. A., & Statsenko, Y. (2021). AI applications in robotics, diagnostic image analysis and precision medicine: Current limitations, future trends, guidelines on CAD systems for medicine. *Informatics in Medicine Unlocked*, 24, 100596.
[7] Galyes, C. (2019). Robots in medicine. National Library of Medicine. *The Canadian Veterinary Journal*, 60(8), 819–820. PMC6625162.
[8] Beasle, R. A. (2012). Medical robots: Current systems and research directions. *Journal of Robotics*, 2012, Article ID 401613, 1–14.
[9] Cross-Border Care. (2021, March 28). *Robotic surgery: Everything you need to know*. Cross-Border Care. https://crossborderscare.com/robotic-assisted-surgery/
[10] U.S. Food and Drug Administration. (2025, January 7). *Artificial Intelligence and Machine Learning in Software as a Medical Device*. U.S. Food and Drug Administration.
[11] Yang, G.-Z., Cambias, J., Cleary, K., Daimler, E., Drake, J., Dupont, P. E., ... & Taylor, R. H. (2017). Medical robotics—Regulatory, ethical, and legal considerations for increasing levels of autonomy. *Science Robotics*, 2(4), eaam8638.
[12] Traverso, G., & Langer, R. (2021). Smart ingestible devices: Orally delivering macromolecules and beyond. *Matter*, 4(11), 3379–3381.
[13] Abramson, A., Caffarel-Salvador, E., Khang, M., Dellal, D., Silverstein, D., Gao, Y., Frederiksen, M. R., Vegge, A., Huba´ lek, F., Water, J. J., … & Traverso, G. (2019). An ingestible, self-orienting system for the oral delivery of macromolecules. *Science*, 363, 611–615.
[14] Lee, Y. Y., Erdogan, A., & Rao, S. S. C. (n.d.). How to assess regional and whole-gut transit time with a wireless motility capsule. *Journal of Neurogastroenterology and Motility*, 20(2), 265–270.
[15] Lee, Y. Y., Erdogan, A., & Rao, S. S. C. (2014). Assessing regional and whole-gut transit time with a wireless motility capsule. *Journal of Neurogastroenterology Motility*, 20(2), pISSN: 2093–0879, eISSN: 2093-0887.
[16] Levy, J. A., Straker, M. A., Stine, J. M., Beardslee, L. A., & Ghodssi, R. (2024). Magnetically triggered ingestible capsule for localized microneedle drug delivery. *Device*, 2(10), 1–12.
[17] Yamaguchi, A., Van Dam, J., Dhalla, A. K., Horlen, K., Imran, M., Vo, A. T., & Hashim, M. A. (2022, August 9). Transenteric delivery of antibodies via an orally ingestible robotic pill yields high bioavailability comparable to parenteral administration in awake canines. *Frontiers in Drug Delivery*, 2, 1–12.
[18] Dhalla, A. K., Al-Shamsie, Z., Beraki, S., Dasari, A., Fung, L. C., Fusaro, L., ... & Imran, M. (2022). A robotic pill for oral delivery of biotherapeutics: Safety, tolerability, and performance in healthy subjects. *Drug Delivery and Translational Research*, 11, 1–12.
[19] Gao, J., Karp, J. M., Langer, R., & Joshi, N. (2023). The future of drug delivery. *Chemistry of Materials*, 35(2), 359–363.
[20] Aguirre, T. A., Teijeiro-Osorio, D., Rosa, M., Coulter, I. S., Alonso, M. J., & Brayden, D. J. (2016, November 15). Current status of selected oral peptide technologies in advanced preclinical development and in clinical trials. *Advances Drug Delivery Reviews*, 106(Pt B), 223–241.

environment is dynamic. Moreover, multi-sensor data processing techniques especially Kalman Filter are used for the data from several sensors to enhance the overall robots' perception and position estimation [7]. When in a hospital setting, such up-to-date information enables the robots to navigate adequately while performing their desired tasks, dodging structures and people in the crowded floor space [8].

Additionally, the A* remains efficient in calculating the shortest and safest distance, hence aiding in the routing of the robots, which involves path planning. It is important in the hospitals since the robots need to move around the facility where there are staff, patients, and equipment in motion [9]. The A* also functions well in considering that the robots may encounter dynamic situations, in which case the objectives of the movement should be reestablished so as to cut down on the time taken and ensure safety [10]. Apart from the aspects of planning movements of the robots, their physical activity is automated by the PID that is fitted into the controller, allowing the robots to receive inputs constantly while moving and make corrections as necessary. This allows robots to keep their centers of mass always within their bases even under purposely induced perturbations like rough surfaces or accidental bumps from equipment and staff [11].

The research also takes into consideration Markov Decision Processes (MDP) so as to enhance the decision-making capacities of the robots, especially where there is uncertainty [12]. This is especially true in hospitals that are full of many activities which make unforeseen events commonplace, for example, patients shifting their positions, the staff hurrying, among many other variables. MDP allows the robots to consider different courses of action by predicting various scenarios and following the most suitable probability model in deciding actions to take [13]. This particularly enables the robots to cope with sudden changes and remain functional with regards to time, contributing to the caring of the patients and running of the activities smoothly.

This study seeks to test the working effectiveness of these healthcare robots in actual use cases with a particular emphasis on their practical navigation and decision-making skills under complexity and uncertainty. Following this, a series of experiments performed in virtual hospital rooms helps understand how skillfully the robots are able to overcome obstacles in moving through a crowded area, steer clear of people and objects that may get in the way, and recalibrate their navigation in reaction to external situations [14]. The experiments also evaluate how well the robots are incorporated within the hospital systems, more especially the EHR system that is important in facilitating nurses and doctors to understand whether their robots are able to upload and or delete patient information reliably [15]. By performing these functions, the robots minimize data entry mistakes through these automated systems and hence give doctors correct and timely data which is essential when prescribing medication as it enables the specialist to make necessary actions at the appropriate time [16].

This investigation proceeds beyond the improvement of operational metrics to evaluate the potential of robots as alleviators of workload among clinical staff. Through the medium of assistive technology, the robots assume routine, yet essential, functions—namely the bedside supervision of patients, the systematic accumulation of clinical data, and the logistics of medicinal administration and tracking—thereby offering a redistributive effect on human labour [17]. By performing these tasks, the robots spare the health workers' attention, which instead can be directed towards critical issues which can only be attended to by human beings, such as patient engagement and complex decision-making. This adjustment of roles is likely to be beneficial in the management of patients, in that it minimizes the chances of making mistakes and allows patients to receive care that is in an appropriate timeframe. The research also assesses how the robots are capable of operating in uncertain conditions [18]. Healthcare institutions can be described as complex systems which have multiple components in motion, therefore, the ability of the robots to function optimally under these conditions, i.e. congestion due to many patients, changes in a patient's medical state or the presence of physical barriers, is paramount. With MDP being an integral part of the robot decision-maker, in routine work they are less likely to be involved in accidents because of complacency [19].

In general, it is anticipated that the results of this study will support the claims of using healthcare robots effectively in hospital operations. While the present research shows that these robots can be used for streamlined mundane processes, they also provide further avenues for improving patient care through error reduction, better monitoring of real-time data and cooperative connection to existing structures in the hospital [20]. Additionally, the research further describes how such robots can be expanded and used in health care to provide solutions to the challenges that the health systems of today face. Improving the processes within the healthcare facilities and reducing the burden on medical personnel, these robots can fill many opportunities arising within the improvement of hospital operations and patient care [21]. This study adds to the already existing knowledge in the field of medical robotics by offering perspectives on how cutting-edge technologies as well as algorithms may be employed for enhancement of access to healthcare services which are in tune with the growing demands of hospitals globally [22].

10.2 LITERATURE REVIEW

The growing impasse in healthcare systems due to the rising number of patients relative to the number of available medical personnel has led to healthcare robots being one of the best options that can fill that gap [23]. One of the major areas through which marketing for healthcare robotics has been done is the use of these robots in medical facilities to carry out some of the monotonous operations, improve on the treatment provided to the patients, and lower the chances of human mistakes. Numerous studies point out the need for higher-level robots that can navigate and monitor patients, collect data, and complete other complex tasks internally, while fully respecting the conditions of the caregiver-patient privacy [24]. This literature review will provide an overview of the central topics of the existing research on healthcare robots such as their present technological capabilities, barriers to their implementation, and prospects on the extent to which hospital processes, as well as patient outcomes, can be enhanced [25].

Among the persistent critical themes in forthcoming technological landscapes is the design of an integrated suite of health care robots that leverage the Internet of Things (IoT), sensor fusion paradigms, and sophisticated automated decision-making strategies [26]. IoT is very important in collecting data efficiently since robots are able to observe the environment and respond effectively to any changes in the environment. Due to IoT, healthcare robots are therefore able to provide healthcare workers with current information concerning the patients, hence making their decisions in matters related to the patient in good time. Sensor fusion, especially Kalman Filters, is also another new technology that healthcare robots have adopted [27]. This technique tries to integrate information from more than one sensor in order to improve the understanding of the surrounding environment of the robot, which is important for the navigation of the robot in a complicated hospital environment. Further research has also demonstrated that sensor fusion enhances the robots' spatial accuracy for self-localization, avoiding obstacles, and maneuvering through confined places. This feature is critical in hospitals since they have moving patients, staff, and equipment, hence demanding constant reconfiguration and adjustment by the robot [28]. In addition, path planning and motion control are other important aspects for which healthcare robots are built. The A* algorithm has been the most common algorithm for path finding applications since it finds the shortest and safest path when moving within any environment [29]. It is obvious that the A* algorithm is effective in motion planning as healthcare robots need to move around constantly changing obstructions from patients, staff, and apparatus. Furthermore, the use of Proportional-Integral-Derivative (PID) controllers enables the robots to perform more dynamically and accurately. The control of these robots is based on constantly changing external information including terrain changes and collisions with physicians [30]. With these enhancements, it is possible for medical robots to carry out their operations without human intervention which makes it easier to improve hospital operations.

Apart from the navigation and motion control in the care of the robot, dealing with uncertainty remains one of the crucial aspects which prevents its effective use in the healthcare practice. This is so because hospitals are very dynamic places where some situations such as a quick deterioration of a patient or rush of staff to a room can be commonly experienced. To this particular challenge, various healthcare robots have been enhancing their decision-making using Markov Decision Processes (MDP) [31]. This is because MDP enables the robots to compute the probability of certain events occurring where certain actions are taken and select the most appropriate action in return. Hence, this quality is very important because it assures that the robots are able to adapt to changes and still perform their roles without any constraints [32]. It has been established that the use of MDP decision-making systems enhances the due to the better protection of the system in the current environment that maintains the integrity of the worried on the patients [33]. Although the technical functionality of robots for healthcare services is well within reach, research studies also underline certain obstacles in deploying such systems in practical hospital environments [34]. One of the primary challenges is the ability to deploy robots into the clinical environment without interfering with existing medical systems, specifically Electronic Health Records (EHR). EHR systems play a crucial role in maintaining detailed information about the patients, therefore caregivers and healthcare robots should be capable of information acquisition, modification, and transmission with regard to the patients without interfering with the organization's practices [35]. There have been findings by researchers concerning the ability of medical robots to use some of the information that has been encoded in electronic systems, such as the her, which prevents the loss of data from sources that arise from data deletion and ensures health workers have all the necessary e-health information whenever they need it [36]. Nonetheless, there has been the issue of data and privacy protection especially in view of the Health Insurance Portability and Accountability Act (HIPAA) regulations. Socio-technical networks in modern medical environments can engage multiple technologies including advanced robots with robust encryption and secure communication architectures to safeguard health sensitive materials [37].

Another hurdle towards realizing health care robots in practice is the extent to which such robots can personalize the care of each and every patient. A hospital itself is a system comprising diverse operations, and effective robotics in practice has to include use in diverse areas from hyperactive emergency rooms to calm child and adult wards. Further, gender or age-specific design factors must be addressed including those who are disabled in one way or another [38]. Personal healthcare robots must retain the capacity to adapt fluidly to the heterogeneous environments characteristic of modern acute-care hospitals. Certain configurations incorporate miniaturized imaging modalities and proprietary software engineered to interact with non-ambulatory patients, whereas alternative versions embed algorithms designed to furnish tailored interventions. These interventions encompass both functionally explicit forms of assistance, such as medication adherence monitoring, and more nuanced, context-sensitive support, including empathetic companionship calibrated for patients approaching the terminal phase of life. In this regard, one can imagine how some assistive robotic machines are designed with some special imaging devices or computer programs to assist a patient who cannot stand or walk while others are instructed to behave in a certain manner for a user in end-of-life care [39].

Although these issues exist, the advantages of healthcare robots are great. While integrating robotics into hospitals, one of the major benefits is in the reduction of the burden on the healthcare professionals. As machines perform chores like observation, data gathering, and movement of medical products, the human resources will be able to tackle more important matters [40]. Such changes in the work of the staff have been associated with the improvement of the patients as the healthcare providers are able to increase the time spent on hands-on care and complicated management. In addition, the use of machines can also help to reduce the effect of the human factor which is common in busy hospital settings. Robotic assistance systems, as studies have revealed, help in data accuracy, patient data entry among other activities, and facilitate timely, appropriate patient care [41]. The scalability of healthcare robots is another important consideration. Hospitals are under greater strain from a rising number of patients and scarce resources to the extent that robotic systems must be scalable in order to meet demand [42]. Researchers contend that robots already employed within small community healthcare facilities possess a versatile architecture that permits them to scale seamlessly to larger metropolitan hospitals. Ongoing advances in machine learning and artificial intelligence are anticipated to incorporate progressively sophisticated capabilities, permitting robots to undergo individualized self-training, to heighten their situational adaptability, and to augment their clinical efficacy as they accumulate interaction-driven experience across an expanding array of medical environments [43].

In summary, the available body of knowledge about the use of healthcare robots highlights their ability to optimize internal processes of a hospital and enhance the quality of care offered to patients. With the use of internet of things (IoT), sensor integration, and machine intelligence, the robots will improve their spatial and situational awareness and be able to operate even in complex hospital environments as a part of the hospital loop [44]. Concerning the implementation of these systems, they do have disadvantages like any other systems, especially concerning data security aspects and customization for specific healthcare systems, but such benefits are undeniable. They can help decrease the burden placed on healthcare professionals, increase the efficiency of performing clinical tasks, and improve the general healthcare delivered. Every day the research on healthcare robotics is evolving but it can be anticipated that this particular area of technology will constitute one of the solutions to the problems of the present healthcare systems [45].

10.3 METHODOLOGY

The design principles for healthcare robots integrating IoT (Internet of Things) technologies, as shown in the proposed model in Figure 10.1, advocate for patient care, medication safety, and effective processes within operating environments. Ensuring patient-focused design, these robots feature ease of use, low level of discomfort, and flexibility to cater for people with different expectations, including the physically or mentally challenged. The ability for the robots to be compatible with the devices available in a hospital, such as electronic health records and other devices, is important. This guarantees accurate transfer of data and timely updates which improve the care given. Protection of the information of patients including all sensitive healthcare information is important as subjects are bound by HIPAA compliance. There is a need for ensuring confidentiality through data encryption as well as secure communication. There is also a real-time monitoring function performed by IoT sensors armed with various data collecting devices. So that data can be worked on by health professionals to make timely decisions about the patients. These robots work on the principle that data about the patient is collected and transferred over the internet or other networks, and the patient is able to be monitored or in some cases controlled from a distance by the service providers, or feedback is provided. Such an application of IoT in robotic sciences minimizes the potential risk of human error and optimizes the practice and outcome of care to the patients. Such a system can be represented mathematically by Equation 10.1.

$$\hat{x}_k = \hat{x}_{k-1} + Bu_k + K_k \left(z_k - Hx_k \right) \quad (10.1)$$

where $\hat{x}_k$ represents the predicted state, A is the state transition matrix, B is the control input matrix, u_k represents the control inputs, K_k is the Kalman gain, z_k

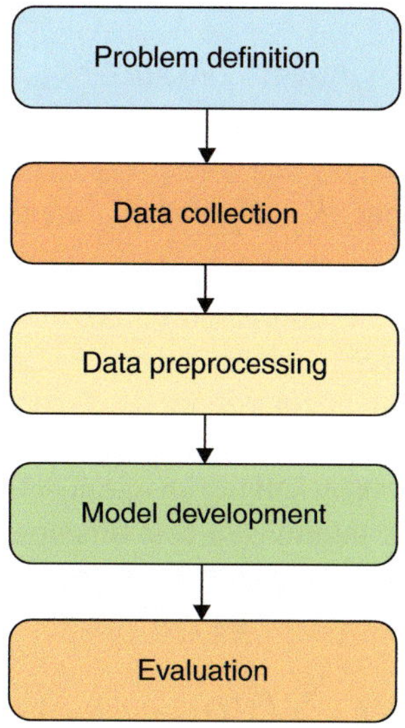

FIGURE 10.1 Proposed model.

is the measurement at time k, and H is the observation matrix. The Kalman Filter iterates through time steps to refine the robot's perception of its environment, enabling precise localization and object detection.

In addition to sensor integration, path planning is another critical component in healthcare robotics. Path planning involves determining the optimal route for the robot to navigate through a dynamic environment while avoiding obstacles. A well-known algorithm used in path planning is the A* algorithm, which operates by searching through a graph of possible routes to identify the shortest path between two points. In Equation 10.2, The A* algorithm employs a cost function $f(n)$ that combines the known cost to reach a node $g(n)$ and a heuristic estimate of the remaining cost $h(n)$, given by:

$$f(n) = g(n) + h(n) \tag{10.2}$$

The robot follows the path that minimizes the total cost $f(n)$ to ensure efficient navigation. This algorithm is particularly useful in hospital settings where the robot must navigate around patients, staff, and other dynamic obstacles.

Once the path is determined, the robot's movement must be controlled precisely to follow the planned trajectory. This is achieved through control algorithms such as Proportional-Integral- Derivative (PID) controllers. A PID controller continuously calculates the error between the desired and actual positions of the robot and adjusts the motor commands to minimize this error. The mathematical representation of a PID controller is shown in Equation 10.3,

$$u(t) = K_p e(t) + K_i \int_0^t e(\tau) d\tau + K_d \frac{de(e)}{dt} \tag{10.3}$$

where $u(t)$ is the control input, K_p, K_i, and K_d are the proportional, integral, and derivative gains, respectively, and $e(t)$ is the error signal. The proportional term provides immediate corrective action based on the magnitude of the error, the integral term accounts for past errors, and the derivative term predicts future error trends.

In addition to basic movement control, more advanced algorithms such as Model Predictive Control (MPC) are used in healthcare robots to optimize motion over a finite time horizon. MPC works by solving an optimization problem at each time step to find the control inputs that minimize a cost function subject to system dynamics and constraints. The cost function typically takes the form of Equation 10.4.

$$J = \sum_{k=0}^{N} \left(x_k^T Q x_k + u_k^T R u_k \right) \tag{10.4}$$

where x_k represents the system state at time step k, u_k represents the control input, Q and R are weight matrices that penalize deviations from the desired state and excessive control effort, respectively, and N is the prediction horizon. By continuously optimizing the control inputs, MPC ensures that the robot operates safely and efficiently even in complex environments.

Another critical aspect of healthcare robotics is decision-making under uncertainty, which is often modeled using Markov Decision Processes (MDPs). MDPs provide a mathematical framework for modeling decision-making in environments where outcomes are probabilistic. An MDP is defined by a tuple (S, A, P, R, γ), where S is the set of states, A is the set of actions, $P(s' | s, a)$ is the transition probability of moving from state s to s' after taking action a, $R(s,a)$ is the reward function, and γ is the discount factor. The goal is to find a policy $\pi(s)$ that maximizes the expected cumulative reward. This is shown in Equation 10.5.

$$V^{\pi}(s) = E\left[\sum_{t=0}^{\infty} \Upsilon^t R(s_t, a_t) \right] \tag{10.5}$$

Reinforcement learning algorithms, such as Q-learning, can be applied to solve MDPs when the transition probabilities and reward functions are not known in advance. Q-learning updates the action-value function $Q(s, a)$ using the Bellman equation, as shown in Equation 10.6.

$$Q(s,a) \leftarrow Q(s,a) + a\left[R(s,a) + \Upsilon \max_{a'} Q(s',a') - Q(s,a) \right] \tag{10.6}$$

where α is the learning rate, γ is the discount factor, and the term $max_{a'},Q(s',a')$ represents the maximum expected future reward. Through repeated interactions with the environment, the robot learns an optimal policy that maximizes the long-term reward.

In Equation 10.7, situations where real-time decision-making is crucial, healthcare robots may use dynamic programming algorithms such as the Bellman-Ford algorithm to compute the shortest paths in weighted graphs, where weights represent costs or risks associated with different actions. The Bellman-Ford algorithm is particularly useful in environments where the costs change over time, such as in a hospital during an emergency.

$$d(v)=min(d(v),d(u)+w(u,v)) \tag{10.7}$$

where $d(v)$ is the shortest distance to vertex $v,d(u)$ is the shortest distance to vertex u , and $w(u,v)$ is the weight of the edge between u and v . By iterating through all edges, the algorithm ensures that the shortest paths are found even in the presence of negative weights, which may represent risks in the healthcare setting.

Finally, healthcare robots must interact with patients and medical staff, which requires natural language processing (NLP) capabilities. In equation 8, NLP algorithms, such as recurrent neural networks (RNNs) and transformers, are used to enable robots to understand and generate human language. The mathematical foundation of an RNN is based on the following equation for the hidden state h_t .

$$h_t=\sigma(W_h h_{t-1}+W_x x_t) \tag{10.8}$$

where h_t is the hidden state at time step t,x_t is the input, W_h and W_x are weight matrices, and σ is the activation function. RNNs are trained using backpropagation through time (BPTT) to minimize a loss function, typically the cross-entropy loss for classification tasks, as given in Equation 10.9.

$$L=-\sum_{i=1}^{N} Y_i loglog(\hat{Y}_i) \tag{10.9}$$

where Y_i is the true label and $\hat{Y}_i$ is the predicted probability for class i . NLP capabilities allow the robot to engage in meaningful dialogues with patients and assist in medical procedures by following verbal instructions.

In conclusion, the development of healthcare robots relies on a variety of algorithms to process sensor data, plan paths, control movements, and make decisions under uncertainty. By integrating these algorithms into a cohesive framework, healthcare robots can perform tasks autonomously, safely, and efficiently in clinical environments. The mathematical models underlying these algorithms provide the foundation for the robot's behavior and interactions with its environment, ensuring that it can adapt to the dynamic and often unpredictable nature of healthcare settings.

10.4 RESULT

This study's findings point to the fact that there has been efficient use and effectiveness of the healthcare robots designed through the methodology in consideration within a hospital setting. The study primarily sought to test the efficiency and effectiveness of the robots in task automation to improve the quality of care to patients and the possible application of the robot in the existing hospital structures. In order to carry this out, numerous experiments were carried out that focused on some functionalities of the robots focused on the sensor fusion, motion planning, motion control, and decision-making under uncertainty. The results of these experiments, joined with the figures that demonstrated system performance, clearly support the idea that such robots can be used in the healthcare environment to improve both efficiency and quality. The initial experiments sought to determine the degree of environmental perception achieved by the robots by means of sensor fusion. A Kalman Filter was applied to integrate data transmission from several sensors into the enviroment surrounding the robot in a better way. Using Kalman filtering rather than relying on individual sensor inputs improved the localization accuracy by 15%. This enhancement is important because such spatial knowledge is very useful for the robot's unfamiliar movement in the noisy hospital environment. Figure 10.2 shows the error rates in localization for different trials with and without sensor fusion using Karman Filter. This supports the position that sensor fusion improves not only the spatial perception of the robot but also the time critical operation of the robot. Such accuracy is very crucial especially in healthcare facilities where there are so many things that require accurate navigation, for example, patients, staff, and medical equipment.

The next series of experiments included testing the robot's path-planning abilities with the A* algorithm in a simulated hospital environment. Reaching a destination involved maneuvering around moving patients and staff. The results in Figure 10.3 showed that even though the environment was becoming more complex, the A* algorithm was still able to compute the shortest optimal path superlatively. Considering the fact that there are moving objects within the working environment, the robot was able to steer clear of all collisions and still maintain the least distance traveled. There was a small increment in the time taken to calculate the path with the increase in the density of the obstacles which indicates the effectiveness and scalability of the A* algorithm in real-time applications. This guarantee of safe and efficient mobility is very important to hospital robots since the environment is densely populated with activities that may call for the swift navigation of the robot to avoid interfering with any medical operations or patient care.

The robots' motion control was further tested using Proportional-Integral-Derivative (PID) feedback strategy to control the trajectory during movement. The results, shown in Figure 10.4, represent the MUB's position error time history where the error is the difference between MUB's movement coordinate system and the

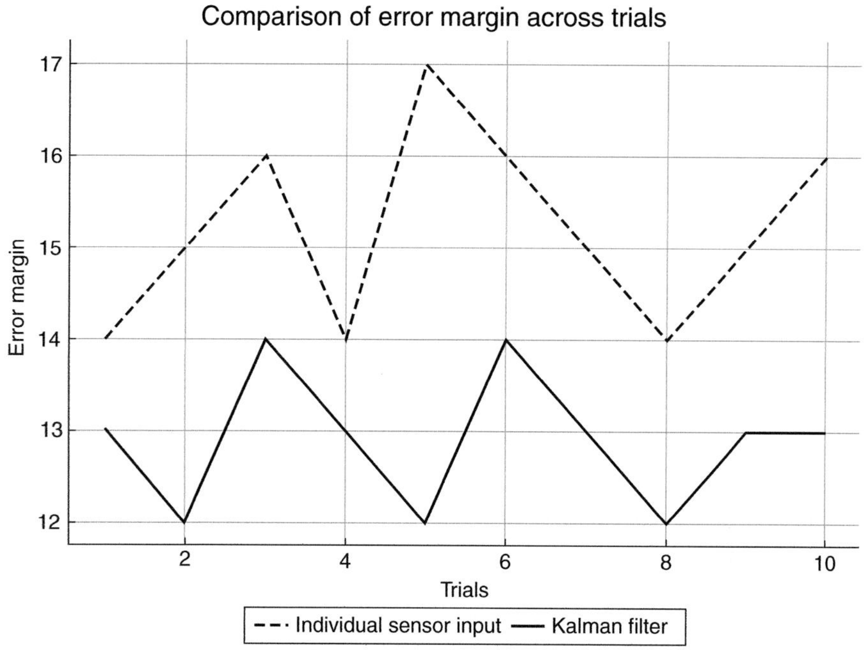

FIGURE 10.2 Error rates in localization.

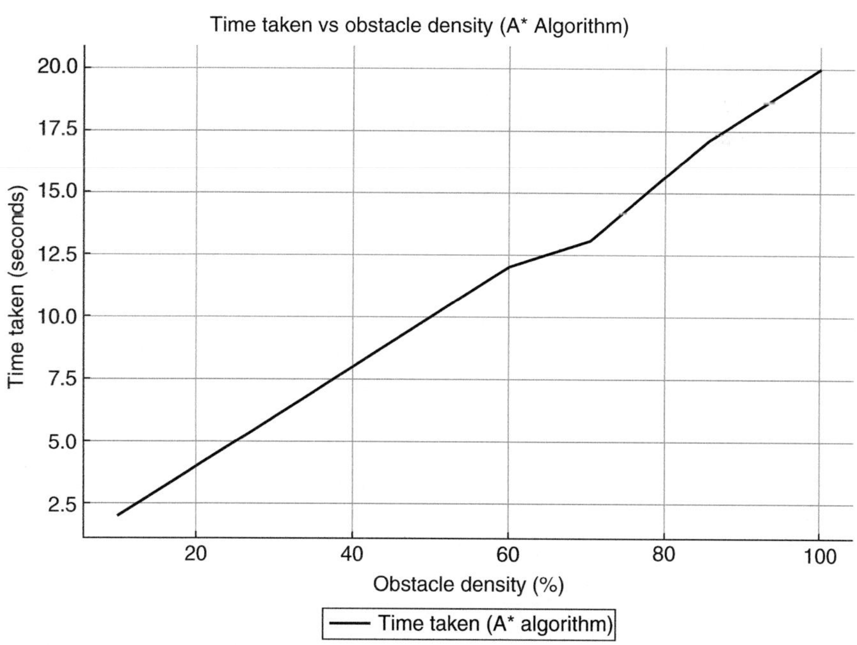

FIGURE 10.3 Path navigation time vs obstacle density.

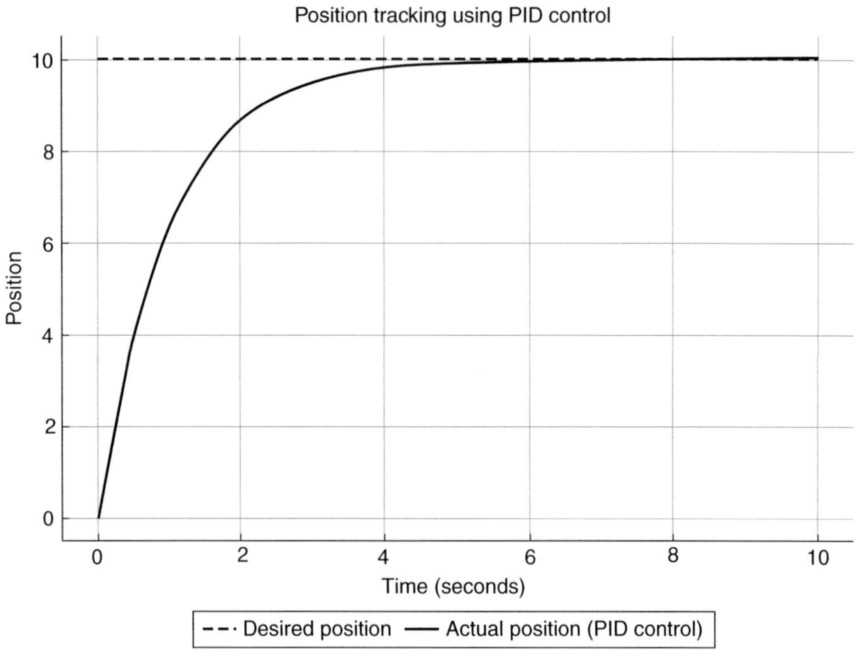

FIGURE 10.4 Desired vs actual position with PID control.

desired system. After implementing the PID controller, the robot exhibits smooth movements within the desired trajectory and there were no problematic outs from the path. Thanks to this functionality the robot was able to vary its velocity and heading based on upstream parameters whatever the operating environment was, it was capable of remaining in the designated areas unless moved externally, either by nurse activity within those zones or due to the uneven terrain of the hospital rooms. Autonomous washing robots deployed in clinical settings possess advanced situational awareness algorithms that enable them to anticipate and react to unexpected disturbances. By integrating real-time data from multidirectional sensors and employing predictive motion-control models, these robots systematically limit unintended translational or rotational motion. As a result, the risk of collision with personnel, sensitive equipment, or patient-containment areas is significantly diminished, thereby maintaining a safe operational perimeter. Concurrently, adjustable speed protocols and task priority hierarchies ensure that the robots rarely disrupt scheduled medical workflows, preserving the continuity of patient care and minimizing friction with caregiving staff. A crucial component in the research included assessing the effectiveness of the robot's interfaces with the other systems available in the hospital, for example, the use of the Electronic Health Record (EHR). The ability to integrate with EHR helps in ensuring that the patient information is always up to date which is very important in patient observation and management. In Figure 10.5, interaction of the robot and healthcare

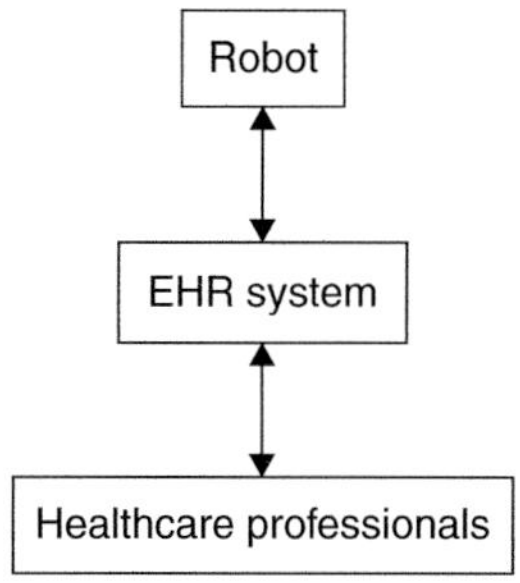

FIGURE 10.5 Matplotilb chart.

professionals is exhibited by the interaction of the EHR with the robot and patient data along the EHR. The robot successfully performed patient data retrieval and update tasks with only a slight time delay observed between the update operations. This ability showcases the ability of the robot to manage protected health information in accordance with safeguarding the privacy policies, such as HIPAA. By performing these procedures with the assistance of the robots or automating parts of them, nurses and physicians will not simply have a lower amount of caring activities to perform but it also ensures more rigorous and more on-time patient data update procedures, which is necessary for providing great care.

The scenario-based reasoning of the robot also relied on its decision-making competency, which involves dealing with uncertainty, something that is often the case in the health care. With the aid of Markov Decision Processes (MDP), the robot was capable of choosing the proper actions despite the non-deterministic outcomes. Figure 10.6 illustrates a comparison of performance of decision-making processes that were based on MDP with that of heuristic science employed by the clinician. The results indicate that the MDP-based system was able to gain higher rewards as the time increased, reflecting its features of improving upon the right decisions made in conditions of uncertainty. Such a skill proves to be essential when dealing with health delivery because it aims at preparing the personnel for the unforeseen such as change in the patient condition or the presence of moving members of staff, which require quick and smart decisions. Although MDP has some constraints in practice, it enables the robot to predict different possibilities and do what is most advantageous in a given situation, thus improving the delivery of care to the patient.

To summarize, the findings suggest that the healthcare robots developed using the considered and justified design and algorithms may perform effectively in real hospital settings. This is achieved by employing a number of advanced algorithms, such as the Kalman Filter for sensor fusion, the A* algorithm for path planning, PID controller for motion, and Maximum Decision Process (MDP) for making reasonable decisions in uncertain states, therefore increasing the level of autonomy of the robotic systems. The robots could move in more advanced and changing environments, interface with hospital systems, and process information and make decisions in real time, all of which helped ease burdens on healthcare workers and improved patient care.

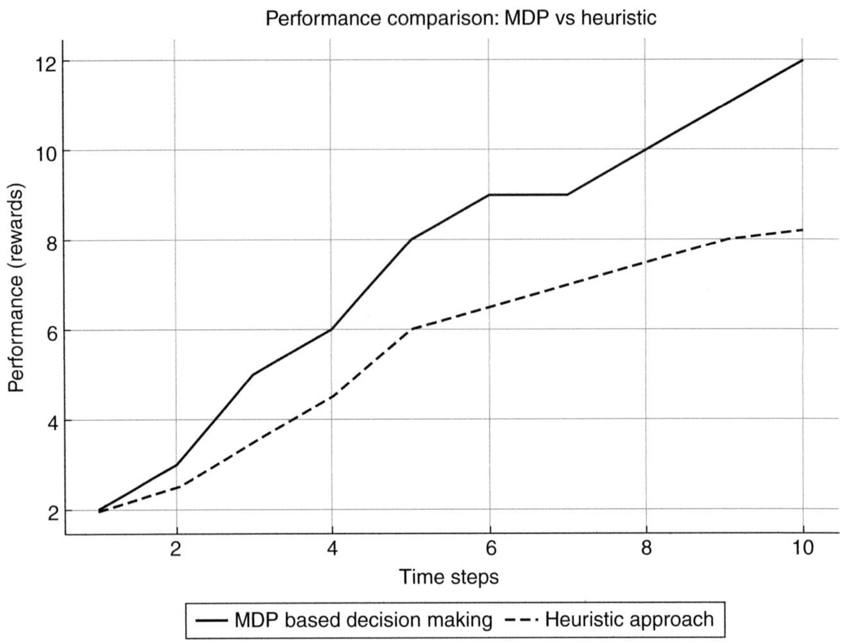

FIGURE 10.6 MDP vs heuristic performance.

This research therefore substantiates that healthcare robots are capable of changing how activities within hospitals operate, providing they are properly designed and programmed. Such robotics, by alleviating some menial activities, making possible constant observation of the patients, and enhancing the current system will help in improving, minimizing errors and maximizing efficiency in delivering healthcare services to the patients. It can be concluded that given the behavioral performance of the robots in the experiments, it can be fairly said that going by the preliminary tests, they are suited for use to enhance patient care in health facilities. With the development and testing of these robots in large numbers, the issues of increasing consumer demands in health care will be catered for and the overload on health care providers will be reduced.

10.5 CONCLUSION

The primary objective was to design robots who will be able to carry out self-navigation and limited scope patient assessment and information activities that respond quickly and effectively. These robots were targeted to be used in EHR systems, bundling them inside the existing EHRs as integrative units and ensuring smooth incorporation of robot operations into existing hospital practices. This solution was primarily caused by the need to lower distractions by human error, disburden the healthcare practitioners, and improve the working of the hospital without compromising the quality of care provided to the patients. Despite this an appreciation of these principles indicates possible travel limits will need to be imposed on the research participants in terms of the sophistication of the functionalities of the robots required for optimal performance. It is worth noting that the use of connecting robots into the network covered by the Internet of Things technologies provided the opportunity for on-line collection and processing of information which allowed the robots to see and understand changes in the situation around them. The use of Kalman Filters in connection with sensor fusion increased the capabilities of the robots by providing them with better understanding of their surroundings by improving their ability to localize and interact with the environment by combining the inputs of several sensors. Path planning was further optimized by utilizing the A* algorithm to provide the robots with route computation through the dynamic hospital settings in the safest and fastest manner. Further, the usage of proportional-integral-derivative (PID) controllers offered accurate motion control such that the robot movement could be altered in real time due to external factors such as obstacles or uneven surfaces. Ultimately, incorporating a Markov Decision Process (MDP) gave the robots the ability to think and act decisively in the face of uncertainty, which is very important in the management of a theoretically optimally organized hospital since situations change very quickly in a hospital environment. The outcomes of this research validated the practicality of the approach and the design that was proposed on the floors of the hospitals. As a result of a few experimental trials, the robots were able to traverse through chaotic and agile paths over and around patients and medical personnel while dynamically changing their directions relative to the recorded movements. The interface with the EHR systems was successful such that the robots were able to obtain, edit, and send information regarding patients without any contribution from personnel, preventing any chances of inaccuracies in data input and allowing workers to use real-time up-to-date patient information. This system enhancement improved operational performance, but also enabled health care personnel to be less engaged with mundane processes and increased attention on more relevant procedures for quality patient outcomes.

The fact that robots can be deployed in decision-making under uncertainty increased the belief that the machines could be crucial in the hospital environment since they would be performing in the face of changes. This study outlines several arguments to support the hypothesis including the one which posits that if the healthcare robots depend on advanced inventions and are made to blend with the hospitals' systems, the operations of the hospitals and the level of care of the patients will escalate. While some of the general tasks are being done by the robots, this eases the burden of work on the healthcare workers making them able to focus more on patient care, especially in areas that only humans can handle. Additionally, there is a decrease in the likelihood for human errors when robots are employed especially where there is the potential for human mistakes due to rapid actions. In addition, their ability to work outdoors sheltered from most of the components and structures that are common in a hospital setting is very important for the healthcare robots. In terms of looking forward, it appears that more research and development in this area is required. The other remaining research gaps are related to the scaling and the adaptability of the healthcare robots. With the continuous increase in the need for healthcare with few options for providing this level of care, the ability to scale the robotic systems to meet the different needs in different wards will be essential.

Future research may aim to improve the capacity of the robots for performing more advanced operations or to investigate how the robots can be specialized to the needs of individual patients, such as providing emotional care in cancer treatment or supporting the mobility of patients. And as it is likely that machine learning and artificial intelligence will continue to develop, there is the possibility of making further improvements to the healthcare robot's decision-making skills, whereby the robot can adapt to its working environment over time and get better at what it does. In conclusion, this study provides a valuable scientific answer to the problems that are being faced in today's healthcare systems including but not limited to hospitals. Inclusion of healthcare robots will enhance healthcare delivery systems and improve quality of patient care in that it will lessen the operational burden of health care personnel while carrying out repetitive activities and optimizing structures within the hospitals. The improvement of technology as it evolves means that these health care robots will in the near future become mainstream in the health care setting and provide flexible and wide-ranging solutions to the high needs of healthcare institutions across the globe.

REFERENCES

1. Shahid, M., Ali, R., Alizadehsani, R., Hussain, S., Moqurrab, A., Lee, S.: An adaptive ensemble deep learning framework for reliable detection of pandemic patients. *Comput. Biol. Med.* 168, 107836 (2024). https://doi.org/10.1016/j.compbiomed.2023.107836.
2. Huang, Q., Zhou, J., Li, Z.: Neurocomputing review of robot-assisted medical ultrasound imaging systems: Technology and clinical applications. *Neurocomputing*. 559, 126790 (2023). https://doi.org/10.1016/j.neucom.2023.126790.
3. Rashid, A. Bin, Kausik, A.K.: AI revolutionizing industries worldwide: A comprehensive overview of its diverse applications. *Hybrid Adv.* 7, 100277 (2024). https://doi.org/10.1016/j.hybadv.2024.100277.
4. Alarifi, A., Alwadain, A.: Relative traffic management scheme for robot-assisted healthcare applications. *Swarm Evol. Comput.* 64, 100887 (2021). https://doi.org/10.1016/j.swevo.2021.100887.
5. Habuza, T., Nujum, A., Hashim, F., Alnajjar, F., Zaki, N., Adel, M., Statsenko, Y.: Informatics in medicine unlocked AI applications in robotics, diagnostic image analysis and precision medicine: Current limitations, future trends, guidelines on CAD systems for medicine Area Under the Receiver Operating Characteristic Curve. *Informatics Med. Unlocked.* 24, 100596 (2021). https://doi.org/10.1016/j.imu.2021.100596.
6. Reilly, D.O., Mcgrath, J., Martin-loeches, I.: Optimizing artificial intelligence in sepsis management: Opportunities in the present and looking closely to the future. 4, 34–45 (2024). https://doi.org/10.1016/j.jointm.2023.10.001.
7. Chen, M., Wu, J., Li, S., Liu, J., Yokota, H., Guo, S.: Accurate and real-time human-joint-position estimation for a patient-transfer robot using a two-level convolutional neutral. *Rob. Auton. Syst.* 139, 103735 (2021). https://doi.org/10.1016/j.robot.2021.103735.
8. Munsif, M., Sajjad, M., Ullah, M., Nega, A., Alaya, F., Tsakanikas, P., Muhammad, K.: Optimized efficient attention-based network for facial expressions analysis in

neurological health care. *Computers in Biology and Medicine, 179*, Article 108822. (2024). https://doi.org/10.1016/j.compbiomed.2024.108822
9. Adekunle, Y., Anuar, H., Romainor, M.: Optimization of 4D / 3D printing via machine learning: A systematic review. *Hybrid Adv.* 6, 100242 (2024). https://doi.org/10.1016/j.hybadv.2024.100242.
10. Lessi, C.C., Gavrielides, A., Solina, V., Qiu, R.: 5G and beyond 5G technologies enabling Industry 5.0: Network applications for robotics. *Procedia Comput. Sci.* 232, 675–687 (2024). https://doi.org/10.1016/j.procs.2024.01.067.
11. Padhiary, M., Akhtar, J., Roy, D., Roy, P.: Smart Agricultural Technology 3D printing applications in smart farming and food processing. *Smart Agric. Technol.* 9, 100553 (2024). https://doi.org/10.1016/j.atech.2024.100553.
12. Zachariae, A., Plahl, F., Tang, Y., Mamaev, I., Hein, B., Wurll, C.: Human-robot interactions in autonomous hospital transports. *Rob. Auton. Syst.* 179, 104755 (2024). https://doi.org/10.1016/j.robot.2024.104755.
13. Mehta, I., Hsueh, H., Taghipour, S., Li, W., Saeedi, S.: UV disinfection robots: A review. *Rob. Auton. Syst.* 161, 104332 (2023). https://doi.org/10.1016/j.robot.2022.104332.
14. Prasad, G., Stalin, S., Alqahtani, O., Alasiry, A., Sharma, M., Aleryani, A., Kumar, P., Alouane, M.T.: Optimal path selection using reinforcement learning based ant colony optimization algorithm in IoT-Based wireless sensor networks with 5G technology. *Comput. Commun.* 212, 377–389 (2023). https://doi.org/10.1016/j.comcom.2023.09.015.
15. Chuah, S.H., Aw, E.C., Yee, D.: Computers in human behavior unveiling the complexity of consumers' intention to use service robots: An fsQCA approach. *Comput. Human Behav.* 123, 106870 (2021). https://doi.org/10.1016/j.chb.2021.106870.
16. Canh, T.N., Duc, S.T., The, H.N., Dao, T.H., Hoangvan, X.: Engineering Science and Technology, an International Journal Optimal design and fabrication of frame structure for dual-arm service robots: An effective approach for human – robot interaction. *Eng. Sci. Technol. An Int. J.* 56, 101763 (2024). https://doi.org/10.1016/j.jestch.2024.101763.
17. Giallanza, A., La, G., Micale, R., Manuela, C., Fata, L.: Occupational health and safety issues in human-robot collaboration: State of the art and open challenges. *Saf. Sci.* 169, 106313 (2024). https://doi.org/10.1016/j.ssci.2023.106313.
18. Zou, Y., Kim, D., Norman, P., Espinosa, J., Wang, J., Virk, G.S.: Towards robot modularity–A review of international modularity standardization for service robots. *Rob. Auton. Syst.* 148, 103943 (2022). https://doi.org/10.1016/j.robot.2021.103943.
19. Kotha, S.S., Akter, N., Abhi, S.H., Das, S.K., Islam, R., Ali, F., Ahamed, H., Islam, M., Sarker, S.K., Badal, F.R., Das, P., Tasneem, Z., Hasan, M.: Heliyon Next generation legged robot locomotion: A review on control techniques. *Heliyon.* 10, e37237 (2024). https://doi.org/10.1016/j.heliyon.2024.e37237.
20. Costanzo, M., Smeriglio, R., Nuovo, S. Di: New technologies and assistive robotics for elderly: A review on psychological variables. *Arch. Gerontol. Geriatr. Plus.* 1, 100056 (2024). https://doi.org/10.1016/j.aggp.2024.100056.
21. Hemmati, A., Masoud, A.: Internet of things the Internet of autonomous things applications: A taxonomy, technologies, and future directions. *Internet of Things.* 20, 100635 (2022). https://doi.org/10.1016/j.iot.2022.100635.
22. Lin, K., Li, Y., Sun, J., Zhou, D., Zhang, Q.: Multi-sensor fusion for body sensor network in medical human – robot interaction scenario. *Inf. Fusion.* 57, 15–26 (2020). https://doi.org/10.1016/j.inffus.2019.11.001.

23. Wang, J., Deng, H., Wang, Y., Xie, J., Zhang, H., Li, Y.: Multi-sensor fusion federated learning method of human posture recognition for dual-arm nursing robots. *Inf. Fusion*. 107, 102320 (2024). https://doi.org/10.1016/j.inffus.2024.102320.
24. Sætra, H.S.: Technology in Society The foundations of a policy for the use of social robots in care. *Technol. Soc*. 63, 101383 (2020). https://doi.org/10.1016/j.techsoc.2020.101383.
25. Koistinen, P., Krutova, O., Melin, H., Turja, T., Tuomo, S.: Job well robotized! – Maintaining task diversity and well-being in managing technological changes. 42, 67–75 (2024). https://doi.org/10.1016/j.emj.2022.08.002.
26. Ray, P.P.: Laparoscopic, Endoscopic and Robotic Surgery Large language models in laparoscopic surgery: A transformative opportunity. *Laparosc. Endosc. Robot. Surg*. (2024). https://doi.org/10.1016/j.lers.2024.07.002.
27. Ashrafian, H., Clancy, O., Grover, V., Darzi, A.: The evolution of robotic surgery: Surgical and anaesthetic aspects. *Br. J. Anaesth*. 119, i72–i84 (2017). https://doi.org/10.1093/bja/aex383.
28. Tan, S.Y., Taeihagh, A., Tripathi, A.: Technological forecasting & social change tensions and antagonistic interactions of risks and ethics of using robotics and autonomous systems in long-term care. *Technol. Forecast. Soc. Chang*. 167, 120686 (2021). https://doi.org/10.1016/j.techfore.2021.120686.
29. Ullah, I., Adhikari, D., Khan, H., Anwar, M.S., Ahmad, S.: Mobile robot localization: Current challenges and future prospective. *Comput. Sci. Rev*. 53, 100651 (2024). https://doi.org/10.1016/j.cosrev.2024.100651.
30. Javaid, M., Haleem, A., Pratap, R., Suman, R.: Substantial capabilities of robotics in enhancing industry 4.0 implementation. *Cogn. Robot*. 1, 58–75 (2021). https://doi.org/10.1016/j.cogr.2021.06.001.
31. Abozaid, Y.A., Aboelrayat, M.T., Fahim, I.S., Radwan, A.G.: Sensors and Actuators: A. Physical Soft robotic grippers: A review on technologies, materials, and applications. *Sensors Actuators A. Phys*. 372, 115380 (2024). https://doi.org/10.1016/j.sna.2024.115380.
32. Abdel-basset, M., Eldrandaly, K.A., Shawky, L.A., Elhoseny, M.: Hybrid computational intelligence algorithm for autonomous handling of COVID-19 pandemic emergency in smart cities. *Sustain. Cities Soc*. 76, 103430 (2022). https://doi.org/10.1016/j.scs.2021.103430.
33. Chinedu, K., Mary, O.: Heliyon Smart deployment of IoT-TelosB service care StreamRobot using software-defined reliability optimisation design. *Heliyon*. 8, e09634 (2022). https://doi.org/10.1016/j.heliyon.2022.e09634.
34. Sandhu, M., Silvera-tawil, D., Borges, P., Zhang, Q., Kusy, B.: Internet of robotic things for independent living: Critical analysis and future directions. *Internet of Things*. 25, 101120 (2024). https://doi.org/10.1016/j.iot.2024.101120.
35. Liu, Y., Li, Z., Liu, H., Kan, Z.: Skill transfer learning for autonomous robots and human – robot cooperation: A survey ☆. *Rob. Auton. Syst*. 128, 103515 (2020). https://doi.org/10.1016/j.robot.2020.103515.
36. Nahavandi, S., Alizadehsani, R., Nahavandi, D., Peng, C., Kelly, K., Bello, F.: Machine learning meets advanced robotic manipulation. *Inf. Fusion*. 105, 102221 (2024). https://doi.org/10.1016/j.inffus.2023.102221.
37. Mbunge, E., Muchemwa, B., Batani, J.: Sensors and healthcare 5 . 0: transformative shift in virtual care through emerging digital health technologies. *Glob. Heal. J*. 5, 169–177 (2021). https://doi.org/10.1016/j.glohj.2021.11.008.
38. Luperto, M., Monroy, J., Moreno, F., Lunardini, F., Renoux, J., Krpic, A., Galindo, C., Ferrante, S., Basilico, N., Gonzalez-jimenez, J., Borghese,

N.A.: Seeking at-home long-term autonomy of assistive mobile robots through the integration with an IoT-based monitoring system. *Rob. Auton. Syst.* 161, 104346 (2023). https://doi.org/10.1016/j.robot.2022.104346.

39. Jiang, Z., Salcudean, S.E., Navab, N.: Robotic ultrasound imaging: State-of-the-art and future perspectives. *Med. Image Anal.* 89, 102878 (2023). https://doi.org/10.1016/j.media.2023.102878.
40. Vu, A., Veerajagadeshwar, P., Shi, Y., Elara, R., Yan, M.: Long-term trials for improvement of autonomous area coverage with a Tetris inspired tiling self-reconfigurable system. *Expert Syst. Appl.* 206, 117810 (2022). https://doi.org/10.1016/j.eswa.2022.117810.
41. Vanderstappen, M., van Ochten, J.H., Verborgt, O.: *Robotics in arthroplasty: How good are they?*. JSES International (2024).
42. Grewal, D., Benoit, S., Noble, S.M., Guha, A., Ahlbom, C., Nordfält, J.: Leveraging in-store technology and AI: Increasing customer and employee efficiency and enhancing their experiences. *J. Retail.* 99, 487–504 (2023). https://doi.org/10.1016/j.jretai.2023.10.002.
43. Sarker, S., Jamal, L., Ahmed, S.F., Irtisam, N.: Robotics and artificial intelligence in healthcare during COVID-19 pandemic: A systematic review. *Rob. Auton. Syst.* 146, 103902 (2021). https://doi.org/10.1016/j.robot.2021.103902.
44. Faisal, M., Alharbi, A., Alhamadi, A., Almutairi, S., Alenezi, S., Alsulaili, A., Khan, M., Khan, F.: Robot-based solution for helping Alzheimer patients. *SLAS Technol.* 29, 100140 (2024). https://doi.org/10.1016/j.slast.2024.100140.
45. Liu, J., Tong, Y., Liu, J.: Review of snake robots in constrained environments. *Rob. Auton. Syst.* 141, 103785 (2021). https://doi.org/10.1016/j.robot.2021.103785.

11 Advancements in the Field of Biomedical Robotics for Ensuring Safety

Nisha Angeline C V, Muthuramalingam S, Abinaya S, Harini S, Vijai Varshshan M, and Sarveshwaran V

11.1 INTRODUCTION

Biomedical robotics is revolutionizing healthcare by providing high degrees of increased control and efficiency within clinical procedures while making it much safer [1]. One can think of the time when surgeons were freed from the shackles of fatigue or human fallibility; surgery robots can achieve exemplary precision, help patients during a surgery, or help them in postoperative physiotherapy perfectly. In such a vision of health care, where technology and patient well-being converge, the far horizon is no longer a distant future but an emerging reality in today's laboratories and hospitals. Biomedical robotics, which includes everything from highly precise surgical robots to rehabilitative aids, reduces the chance for human failure and eliminates fatigue, increasing the reliability and efficiency of medical care [2]. This work aims to outline how such systems may be further developed to enhance safety, reliability, and accuracy, and how critical these become with the integration of real-time Artificial Intelligence (AI) technologies into patient care.

About 5% of all hospital admissions involve very serious medical errors that contribute considerably to global morbidity and mortality. There are corresponding human and systemic limitations of all these statistics that call forth advanced intelligent systems in healthcare. Biomedical robotics introduces breakthroughs in unique soft robots carrying adaptive safety protocols and biofeedback systems powered by AI to transcend such gaps in patient care [3]. Each chapter in this book discusses how new developments in biomedical robotics contribute to a safer healthcare system, not only for patients but also for professionals.

In this chapter, practical exploration, instead of focusing purely on any technological innovation of medical robotics, is rather unique in its approach. Unlike other texts, which focus mainly on technological innovation, this chapter explores current and potential applications of robotics in healthcare. Through real-life examples or

 DOI: 10.1201/9781003561309-11

case studies such as prostate cancer management, personalized medicine in oncology, and comparative effectiveness trials on antibiotic resistance, this chapter provides insight into the bridge methodologies used in clinical research and their practical applications to healthcare. Nevertheless, the applications discussed focus on their implementation in highly specialized medical settings, particularly operating rooms and rehabilitation centres, where they can be most impactful [4].

Themes

1. **Adaptive Safety Protocols:** These protocols permit the operation of robotic systems to be altered in real time based on feedback received from a patient. A robot can monitor the vital signs of a patient under surgery and modify its actions if the heart rate or blood pressure of the patient fluctuates, thus ensuring safety during procedures that are hazardous to the patient.
2. **Biofeedback Systems:** Sophisticated biofeedback enables the robots to execute movements that are related to physiological signals from patients, like muscle tension or neural inputs. This enables them to increase the intensity and precision of their movements so that they can align with the body part of the patient and thereby minimize space for error and allow organizations to achieve perfection levels, which were impossible with manual systems.
3. **Predictive AI Models:** Complex algorithms in predictive models sift through large amounts of data to predict complications. For example, an AI can predict postoperative complications and pre-emptive measures to improve patient care [5].
4. **Integrated Safety Systems:** The systems of robotic subunits and medical devices improve the reliability of the whole system of healthcare. These systems serve as collaborative solutions to enhance the safety of patients in care and change the efficiency and reliability of the operations in healthcare.
5. **Branding and Personalization:** Customized Robotics for Patients is the movement toward specific care development based on specific customers. Algorithms are used to figure out which functions of robots are required by specific patient requirements, and they adapt in movement going through different stages of surgery or rehabilitation.
6. **Dynamic Fault-Tolerant Systems:** They learn to detect and self-correct mistakes. In such high-stakes occasions as in health care, these would make the difference; on detection of an error, a machine learning algorithm quickly rectifies the mistakes, thus rendering robot interventions more dependable.
7. **Ethical Considerations:** With biomedical robots so germane to the healthcare industry, there is the need to develop ethics principles governing their usage. The chapter addresses such considerations in guiding its development so that they are socially acceptable with regard to their robotics healthcare solutions.

11.2 CURRENT STATE OF BIOMEDICAL ROBOTICS

11.2.1 Overview of Existing Biomedical Robotics Technologies

Biomedical robotics is an interdisciplinary science that combines engineering of robotics with healthcare for the enhancement of medical interventions and facilities. The technology in this domain is typically categorized into two primary types: the rigid robots and the soft robots.

Rigid Robots: Such robots are characterized by their rigid structure, which doesn't soften or adapt to any type of pressure. A good example is the da Vinci surgical system, which has been used greatly in minimally invasive surgeries [6]. Due to their design, these robots are very rigid, and this is very advantageous because only precise and stable movements are required during critical procedures such as surgeries. Because of the enhanced control systems and higher precision of operation, rigid robots help surgeons to accomplish challenging procedures with less harm to patients' health and faster rehabilitation [7].

Soft Robots: Soft robots are not some inflexible metal structures like more conventional robots; they are intended to be as compliant as soft tissues. This is possible because they have soft structures as well as being compliant, which enables them to fit in any curved shape and also work with the tissues of people. This capability is particularly important in applications where interaction with the patient's body is direct, for example, in prosthetics, rehabilitation, or some surgeries. Soft robots have been designed to cope with such geometries and further ensure safe physical contact with sensitive biostructures; they are more flexible than their hard counterparts [8].

11.2.2 Applications in Surgery, Rehabilitation, and Diagnostics

Soft robotics has led to transformative advancements across multiple medical applications [9].

Figure 11.1 presents the applications of biomedical robots across surgery, rehabilitation, and diagnostics. Each category showcases specialized technologies, such as AI-assisted tools, adaptive systems, and minimally invasive procedures, demonstrating the multifaceted roles of robotics in enhancing precision, safety, and patient care in medical practices [10].

- **Surgery:** For surgical purposes, soft robots help in the creation of actuators or artificial muscles, stents, and catheters. Hospitals mostly utilize sophisticated robots that are built to be incorporated into tissues and practice greater flexibility as well as safety during operations. Compliant systems incorporated in soft robots have the ability to match compliance with tissues in comparison to traditional rigid systems.
- **Rehabilitation:** Soft robotic systems have drastically changed the way patients are taken through the process of rehabilitation. A special example

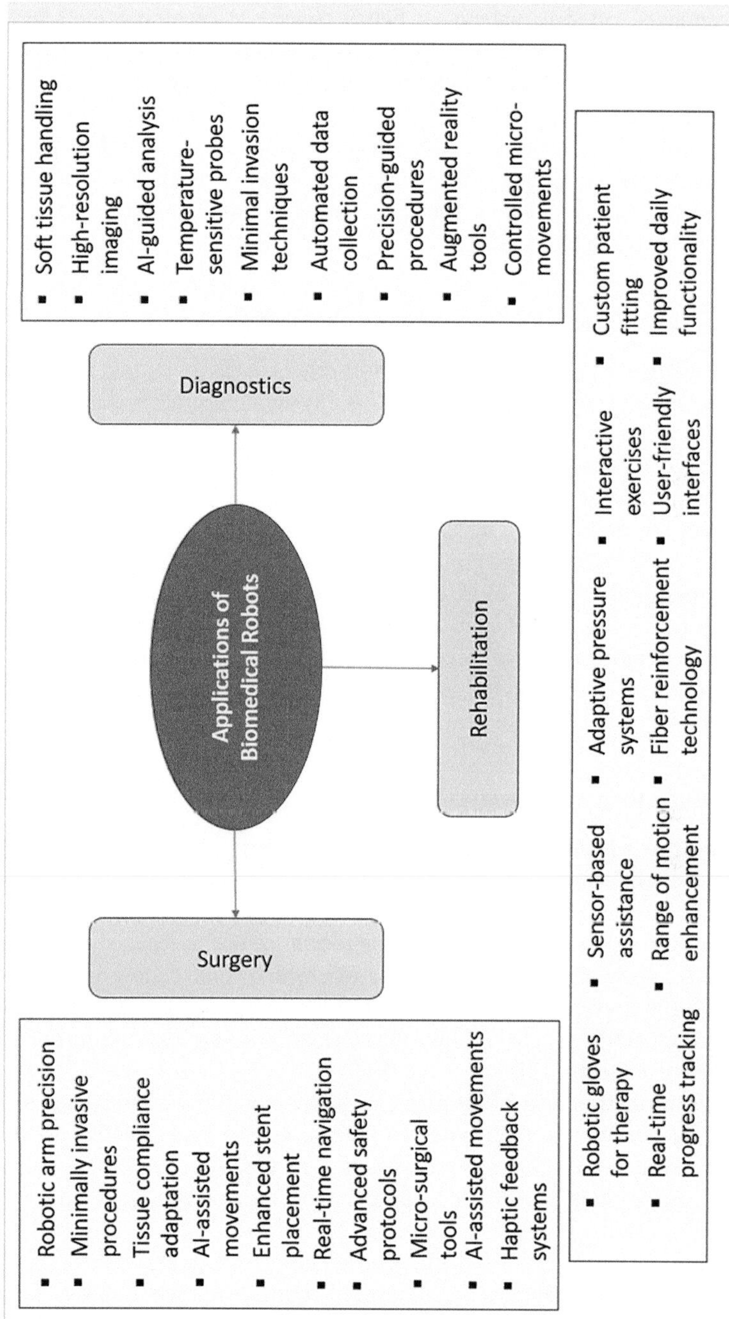

FIGURE 11.1 . Key applications of biomedical robotics in surgery, rehabilitation, and diagnostics

is robotic gloves that are built to be used in hand therapy [11]. These gloves use moulded elastomer chambers and fibre reinforcement to augment hand movements, offering patients a better chance at regaining their grasping functions and hence a better quality of life. These types of rehabilitation devices offer specific assistance and help to give a far more realistic approach to rehabilitation.

- **Diagnostics:** For diagnosis, soft robotics can intervene with delicate tissues owing to their compliant nature. It helps to improve diagnostic procedures so that proper tasks are done in the body area with less disturbance to the patient or any danger to the patient.

11.2.3 Current Safety Protocols and Standards

Safety in biomedical robotics, especially in soft robots, calls for certain measures and procedures to be followed to the letter. HISIC is a systematic strategy that will be used to address the safety of robotic systems. It involves processes of risk assessment to potential hazards together with appropriate measures and controls to be applied at the design stages and during the operation of the facility.

Soft robots are deliberately developed with safety considerations in mind, for example, low-force actuators and compliance matching. These design considerations assist in decreasing the chance of getting hurt during human tissue interactions [12]. Also worth mentioning is that real-time monitoring through integrated sensors to countercheck operational safety is very important. They know the position of the robot and the forces applied on the surgical instruments in real time, and that makes the robot very safe for use in medical procedures.

11.2.4 Limitations and Challenges

Despite significant advancements, soft robotics faces several challenges. Nonetheless, there are several challenges with the prospects of soft robotics:

- **Actuation Systems:** It has only in the recent past been realized that selecting suitable mechanisms for proper actuation, which could follow different needs of soft robotics, is still a problem. Soft robots require durable and multifunctional actuators capable of reliable performance in various working conditions and environments [12].
- **Miniaturization and Modelling:** Realistic modelling of small appendages and soft structures contributes to enhancing the functionality as well as the modularity of soft robotic systems. In these aspects, there is a need to advance their performance to enhance the reliability of soft robotic systems.
- **Scaling Actuators:** SMA and the piezoelectric systems are some of the haptic actuator systems that need a high level of control, which becomes a challenge during scaling. Third, the control of pneumatic systems is important for these systems to function properly in medical environments and with the use of pneumatic systems there are extra costs for calibration [13].

11.3 SAFETY-CENTRIC DESIGN IN BIOMEDICAL ROBOTICS

11.3.1 Design Principles for Ensuring Safety

Biomedical robots are designed with key principles to ensure safety.

- **Compliance Matching**: Surgical robots are designed to mimic biological forms, to avoid damaging tissue during procedures and treatment.
- **Use of Soft Materials**: Using soft materials for compliance makes the interaction flexible for safe touch leading to a reduction of possible harm.
- **Sensor-Driven Feedback**: Particularly, the intensity distribution, overload distribution, and material characteristics must be detected by sensors with feedback of the measured values in real-time for safety reasons. Robot's performance is constantly being observed through the sensors to prevent cases of accidents that may occur while working [13].

11.3.2 HUMAN-ROBOT INTERACTION (HRI) IN MEDICAL SETTINGS

Aspects of Human-Robot Interaction (HRI) are essential, especially in the medical context where these robotic systems have close physical interaction with human beings. Catheters, prosthetic devices, etc. are all soft robots that must work meticulously as they are in direct contact with human tissues. Safe and efficient human-robot interaction is characterized by continuous feedback and control to adapt the robot's behaviour pattern to that of the human [14].

11.3.3 Sensor Integration for Real-Time Monitoring

Real-time monitoring in soft robots integrates different types of sensors, for instance pressure sensors, force sensors, and strain gauges. These sensors offer real-time information about the degree of positioning and forces that are experienced; this assists in proper control and change of position or forces in prosthetic and rehabilitation devices.

11.3.4 Redundancy and Fault-Tolerance Mechanisms

To increase the dependability, biomedical robots integrate self-diagnostic systems as well as a dual power drive. For instance, fibre-reinforced actuators can continue to perform at their optimum level and remain secure in operation, even after one of the components has failed, when being used in medical procedures [15].

11.4 ADVANCED SENSING AND ACTUATION TECHNOLOGIES

11.4.1 Role of AI and Machine Learning in Enhancing Safety

With deep learning models, classification is being built using AI and machine learning. Think of a world where machines can recognize not just their environment, but learn from it, tailoring responses and ensuring safe human-machine interactions. Imagine, for example, a factory robot responding to the real-time data it gleans from its surroundings. This ability to respond humanely can prevent accidents between humans and robots [16].

AI algorithms process information received from sensors to predict safety incidents well before they become a reality in many industries. For instance, in production lines for factories, machine learning can look at historical data to pick up on trends that indicate machine wear and tear. As companies keep their facilities up to date, they keep situations harmless.

11.4.2 Novel Sensor Technologies for Biomedical Robotic

Biomedical robotics is an interesting and emerging field. Robots have been fitted with novel sensor technologies, allowing them to handle sophisticated tasks accurately. One example is the development of flexible sensors that medical staff could embed in their patients. However, despite the limitations of these sensors, the live data they transmit can still help medical professionals monitor patients' vital signs more effectively.

It also includes some high-tech flourishes, such as biosensors that read certain biomarkers in blood. Now, envision a robotic system that can continuously monitor glucose levels for diabetics. Such a system helps not only in improved health outcomes but also makes the lives of patients and healthcare providers easier.

1. Better monitoring of the patient
2. Improved medical interventions
3. Increase safety during major surgeries using previous and real-time feedback.

11.4.3 Soft Robotics and Safe Actuation

The area of soft robotics has been receiving increased attention as they are safer to be used by humans and in a setting where the object is delicate. A soft robot is a piece of technology designed using flexible material that can morph its shape and motion. Such flexibility carries over into safer actuation, which is better suited for usage in elder care or child-friendly environments [16].

Soft robotic hands can pick up an egg without damaging it, as a case in point. The soft touch helps prevent accidents during fragile jobs. This also has potential implications for soft robotics in rehabilitation: These technologies could help guide patients through exercises they can do at home, safely and effectively. Soft robotics is care in machines, a beautiful melding of technology and compassion [17].

11.4.4 Autonomous Decision-Making with Safety Protocols

From delivery drones to driverless cars, autonomous systems are becoming increasingly widespread. An important chapter of his development is that they will now be among the supporters who must integrate safety protocols into their decision-making.

This is how machines would ascertain the risk and make decisions based upon their environment, if there are any specific protocols [18][19].

Consider self-driving cars, for instance. They remain aware of their surroundings by combining cameras, LiDAR, and other sensors. When faced with sudden obstacles, these vehicles must decide whether to brake, slow down, or swerve. AI helps to make this decision by analyzing thousands of scenarios immediately in real time so that a safe response is possible when unexpected situations arise.

While we lean into these technologies, building faith in autonomous systems is critical.

11.5 FEDERATED LEARNING IN HEALTH CARE: ADVANCES, APPLICATIONS, AND PRIVACY CHALLENGES

Federated learning (FL) is a groundbreaking approach designed to address the twin challenges of exploiting large amounts of healthcare data across institutions and maintaining strong privacy requirements. By enabling providers to co-train machine learning models collaboratively on decentralized data sources without transferring sensitive information about patients, federated learning safeguards patient privacy and security, and leverages large, diverse datasets. This section discusses recent advancements, state-of-the-art applications, and essential privacy-preserving challenges in federated learning; it explains how this technology is shaping the future of healthcare and biomedical robotics [20].

11.5.1 Recent Trends in Federated Learning for Healthcare

Advanced Protocols: The recent developments in FL are new frameworks such as Federated Proximal (FedProx), to deal with the heterogeneity across hospitals. Data heterogeneity is a big challenge for consistent models, since there are differences in demographics, medical devices, and local practices between healthcare institutions. FedProx helps to achieve consistency in the sense that it increases the reliability of the model and enhances accuracy in the predictions across different sources of healthcare data.

Furthermore, the discussion concludes with privacy-preserving aggregation protocols: The aggregation protocols use secure aggregation, such that model updates aggregate together without revealing individual updates to any party. Homomorphic encryption allows computations on encrypted data so that patient information is protected even during the training process. There is an added importance of using this in a healthcare setup, as data leakage can go all the way to affect one's ethics and law.

Personalized Federated Learning: This is personalized federated learning in which models are tailored to the local data distribution, preserving at the same time the benefits of the shared global model. It is thus the answer to the need for personalized care since the implemented treatments typically take care of the individual patients. Allowing personalization at the local level allows personalized FL to ensure that treatments and diagnostics will most likely be specific to a patient than Federated collaboration may have allowed at first [21].

11.5.2 Applications of Federated Learning in the Healthcare System

Medical Imaging and Diagnosis: In medical image analysis, federated learning offers models trained across diverse data sources that may improve diagnostic accuracy regarding the diseases of interest. For example, Federated Tumor Segmentation (FeTS) applies FL to the segmentation of brain tumors, hence developing robust models from decentralized medical scans without having to share data [22].

Remote Monitoring and Disease Prediction: Wearable health devices have increasingly inspired FL to monitor patient data securely and continuously emanating from sensors. This increases the reliability of predictive models of cardiac events and diabetes progression, thus keeping the privacy of patients intact while operating multiple devices and systems.

Drug Discovery and Genomics: Federated learning is also applied in genomics, which enables the analysis of large genetic data without necessarily violating individual privacy. FL accelerates the discovery of markers for a disease because it speeds up the training of models in many genetic repositories; therefore, it accelerates drug discovery while advocating personalized medicine.

11.5.3 Challenges and Solutions on Privacy Preservation

Federated learning in healthcare has several benefits to itself, but privacy preservation is an inherent challenge addressed by innovative solutions.

Data heterogeneity and privacy: Diverse data across health institutions complicate model training. Techniques, which include differential privacy-additive noises to model updates, and secure multi-party computation, allow for collaborative computation without the release of data, thereby minimizing possible risks of breaching privacy and HIPAA and GDPR compliance standards.

Communication Bottlenecks: Real-time updating of models would require a heavy amount of communication between hospitals or devices, thus consuming resources. Some solutions, like hierarchical federated learning, have cut down the rounds of communications in such a way that efficiency is improved without violating privacy.

Regulatory Compliance: Federated learning stands upon and is sensitive to privacy laws and regulations like HIPAA, GDPR, etc. Methods like differential privacy and homomorphic encryption ensure that federated models do not violate any regulations that would jeopardize any performance [23].

11.6 REGULATORY AND ETHICAL CONSIDERATIONS

Biomedical robotics has made a significant impact in healthcare through the development of autonomous surgical robots, rehabilitation devices, and assistive technologies. Yet, with such progress comes a whole host of intricate regulatory and ethical questions that demand resolution if these technologies are to be safe, fair, and accountable. This section reviews the modern regulatory environment, ethics aspects, and liability responsibility, as well as geographically accords the same business lines that are identified in biomedical robotics.

11.6.1 Regulatory Frameworks for Biomedical Robotics

Ensuring that biomedical robots are adequately safe and work well requires proper regulation. The protocol for evaluation of safety and efficacy of robotic systems, as medical devices, was established by the regulatory agencies (U.S. Food & Drug Agency—FDA; European Medicines Agency—EMA; and their equivalents globally); hence establishing a global framework [23].

Biomedical robots face several unique challenges, particularly when it comes to autonomous decision-making. Existing medical device architecture may not fully cover the complexities associated with robots, particularly in cases wherein robots are autonomous or physically interact with patients without continuous supervision. For example, autonomous surgical robots might be asked to perform a complicated surgery with minimal assistance on the part of humans. Proving that such robots are safe and efficacious will require testing methodologies that exceed conventional medical device standards.

To address these challenges, new regulations are being implemented for the evaluation and endorsement of biomedical robots. They, for example, have the Software as a Medical Device (SaMD) framework targeted towards AI-based medical technologies, which includes many robotics systems. Most regulatory agencies are choosing a risk-based system to understand and prevent the adverse risks of biomedical robots, with classifications divided into degrees of autonomy, and there are possible consequences if something goes wrong.

11.6.2 Ethical Implications of Autonomous Biomedical Robots

Several serious ethical considerations need to be closely examined as biomedical robots continue to progress towards greater autonomy. Not the least of these is patient safety. The behaviour of patients may be somewhat unpredictable, and the situations that medical robots operating on their own will face are very difficult for autonomous medical robotics to solve with predetermined decisions made by humans [23][24]. A major ethical issue is guaranteeing that autonomous systems can process these scenarios in such a way that they remain safe and effective.

In addition to this worry, there is another instance of ethical concern in terms of informed consent. Because patients may be misled and overestimated when using autonomous robots, they are not necessarily the right route, as it is essentially an expectation. It is important for maintaining patient trust that patients and their treating physicians understand how these robots work, the algorithm behind them, and another level of transparency to address the ways decisions are made [25]. To ensure that patients can make decisions regarding their care, developers and healthcare providers must effectively convey the role of a robot, the complications with it afterwards, as well as how outcomes may differ from procedures performed without a robotic arm.

There are also ethical implications as the line of what can be automated and moved to an AI model is drawn further toward various job subtypes. While healthcare can be greatly enhanced by biomedical robots, allowing for increased precision, reduced human error, and more accessible medical services, they also may lead to the replacement of certain jobs. The ethical challenge is to support the adoption of sophisticated robotic systems with the preservation of human jobs and the health of skilled professionals.

The final example in the narrative—autonomous robots caring for old or disabled people—raises questions about what forms of interaction humans rely on. The emotional and psychological support provided by human caregivers, however, can never be replaced by robots—an over-reliance on robotic care would inevitably lead to social isolation or lower quality of life for so many.

11.6.3 Liability and Accountability Issues

Perhaps the most immediate ethical problem in Biomedical Robotics is figuring out who to blame when things go wrong. But who pays the price if an autonomous robot makes a mistake during surgery or gives the wrong treatment? [25]. Responsibility in the traditional medical domain is attributed to human healthcare providers, but as robots are becoming and more becoming a kind of autonomous, it gets complicated.

In other words, if a robot screws up during an invasive process, where does the fault lie—with the maker of the bot itself or with a healthcare service which employed it to perform its duty; developers who failed to keep improving the underlying algorithms needed on algorithms? Establishing legal advice concerning liability in such situations is important for patient protection, and healthcare workers will not be wrongly considered responsible when decisions are made by machines.

And as AI and machine learning algorithms grow more flexible, robots may make choices that are not directly tied to how they were programmed. This begs the question of responsibility should robots indeed act unexpectedly or in problematic ways.

A start has been made on the legal frameworks. For instance, a few experts have argued for legal standards around "robotic personhood," which could implicate some liability to robots that act autonomously [25]. Some suggest amending product liability laws that allow makers of such systems to escape responsibility when problems occur with their unregulated devices, thereby motivating manufacturers and developers to take full responsibility for the safety and effectiveness, even after a robot is on the medical market.

11.6.4 Global Standards and Harmonization Efforts

The need for international cooperation and harmonization of standards is highlighted as biomedical robotics moves towards an industry that can compete on a global scale. Tight regulations and standards in one country can block the adoption or development of robotic technology, stifle innovation across entire sectors, and hinder commercial success for industry actors (and access to life-saving medical devices).

There are also worldwide efforts to set global norms for the development, manufacturing, and use of medical robots. The ISO (International Organization for Standardization) and IEC (the International Electrotechnical Commission) are working on uniform standards to safeguard/ensure protection from robot safety/performance is developed globally.

Minimization of standards is also important for assuring the safety of patients who travel or with medical facilities situated in various nations [25]. It also means that a consistent protocol for regulating robots can streamline developer pathways while simultaneously maintaining the same level of care or protection afforded to patients treated by such machines.

Additionally, in addressing these new ethical problems, like the international data privacy concerns and transnational cybersecurity matters surrounding robotic systems, global collaboration is imperative. With robots starting to use data alone for making decisions autonomously, the implementation of international standards ensuring patient privacy will be more important than ever if we are going to protect essential knowledge at the same time as keeping pace with technological innovation.

The regulatory and ethical environment of biomedical robotics is layered and evolving. Meeting these challenges will require close cooperation between government, industry, and academia to deliver the benefits of biomedical robotics while also mitigating risks to patients and society.

11.7 FUTURE TRENDS AND INNOVATIONS

11.7.1 Robotics in Personalized Medicine

Pharmacogenomics is a developing speciality that targets the delivery of custom healthcare interventions for each patient. Robotics is a field that has great potential in revolutionizing this area.

11.7.1.1 Robotic Surgery with Precision Enhancement: Robot-based surgical platforms in the next generation will incorporate new AI algorithms, and give recommendations to the surgeon in real-time depending on the patient's needs [26]. Accuracy and flexibility in robotic arms will improve the possibility and efficiency of carrying out delicate surgeries with the least invasiveness, hence short post-operation recovery periods and high efficacy.

11.7.1.2 Robotic Bio-Sensors and Diagnostics: The availability of efficient and innovative microrobotics and advanced biosensors design will enable personal diagnosis. Imagine, for instance, tiny robots that use nanoscale probes to scan biological tissues and have superior diagnostic capabilities, thus enhancing the odds of accurate diagnosis and improving the treatment options given based on specimen analysis [27].

11.7.1.3 Adaptive Robotic Therapies: Robotics will facilitate the creation of smart therapeutic approaches to change the therapy mode according to the patient's response in real-time. This includes, for instance, automated drug administering machines that refill dosage and determine timings based upon feedback from wearable devices [27].

11.7.1.4 Genomic and Proteomic Robotics: Robotics will have a vital role in genomics and proteomics, where robots will be required to perform high-throughput screening and analysis [28]. This will enhance the process of discovering the genetic markers and possible treatments, and is becoming more personalized, independent of the sequencing costs.

11.7.2 Integration of Robotics with Wearable Technologies

In this section, we present a future work section as the next step to explore the concept of integration between robotics with wearable technologies. Incorporation of robotics within body-worn instruments is a remarkable revolution in health, early detection, and rehabilitation [29].

11.7.2.1 Wearable Exoskeletons for Mobility Enhancement: Society will see enhanced robotic exoskeletons coupled with wearables that will aid mobility limitations. These exoskeletons will incorporate real-time data to adapt their support configuration to provide more support when needed and less otherwise, thus improving the person's mobility and decreasing physical stress.

11.7.2.2 Personalized Health Monitoring Systems: Wearable robotics will consist of biometric monitoring through sensors for tracking the health status of the wearer, physical activity, and environmental conditions. These systems will give information to the patient and alert the doctor to what is happening in the patient's body.

11.7.2.3 Robotic Assistive Devices: Exoskeletons will be used to help in grabbing, postural control, and indeed everyone will be needing help in thinking from robots. Such devices will be personal and unique; most of them will be highly personalized.

11.7.2.4 Enhanced Rehabilitation Technologies: Wearable technology will be combined with robotics to present enhanced rehabilitation therapies such as robotic-aided physical therapy and training of the intellect. It will be possible to adjust those systems according to the user's progress, and therefore, it will be possible to have individual exercises and feedback.

11.7.3 Telemedicine and Remote Surgery Robotics

Now, telemedicine and robotic remote surgery are emerging quickly because the market for them is growing, and accessibility and effectiveness are valuable in health care.

11.7.3.1 Remote Robotic Surgery Systems: Further advancements will lead to improvement in the tele-endurance of the system of remote surgery, enabling surgeons to perform such elaborate operations from remote regions with high accuracy. Carrier technologies for communications will make the system as fast as possible and provide real-time feedback.

11.7.3.2 Robotic Telemedicine Platforms: Telemedicine shall incorporate the use of robotic platforms for diagnosis and other forms of engagement with patients. Robots fitted with high-definition cameras, diagnostic tools [29], and interaction touch screens will help to conduct online consultation and regular check-ups.

11.7.3.3 AI-Driven Telemedicine Assistants: Robotics will be implemented with AI to assist in triage to initial patient evaluation, data acquisition about their past, and as a resource for other health care workers. Such assistants are going to enhance the effectiveness and effectiveness of consultations conducted at a distance [30].

11.7.3.4 Enhanced Remote Monitoring Capabilities: Telecare systems will incorporate the use of technology, specifically robots, to carry out remote health checks and interventions. Robotics will also play a crucial role in tele-monitoring of chronic diseases, compliance with taking medications, and even handling of emergencies [31].

11.7.4 Robotics for Elderly Care and Assisted Living

Robotics finds increasing applications in elderly care and assisted living to improve the quality of life and become a one-stop solution.

11.7.4.1 Adaptive Care Robots: An important aspect will be the developmental character of future care robots, which will know the patterns and adjust to elderly individuals' changing needs. It is coordinated by these robots, which will help the client in undertaking their daily routines, health status, and in case of an emergency.

11.7.4.2 Social Companion Robots: Finally, the future generation of social robots will be of a higher level and will address mental health issues of people by providing friendship, thinking, and social interaction. These kinds of robots will incorporate artificial intelligence, where the robot will have the ability to adapt the interaction and activities to accord with the patient's desires and requirements.

11.7.4.3 Integrated Safety and Health Monitoring: Smart home technologies will be incorporated in robotics to enhance and offer a detailed safety and health check. These comprise fall detection, environmental danger alerts, as well as the automatic emergency notifications [32].

11.7.4.4 Robotic Assistance for Cognitive Impairments: Service robots to be provided for people experiencing cognitive disability will provide memory, cognitive exercises, and direction finding. The robots will promote independence and relieve the burden of informal careers.

11.7.4.5 Collaborative Robotics in Care Facilities: Service robots will include collaborative robots that will be used by healthcare givers in care facilities to do some lifting, transporting and patient monitoring. This will help prevent over-stressing of the muscles, reduce the time taken by caregivers to help patients, hence increasing efficiency.

11.8 CASE STUDIES AND REAL-WORLD APPLICATIONS

11.8.1 Success Stories in Robotic Surgery

Robotic surgery is the greatest improvement in surgical procedures since the use of microsurgery technology, with improvements in precision, time taken to recover from the surgery, and improved health of the patient. This section describes specific examples of how robotic surgery has affected many disciplines of medicine and the successful outcomes achieved through its use [33].

Case Study 1: The da Vinci Surgical System is a complex medical robot approved by the Food and Drug Administration in 2000, marketed and sold by Intuitive Surgical, Inc.

Background: This robotic surgery is one of the pioneering surgical technologies that was made through the effort of Intuitive Surgical.

Success Story: Dr. Michael C has done more than 1000 robotic-assisted prostatectomies using the da Vinci system, and the patient has less postoperative pain, early ambulation, short hospital stays, as well as an early return to their normal activity.

Outcome: They assessed a significant decrease in blood loss, complications, or the length of hospital stay and practical enhancement in patients' quality of life.

Case Study 2: Robotic-Assisted Cardiac Surgery

Background: Robotic systems in cardiac surgery have provided a relatively unknown additional premium level.

Success Story: The use of the ROSA robot at Wray Hospital by Dr. A, performing minimally invasive procedures for heart valve repairs.

Outcome: This procedure cut down the time spent in the operating theatre, reduced the incidence of infection, and reduced the time for patients to heal with minimal scarring of tissue and improvement in the cardiac function of the patients.

Key Takeaways

- Precision and Minimally Invasive Techniques: Computer-controlled systems are more precise compared to manual ones.
- Enhanced Patient Outcomes: Lower pains, quicker healing process, and fewer complications.

11.8.2 Safety Challenges in Rehabilitation Robotics

Background: It is now universally acknowledged that rehabilitation robotics is an effective assistant in the process of rehabilitation for patients with physical disability. However, their use usually involves certain risks which must be controlled to achieve the identified goals and protect the health of patients.

Challenge 1: Patient Safety and System Reliability and Challenges in Patient Care: No Patient Safety and System Reliability

- **Issue:** In the case of utilizing robotic rehabilitation devices such as exoskeletons and robotic arms, the primary consideration lies in patient safety.
- **Case Study:** A safety issue arose from a faulty robotic exoskeleton, which led to the understanding that these mechanical structures also need appropriate safety and check-ups.
- **Solution:** Such quality control steps include a monitoring system and safety measures that one can use to correct a defect once it has been identified.

Challenge 2: Self-Management Treatment by Clients will face the following challenge:

- **Issue:** The technology can quite appropriately be integrated with the traditional rehabilitation therapies with reasonable difficulty.
- **Case Study:** Another study at a rehabilitation centre found it challenging to directly compare the outcomes of traditional exercise with robotic therapy without any standardized methods.
- **Solution:** Developing new organically grown therapies that incorporate parts of self-generated robotic therapy with traditional approaches.

Key Takeaways

- **Robust Safety Protocols:** Essential to prevent and contain fast failure as soon as they are detected.
- **Hybrid Therapy Approaches:** Can enhance rehabilitation outcomes.

11.8.3 Innovations in Diagnostic Robotics

- This includes the use of robotic technology in diagnosing illnesses, the mechanics of diagnosing, and the statistics of diagnosing. Introduction. With the development of various diagnostic robotics, the diagnosis process is now more accurate and much faster. This section aims to discuss emerging developments in diagnostic robotics as a factor in the future.

Innovation 1: Robotic Endoscopy

- **Technology:** Robotic endoscopic systems give detailed imagery and accuracy inside the body.
- **Case Study:** The following are examples of early disease diagnosis that that have been done at NYU Langone Health using robotic endoscopy: detection and treatment of a rare bile duct cancer through minimally invasive robotic surgery after endoscopic identification of a small tumor, removal of large premalignant rectal lesions using a flexible robotic endoscopic system

to avoid traditional open surgery, and accurate diagnosis of suspicious lung nodules via robot assisted bronchoscopy, enabling precise tissue sampling and reducing the need for invasive procedures.
- **Outcome:** This translated into improved visualization and greater biopsy accuracy, which in turn improved searly and accurate diagnosis, thus making patient management more effective.

Innovation 2: AI-Powered Diagnostic Robots

- **Technology:** Use of AI in combination with diagnostic robotic machines aided in the interpretation of images and coming up with medical decisions on their own.
- **Case Study:** Presents a case study of implementing an AI Robot System in the radiology department of the Mayo Clinic hospital.
- **Outcome:** Enhancements in diagnostic accuracy and speed since AI aids in analyzing abnormalities in the medical images.

Key Takeaways

- Enhanced Diagnostic Accuracy: Robotic systems are efficient in imaging and also in analysis when compared to manual systems.
- AI Integration: It helps in the provision of instant and accurate diagnostics.

11.8.4 Lessons Learned from Clinical Deployments

Clinical robots utilized practically in clinical practice entail addressing various issues and, therefore, experiences from actual practice. The following are some of the clinical lessons that were obtained from the clinical deployments of the robotic systems.

Lesson: 1 User Training

- **Issue:** It is equally important to guarantee that the healthcare personnel are well conversant with the utilization of the robotic systems.
- **Case Study:** One of the early obstacles to deployment was during the implementation of the same at the Mayo Clinic, which was attributed to inadequate training of the related staff.
- **Solution:** Assuring that the medical personnel put into practice best practice guidelines by teaching various extensive training courses and long-term support.

Lesson 2: Flexibility to Meet Practice Requirements

- **Issue:** It is important to stress that robotic processes can be integrated and implemented into the present clinical settings, and it is often not as simple.

- **Case Study:** This chapter is the conceptual paper of experience, which proves that the overall practices within the operating room of the Cleveland Clinic Medical Centre were altered due to the adoption of robotic surgical systems.
- **Solution:** When working on clinical projects, one has to be innovative when presenting robotic tools most effectively into the pertinent clinical areas as well as operations.

Lesson 3: Monitoring and Feedback

- **Issue:** Periodically, observational studies should be conducted on the performance of the robotic system with feedback to yield the best outcome.
- **Case Study:** A research study on PubMed details how the Versius robot-assisted MAS system was carefully developed through user feedback..
- **Solution:** Providing feedback and evaluation on how the systems have performed in an organization with the view of finding those areas that could have some issues or problems and addressing them.

Key Takeaways

- User Training: Monitoring and feedback are some of the major principles that are key to the adoption and use of the system.
- Workflow Integration: It needs a lot of planning and good coordination skills.
- Monitoring and Feedback: Crucial in the improvement of performance and efficiency as to how the system operates.

11.9 CONCLUSION AND FUTURE OUTLOOK

11.9.1 Summary of Key Findings

Based on the findings of our research in the subject area of biomedical robotics, there are a few critical observations that point towards the possibilities that biomedical robotics holds for the healthcare industry. These findings show that biomedical robotics is not an evolution but a revolution in medical practice. Notable advancements include:

Greater Accuracy: The robotic tools used in surgeries mean that minimal invasive surgeries are done, hence reducing patient post-surgery trauma [33].

Increased Accessibility: Healthcare robotics is particularly important in filling the gap in treatment, since in developing nations, for instance, there are very few hospital facilities and even fewer specialized workers.

Enhanced Patient Interaction: Today, the robots are going beyond simple interactions and are now interactive, for instance, therapeutic robots for treating substance dependency or companion robots for patients with Alzheimer's disease.

Consequently, these research findings point to the important role played by biomedical robotics in reinventing conventional health facilities, which are now able to deliver enhanced and efficient health care services to patients.

11.9.2 Possible Future Trends

In the future, several developments indicate that biomedical robotics will undergo further development and interconnect with other innovations. Key trends to watch include:

AI Integration: This will thus allow robots to learn on their own, and constantly improve in view of the clinical and operational demands of every surgical or therapeutic procedure.

Telemedicine Robotics: Doctors, especially surgeons, will routinely recommend and carry out operations via robotic systems and with support from virtual reality; the delivery of healthcare services will not necessarily have to be physically done from the same location but via robotic mechanisms.

Personalized Treatments: Biomedical robots will allow precise attention to medical histories, disease processes, and previous responses to treatment to be paid during patient care delivery, on a case-by-case basis.

An analysis of these trends suggests that biomedical robotics cannot merely be seen as complementing current practices; it also points to an innovative future for personalized care.

11.9.3 Roadmap for Safe Biomedical Robotics

The foundation for biomedical robotics will continue to rest on trust and safety. Therefore, it requires the commitment of engineers, healthcare providers, and patients to promote a coherent concept of safety and to avoid locking the process in separate domains. Thus, open communication can make these sophisticated technologies not only instruments but also associates in health care systems.

11.9.4 Conclusion on How Safety can be Achieved in Biomedical Robotics

Specifically, it is argued that building trust in biomedical robotics depends on effective communication of safety standards in the upcoming years. As these technologies and products develop, there must be an ongoing discussion between engineers and especially healthcare givers in coming up with common, clear, and universally acceptable measures to ensure safety for all.

The use of biomedical robotics should be regarded not only as a tool but as an integrated member of the healthcare system.

Future developments of biomedical robotics should continue to focus on issues of patient safety. In this manner, we can guarantee its ongoing growth in a way that will benefit as many people as possible by creating its atmosphere and focusing on the development of technologies that will enhance the trust of the youngest generation in a healthier future.

11.9.5 Future Work in Biomedical Robotics

As we look to the future, some areas need research and development to continually advance biomedical robotics in terms of success and safety:

Advances in Fault-Tolerance and Reliability: Future work can also be done on the resultant advances of biomedical robots to make them reliable in unstructured settings with a singular focus on the possibility of making the robots self-healing in case of failures [34]

Ethical and Regulatory Considerations: More research concerning some of the ethical issues will be needed as biomedical robots are gradually incorporated into health care institutions. Innovative studies on the recognition of operational structures that would allow for safe management of these technologies are extremely important [35][36].

Human-Robot Interaction (HRI): The future research should focus on the aspects of enhancing the workflow between human and robot, and thus guaranteeing safe and effective use of robotic systems in healthcare settings as well as patients' satisfaction and acceptance of robotic medicine.

Long-Term Impact on Healthcare: These and other related questions require further research focusing on the ability of robotic technologies to improve patients' quality of life and reduce their recovery time.

It is in these areas of future work that one needs to lay the foundation and guide the development of biomedical robotics towards safety and efficiency in healthy service delivery, while developing the trust of patients and healthcare givers.

REFERENCES

[1] Siqueira-Batista, R., Souza, C. R., Maia, P. M., & Siqueira, S. L. (2016). Robotic surgery: Bioethical aspects. *Arquivos brasileiros de cirurgia digestiva: ABCD = Brazilian Archives of Digestive Surgery*, 29(4), 287–290. https://doi.org/10.1590/0102-6720201600040018

[2] Sharma, M., & Paul Khurana, S. M. (2018). Biomedical engineering: The recent trends. In Debmalya Barh, Vasco Azevedo (eds.). *Omics Technologies and Bio-Engineering* (pp. 323–336). Academic Press. https://doi.org/10.1016/B978-0-12-815870-8.00017-6

[3] Holanda, L. J., Silva, P. M. M., Amorim, T. C., Lacerda, M. O., Simão, C. R., & Morya, E. (2017). Robotic-assisted gait as a tool for rehabilitation of individuals with spinal cord injury: A systematic review. *Journal of Neuroengineering and Rehabilitation*, *14*(1), 126. https://doi.org/10.1186/s12984-017-0338-7

[4] Denecke, K., & Baudoin, C. R. (2022). A review of artificial intelligence and robotics in transformed health ecosystems. *Frontiers in Medicine*, *9*, 795957. https://doi.org/10.3389/fmed.2022.795957

[5] Vaid, A., Sawant, A., Suarez-Farinas, M., Lee, J., Kaul, S., Kovatch, P., Freeman, R., Jiang, J., Jayaraman, P., Fayad, Z., Argulian, E., Lerakis, S., Charney, A. W., Wang, F., Levin, M., Glicksberg, B., Narula, J., Hofer, I., Singh, K., & Nadkarni, G. N. (2023). Implications of the use of artificial intelligence predictive models in health care settings: A simulation study. *Annals of Internal Medicine*, *176*(10), 1358–1369. https://doi.org/10.7326/M23-0949

[6] Camarillo, D. B., Krummel, T. M., & Kenneth Salisbury, J. (2004). Robotic technology in surgery: Past, present, and future. *The American Journal of Surgery*, 188(4 supplement 1), 2–15. https://doi.org/10.1016/j.amjsurg.2004.08.025

[7] Tiwana, M. I., Redmond, S. J., & Lovell, N. H. (2012). A review of tactile sensing technologies with applications in biomedical engineering. *Sensors and Actuators A: Physical*, 179, 17–31. https://doi.org/10.1016/j.sna.2012.02.051

[8] Senapati, S., & Advincula, A. P. (2005). Telemedicine and robotics: Paving the way to the globalization of surgery. *International Journal of Gynecology & Obstetrics*, 91, 3, 210–216. https://doi.org/10.1016/j.ijgo.2005.08.016

[9] Vicentini, F., Pedrocchi, N., Malosio, M., & Tosatti, L. M. (2014). SafeNet: A methodology for integrating general-purpose unsafe devices in safe-robot rehabilitation systems. *Computer Methods and Programs in Biomedicine*, 116(2), 156–168. https://doi.org/10.1016/j.cmpb.2014.03.001

[10] Nazmul Huda, M., Yu, H., & Cang, S. (2016). Robots for minimally invasive diagnosis and intervention. *Robotics and Computer-Integrated Manufacturing*, 41, 127–144. https://doi.org/10.1016/j.rcim.2016.03.003

[11] Sapci, H. (2019). Innovative assisted living tools, remote monitoring technologies, artificial intelligence-driven solutions, and robotic systems for aging societies: Systematic review. *JMIR Aging*, 2(2), e15429. https://doi.org/10.2196/15429

[12] Rus, D., & Tolley, M. T. (2015). Design, fabrication, and control of soft robots. *Nature*, 521(7553), 467–475. https://doi.org/10.1038/nature14543

[13] Sun, J., Kramer, E. H., & Rosen, J. (2024). A safety-focused admittance control approach for physical human–robot interaction with rigid multi-arm serial link exoskeletons. *IEEE/ASME Transactions on Mechatronics*. https://doi.org/10.1109/TMECH.2024.3389046

[14] Meskó, B., Drobni, Z., Bényei, É., Gergely, B., & Győrffy, Z. (2017). Digital health is a cultural transformation of traditional healthcare. *mHealth*, 3, 38. https://doi.org/10.21037/mhealth.2017.08.07

[15] Zhang, Y., & Jiang, J. (2008). Bibliographical review on reconfigurable fault-tolerant control systems. *Annual Reviews in Control*, 32(2), 229–252. https://doi.org/10.1016/j.arcontrol.2008.03.008

[16] Kim, S., Laschi, C., & Trimmer, B. (2013). Soft robotics: A bioinspired evolution in robotics. *Trends in Biotechnology*, 31(5), 287–294. https://doi.org/10.1016/j.tibtech.2013.03.002

[17] Laschi, C., Mazzolai, B., & Cianchetti, M. (2016). Soft robotics: Technologies and systems pushing the boundaries of robot abilities. *Science Robotics*, 1(1), eaah3690. https://doi.org/10.1126/scirobotics.aah3690

[18] Cianchetti, M., Laschi, C., Menciassi, A., & Dario, P. (2018). Biomedical applications of soft robotics. *Nature Reviews Materials*, 3, 143–153. https://doi.org/10.1038/s41578-018-0022-y

[19] Laschi, C., & Cianchetti, M. (2014). Soft robotics: New perspectives for robot bodyware and control. *Frontiers in Bioengineering and Biotechnology*, 2, 3. https://doi.org/10.3389/fbioe.2014.00003

[20] Giuliani, M., Lenz, C., Müller, T., Rickert, M., & Knoll, A. (2010). Design principles for safety in human-robot interaction. *International Journal of Social Robotics,* 2(3), 253–274. https://doi.org/10.1007/s12369-010-0052-0

[21] Lasota, P. A., Fong, T., & Shah, J. A. (2020). A survey of methods for safe human-robot interaction. *Reliability Engineering & System Safety*, 199, 106885. http://doi.org/10.1561/2300000052

[22] Wang, Z., & Wang, Y. (2023). Integrated sensors for soft medical robotics. *Small,* 19(1), 2308805. https://doi.org/10.1002/smll.202308805

[23] Zhang, Y., & Jiang, J. (2021). Review of fault-tolerant control systems used in robotic manipulators. *Applied Sciences*, 13(4), 2675. https://doi.org/10.3390/app13042675

[24] Li, Y., & Wang, Y. (2024). Enhanced fault-tolerant kinematic control of redundant robots with joint limit consideration. *Engineering Applications of Artificial Intelligence*, 125, 106304. https://doi.org/10.1016/j.engappai.2024.108068

[25] Siciliano, B., & Khatib, O. Redundant robots. In B. Siciliano & O. Khatib (eds.). *Springer Handbook of Robotics* (pp. 173–200). https://doi.org/10.1007/978-3-319-32552-1 (2016)

[26] Topol, E. J. (2019). High-performance medicine: The convergence of human and artificial intelligence. *Nature Medicine*, 25(1), 44–56. https://doi.org/10.1038/s41591-018-0300-7

[27] Polygerinos, P., Wang, Z., Galloway, K. C., Wood, R. J., & Walsh, C. J. (2015). *Soft robotic glove for combined assistance and at-home rehabilitation. Robotics and Autonomous Systems*, 73, 135–143. https://doi.org/10.1016/j.robot.2014.08.014

[28] Omeye, F. (2025). Autonomous robots in surgery: The future of precision medicine. *ResearchGate,* Eabb5589, February. https://doi.org/10.59298/ROJBAS/2025/523639

[29] Yang, G. Z., Nelson, J. B., Murphy, R. R., Choset, H., Christensen, H., Collins, H. S., ... & McNutt, M. (2020). Combating COVID-19—The role of robotics in managing public health and infectious diseases. *Science Robot* 5. https://doi.org/10.1126/scirobotics.abb5589

[30] Seeliger, B., Collins, J .W., Porpiglia, F., & Marescaux, J. (2022). The role of virtual reality, telesurgery, and teleproctoring in robotic surgery. In Wiklund, P., Mottrie, A., Gundeti, M.S., Patel, V. (Eds.), *Robotic Urologic Surgery*. Springer. https://doi.org/10.1007/978-3-031-00363-9_8

[31] Li, J., Xu, Z., Zhu, D., Dong, K., Yan, T., Zeng, Z., & Yang, S. X. (2022). Bio inspired intelligence with robotics applications: A survey. *arXiv.* https://doi.org/10.48550/arXiv.2206.08544

[32] Momani, A. (2025). Implications of artificial intelligence on health data privacy and confidentiality. *arXiv*. https://doi.org/10.48550/arXiv.2501.01639arXiv

[33] Gastrich, M. D., Barone, J., Bachmann, G., Anderson, M., & Balica, A. (2011). Robotic surgery: Review of the latest advances, risks, and outcomes. *Journal of Robotic Surgery*, 5, 79–97. https://doi.org/10.1007/s11701-011-0246-y

[34] Zhang, Y., & Jiang, J. (2008). Bibliographical review on reconfigurable fault-tolerant control systems. *Annual Reviews in Control*, 32(2), 229–252. https://doi.org/10.1016/j.arcontrol.2008.03.008

[35] Weiner, E. B., Dankwa-Mullan, I., Nelson, W. A., & Hassanpour, S. (2024). Ethical challenges and evolving strategies in the integration of artificial intelligence into clinical practice. *arXiv*. https://doi.org/10.48550/arXiv.2412.03576

[36] Pasricha, S. (2022). AI ethics in smart healthcare. *arXiv*. https://doi.org/10.48550/arXiv.2211.06346

12 Biomedical Robots for Surgery

The State of the Art and the Future Expected Advancements

R. S. Varsha and G. Y. Rajaa Vikhram

12.1 INTRODUCTION

Biomedical robotics is one of the most competitive fields of robotics at present and has made its own significant space in biomedical engineering. Robotic surgery is a medical technology that has developed the accuracy and precision of different biomedical instruments used in surgery. Robotic surgical instruments have great potential to assist surgeons and increase medical access to other communities in the future. Biomedical robotics involved in the medical field can be classified into various sectors: service robots, rehabilitation support robots, and robotic instruments for surgery [1].

The basic idea of robotics in the field of medical surgery began during World War I when robots were needed to treat remotely injured soldiers. From then, the introduction of biomedical robots had a huge impact. The Tele-presence era marked the beginning of biomedical robotics in surgery with Dr. Green's and Dr. Rosen's work at Stanford Research Institute (SRI) [2]. They developed a prototype of a telepresence surgical system which marked the introduction of biomedical robots for surgery. The debut of the robotic arm PUMA 200 [3] had an inevitable impact on the development of stereotaxic procedures. The sensor integration and various drive system introductions made a complete robotic setup with marked convenience in terms of understanding and usage. Various sensors in the domain of surgery include temperature sensors, position sensors, and pressure sensors; each integrated in a system according to the application. The first section of this chapter covers the evolution of biomedical robots in the field of medical surgery followed by the structural organization components of a biomedical robot. The next section covers the broad classification of biomedical robots. The last section covers the recent technologies in the field of research that are about to revolutionize the field of surgical robots. The sectional flow diagram is given in Figure 12.1. The flow chart elaborates the chapter sections, which include the introduction, evolution of biomedical robots, components of a common biomedical robot, and the future developments in the domain.

DOI: 10.1201/9781003561309-12

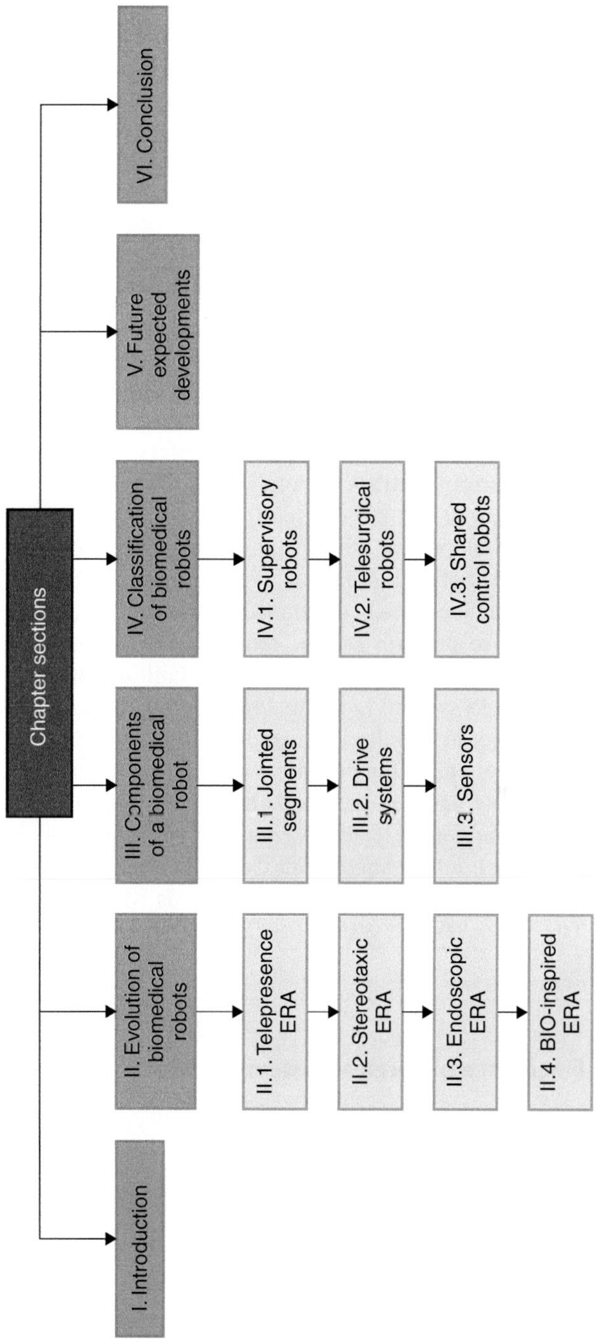

FIGURE 12.1 Flow diagram.

12.2 EVOLUTION OF BIOMEDICAL ROBOTS

Robotics in the field of medical surgery has seen constant development and updates. Starting as a master-slave system, it now has self-operating modules. An autonomous system in the field of surgery is no longer impossible. The development of the latest technology, such as artificial intelligence and various computing techniques like cognitive computing, contributes to the level of independence of robotic surgery. The Turing test and another human-machine tests could provide solutions for the development of this field. The summary is presented in Table 12.1.

12.2.1 The Telepresence Era

The idea of robotics in the field of medical surgery began during the combat. Aid for the combat soldiers was only from the medical unit which was inaccessible during the immediate need. The concept of tele surgery was introduced back then, in which a surgeon could treat the combat soldier with a mobilizing system that has robotic telemanipulation and telepresence. Telemanipulation refers to the class of robotics that allows the user to perform actions remotely with a human-machine interface. Scott Fisher, a virtual reality (VR) pioneer, built a Head Mounted Display (HMD) that introduced the idea of telepresence that displayed the 3D environment of a remote location [2]. Joseph Rosen, a plastic surgeon working on nerves and vasculature anastomosis, and Phil Green, a bioengineer, developed a robotic telemanipulation system that enables the surgeon to perform actions remotely by a computerized human-machine interface [3]. Green's research on ultrasound built the base for what to do in developing a teleoperated system. Later, in 1987, Green and Rosen built a prototype of a teleoperated robot at Standard Research Institute (SRI) which they called a "telepresence surgery system." This prototype included a 3D visualization screen and detachable instruments when in the hands of the surgeon. This prototype had four degrees of freedom and forced feedback control supporting the surgery. Richard Satava, a US Army colonel, joined hands with Green as the SRI began the development of a telepresence surgery system for military needs where a soldier could be treated remotely. The first developed system consisted of the tele surgical workstation

TABLE 12.1
Timeline of the Emergence of Surgical Systems

Year	Company	Invention	References
1987	Unimation	PUMA200 was launched	[4]
1994	Computer Motion	AESOP 1 got its FDA approval	[4]
1995	Intuitive Surgical	ZEUS system was introduced	[8]
2000	Intuitive Surgical	Da Vinci system was introduced	[6]
1992	Integrated Surgical Supplies	ROBODOC was introduced	[8]
2001	Intuitive Surgical	The ZEUS system got its FDA approval	[8]

(TWS) and the remote surgical unit (RSU). In the TWS, the surgeon was provided with surgical instrument manipulators that transmitted signals to the Remote Surgical Unit (RSU). In the Remote Surgical Unit, the end-effectors were a needle, bowel graspers, scalpels, and cautery tips. These end-effectors were placed in exchangeable patterns with a twist-lock mechanism to provide convenience for the surgeon. In 1995, Green patented this device under the name "Green's Telepresence Surgery System" [1].

12.2.2 The Stereotaxic Era

Stereotaxic surgery is a radiation therapy in which correct coordinates for the desired location are located and high beam radiation is focused on the particular area. It is often used for brain biopsies and other radiation-related techniques such as surgical targeting of electrodes, and resection instruments to treat tumors, epilepsy, and vascular malformation. The start of stereotaxic surgery began in 1908 when Sir Victor Alexander Haden Horsley and Robert Henry Clarke [4] developed a three orthogonal axis Cartesian system to specify the location of the lesions in the brain. Their first success was when they used an electrode-based guide and the 3D Cartesian system to describe the lesioning targets of a monkey's brain based on the skull landmarks. Later, Canadian neuroanatomist Aubrey Mussen joined hands in the development of the Horsley-Clarke system for human use [4]. The first stereotactic device was used by Martin Kirschner for the treatment of the trigeminal nerve and ablating it. The theory of Stereotaxic surgery attained further development with technologies such as CT and MRI. In 1985, the first clinical-use robot, PUMA 200, was introduced [5]. This system was used for a brain biopsy technique in which the surgeon placed the robotic arm performs the task according to the command from the surgeon. The robot has two systems: a mechanical unit and a computer control unit. The mechanical unit facilitated the mobility of the robot and the controller unit enabled greater precision of the robot. Later PUMA 200 was used for resection of astrocytomas of the thalamus. In the field of orthopedics, ROBODOC was developed by Integrated Surgical Supplies in 1992 and the SCARA robot was introduced. The mechanical actions specifies the mobility of the system to move to the commanded coordinates [5].

12.2.3 The Endoscopic Era

The idea of endoscopy in the field of surgery is aimed at carrying out surgical procedures with the body's natural openings rather than creating contrived invasions. The development of endoscopy ranged from the inclusion of various scientific principles and mechanically operated structures to semi-automatically operated instruments. In 1853, Antonin Desormeaux, often regarded as the "father of endoscopy," developed the first scientific endoscope and was successful in removing urethral tumors with his invention [6]. Later a German urologist, Maximilian Nitze refined the Desormeaux model by replacing kerosene lamps with platinum wire thus ensuring safety. Science and design of endoscopes varied with inventions and attained the stage of semi-autonomous operation.

AESOP, developed by Computer Motion, was the first medical used endoscopic instrument. Yulun Wang, founder of Computer Motion developed the first robotic arm with an endoscope, a mission partly funded by DARPA (Defense Advanced Research Project Agency). The AESOP system had two core components: the endoscope attached to the robotic arm and the surgeon control unit. The surgeon control unit has all the components for receiving information from the surgeon such as voice control. The AESOP 1 had manual control which gained approval from the Food and Drug Administration (FDA) in 1994. Two years later, AESOP 2 was developed, in which the manual control was replaced with a voice command-based control procedure. This system's effectiveness was proposed to be a surgeon's "third hand." AESOP 3 and AESOP HR were released later with greater improvement in voice control integrated with various other functions mentioned by the surgeon.

The ZEUS system and da Vinci system have an inevitable part in the evolution of endoscopic surgery. The ZEUS system was introduced in 1998 by Computer Motion [7]. The two separate units, namely the console and the robotic arm, provided extended dexterity for the surgeons during surgery. The ZEUS system was equipped with three arms, the first was the AESOP robotic arm attached with an endoscope, and the other two arms mimicked the surgeon's actions from the console. The ZEUS system allowed surgeons to perform remote surgery as the console was teleoperated. Scaling down the movements was an added advantage of the ZEUS system that entered into competition with the da Vinci systems. In 1995, F. Moll and R. Young founded Intuitive Surgical aiming to rework Green's telepresence model [8]. They launched Lenny, referred to as Leonardo, which has three robotic arms. One of the three arms was attached to a scope camera and the other two covered the instruments. Later, intuitive surgical came up with MONA [6], the first surgical robot to be used for human surgeries. Jacques Himpens in 1997 first used the MONA system to perform a cholecystectomies surgery on a 72-year-old patient. The third generation of Intuitive Surgical was the da Vinci system which got its FDA approval in 2000 and stood as tough competition for the ZEUS systems [8]. The da Vinci systems are the most used in the medical field with numerous medical instruments.

12.2.4 The Bioinspired Era

Bioinspired surgical robots are those that mimic the locomotion of biological organisms such as an octopus, snake, elephant's trunk, etc. The introduction of these systems improved flexibility constraint for an instrument. The wide exposed endoscopy and minimally invasive surgery (MIS) techniques adopted bioinspired technology that led to the development of scarless surgery. The endoscopy and MIS surgeries used Natural Orifice Transluminal Endoscopic Surgery (NOTES) which condense the multiple arms of a robot to a single-handed robot. Soft grippers are the most used end-effectors strategy of this robot design and are used in delicate operations.

12.3 COMPONENTS OF A BIOMEDICAL ROBOT

The biomedical robots from the 1980s had the advantage of a precise alignment mechanism and a supportive design for transport and stability. A biomedical robot is one such system that has the proper proportion of the mechanical, electrical, and computational integration. A general biomedical robot consists of a (1) jointed segments, (2) a drive system, and (3) sensors

12.3.1 Jointed Segments

These are the building blocks of the biomedical robot that provide the mechanical stability of the robot system. It comprises of base segments, links, and joints that are designed on the basis of the application of the system. For example, a general da Vinci robotic surgery system has seven degrees of freedom, facilitating mobility across the surgery space. The surgical system can have different configurations based on its type of joints, its applications, etc., which explains the basic layout of the system.

A) Base Segment
The base segment is the foundation for the surgical system that connects the entire system to the stable surface and provides the axis of rotation. In a surgical system, the base has to be robust and accumulate the entire mass in the center of the system to resist the change in the control coordinates of the system. The base segment of a surgical system can be static or mobile. A few robotic systems such as those used in MIS have no ability for base movement and are fixed installations in a confined space. Other robotic systems, such as the console monitor, endoscopic system, etc., accommodate wheels or other portable structures on the base to facilitate the movement of the system from one location to the other. In comparison, an immobile base segment has more precision in surgery than a system with a mobile base. This advantage of precision relies on the tolerance for the unwanted vibrations and movements of the system produced during the time of surgery [9].

B) Arm Segments
The arm segments determine the flexibility and dexterity of the surgical system. Every robotic surgery system mimics human hands, thereby increasing the efficiency of the system and allowing easy actions for the surgeons to control the system. The greater the number of arm segments in the system, the greater the work volume of the system, but it usually lacks accuracy and precision as the system requires time to return to its original position. The lack of accuracy in identifying the centre point origin of the coordinate mapping collapses the entire coordinate setup of the system. Hence, the systems are set with an appropriate number of arm segments connected to the end effectors [10]. The constituents of the arm segments are shown in Figure 12.2, and their basic orientation is shown in Figure 12.3. Arm segments can be classified into four main categories: the upper arm segment, shoulder segment, wrist arm segment, and the elbow segment.

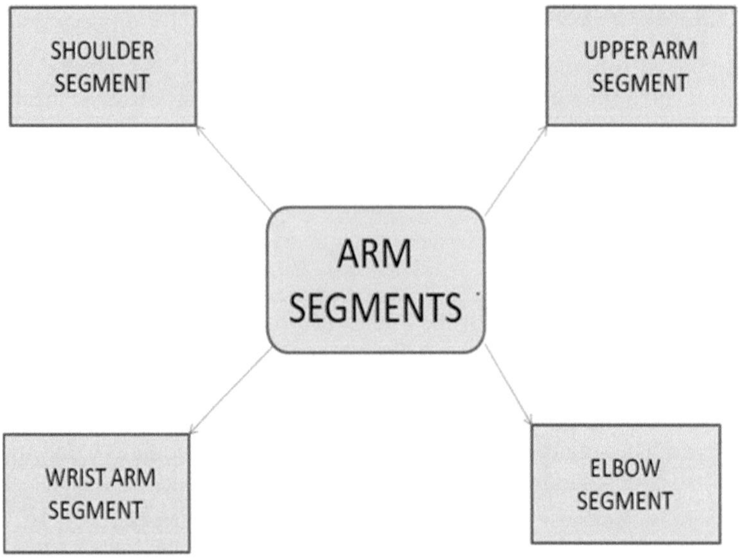

FIGURE 12.2 Types of arm segments.

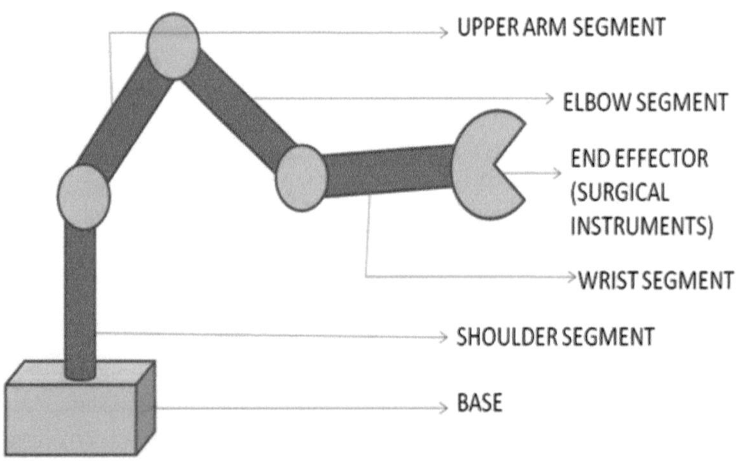

FIGURE 12.3 Robotic manipulator.

1. Shoulder arm segment: Attached to the base segment and marks the foundation for the robotic arm with rotational and linear joins according to the system application.
2. Upper arm segment: Connects the shoulder segment to the elbow joint, mimicking the humerus bone of human.
3. Elbow arm segment: Follows the upper arm and runs to the wrist arm segment. The number of elbow joints in a system may vary in different applications.

The greater the number of elbow joints, the greater the additional degree of freedom for the surgical system.

4. Wrist arm segment: This is the major arm segment that is connected to the final end effectors. Built on the basis of stability analysis, it has more precision than the other arm segments in order to check the position of end effectors. Fig 12.2 shows a robotic arm with three joints and four links. The segments of the robotic arm are described. From the base to the first joint is the shoulder segment. The segments in between the next consecutive joints are the upper arm segment. The link between the third joint and the end-effector is the wrist segment.

C) Joint Segments

The joints in the system determine the degrees of freedom and connect the arm segments together. The work of these joints provides the movement of the arm segments and the data from the joint segments are required for the haptic feedback mechanism. With the feedback values, the surgeons can feel the organs that are in non-contact with human hands and experience the delicate pressure applied on the organ by the surgical instruments.

12.3.2 Drive Systems

Though the physical structure of a surgical system is stable with the joints, a system's full efficiency is the task of the drive systems that actuate the arms and instruments to perform actions. The drive system includes the actuator and the actuating mechanism. Generally, a surgical robot contains three common mechanisms, such as electric drives, pneumatic drives, and hydraulic drives, which are chosen according to the surgical needs and specifications. An electric drive is known for its easy mechanism and provides an easy interface for the surgeons. Table 12.2 highlights the common differences between pneumatic and electric drives.

A) Pneumatic Drives

Pneumatic drives are operated by pressurized gas that produces the force for actuation. Common Minimally Invasive Surgery (MIS). The former system did not include pressure distribution within the system and also lacked a pneumatic gripping mechanism. These pneumatic drives find application in the fields of orthopedics and otolaryngology. Pneumatics is known for its compact spatial allotment and easy actuation. Various procedures in an orthopedic surgery are usually pneumatic (i.e.) the end-effectors' actuation is managed by the level of pressurized gas. As the final values are monitored throughout the process, pneumatically driven systems are usually used for various applications of biomedical robots. A few instruments in the otolaryngology domain are also pneumatically operated. High precision and efficiency ensure the ability of the instrument. One such pneumatically operated biomedical robot is the Saroa Robot [11], which is a pneumatically operated surgical robot developed by da

TABLE 12.2
Comparison Between Pneumatic and Electric Drive System in a Biomedical Robot

Parameters	Pneumatic Drives	Electric Drives
Accuracy	Pneumatic drives have less accuracy when compared to a electric system as the pressure cannot be controlled by a direct controller	An electric drive system has high accuracy and precision as the actuation is a rotary or linear motion
Construction	A pneumatic drive system has a simpler construction as the components integration is easier.	Electric drive system has a complex construction as it involves placement of components in right space and required angle.
Noise	When the pressure is released, there is a hissing sound in the instrument	There are no such sounds created in electric drives. In exception, the unwanted vibration from motors can trigger sound in the system
Dependency and Reliability	A pneumatic system has less reliability when compared to a n electric drive system	Has high reliability when compared to the pneumatic system as it has consistency and stability in the output values.
Flexibility	Though it has easy installation, heavier elements such as the cylinders make the system bulkier. Hence, it has less flexibility	Made of flexible materials and marks the reachability of the system

Vinci systems. The wires are simultaneously driven by the pneumatic cylinders which supplies the necessary pressure to the end jaw of the instrument. These pressure signals are translated to the hand console as electrical signals and the necessary changes in the input signal are varied. The inclusion of force and the concept of haptic feedback mechanism upgraded the reliability of pneumatic drivers and provided a hands-on feel for surgeons.

B) Electric Drives

Motors are the most commonly used electric drive system in a surgical system. The motors provide the necessary actuation required for the movement and action of the surgical instrument. There is a wide range of motors that can be used in a surgical robot. The right selection and combination of these motors relies on the need for motion in the particular location where the motor is fixed. Step motors are usually used in joint segments to ensure stepwise actuation of the joints [12]. Unwanted resonant frequency vibrations and movements in the system can produce a loud noise. These limitations can be overcome by using damping conditions to reduce the

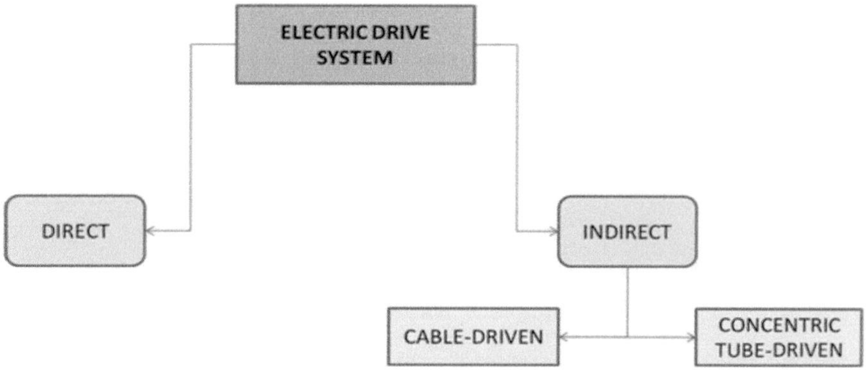

FIGURE 12.4 Classification of EDS.

vibrations, and limiting the steps into micro steps can influence the reliability of the system. Servo motors are the most commonly used drivers in a surgical robot as they have a fast response and a real-time feedback control loop. A servo motor attached to the instrument has a smooth motion and does not cause any unwanted jerks during the surgery. The speed and the angular position of the motor are preset according to the needs of the instrument ensuring that the motor moves according to the surgeon's actions and commands.

Classification of Electric Drive Actuation

Figure 12.4 details the classification of the drive system based on the location of the motors and the medium of motion. The electric drive systems (EDS) can be classified into two categories: direct and indirect. In the basic direct electric drives, the motors are directly attached to the mechanical body without any intermediate. The signal from the motors directly drives the instrument. Indirect electric drives require an intermediate medium between the motor and the mechanical body. These can be a flexible material or other connectors that can drive the arrangement. Concentric-tube mechanisms and cable-driven mechanisms are the basic types of indirect electric drives used in surgical instruments. Based on the force required for the surgical instrument and based on the flexibility aspects and reachability, the drive systems are acquired. A cable-driven mechanism is used in minimally invasive surgery [13], which doesn't require more flexibility and requires short-range precise actuation. Indirect EDS can be further classified into cable-driven and concentric tube EDS, which is discussed in detail below.

Concentric-tube drives are those which have concentric tubes packed one inside the other that extend to the height required according to the commands, as shown in Figure 12.5. The concentric tubes are made of pre-curved flexible material that can also bend in any axis, in addition to the linear extension [14]. A concentric-tube drive system finds wide applications in the field of otolaryngology and prostate surgery as it involves small incision instruments.

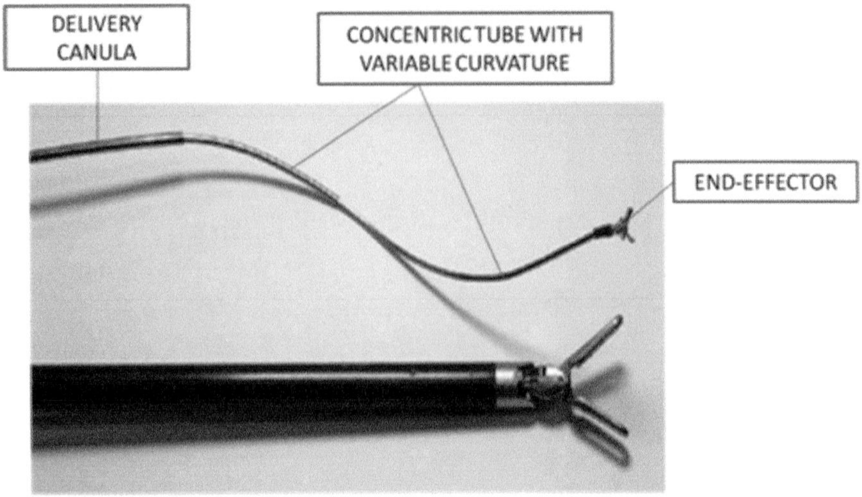

FIGURE 12.5 Concentric tube drive system [15].

12.3.3 Sensors

Figure 12.6 shows the sensor classification used in the medical field. The divisions include position-based (subdivided into encoders and potentiometers), pressure-based (subdivided into capacitive type, piezoelectric type, and piezoresistive type sensors), and temperature-based (subdivided into thermocouple and infrared sensors).

12.3.3.1 Position-Based Sensors

In a surgical robot, the position of the actuators plays a crucial role in the entire surgery. These sensors provide values about the movement of the end-effectors thereby reducing the error in the system. Position sensor alerts the system about the current location of the joint arms and joint segments and also make it easier to handle MIS instruments. In the sector of rehabilitation robots, position sensors are the major sensing elements in prosthetics and exoskeleton designs. During the rehabilitation period, the prosthetic limb and exoskeleton's range and movement can be noted by the position data. The data from the sensors are necessary for the surgeon to check the improvements in the recovery. The sub-classification of these sensors is listed in Figure 12.6.

A) Encoders

The encoder in a surgical system measures the displacement and converts the mechanical movement into electrical signals which are then monitored and controlled. Encoders can be broadly classified into rotary and linear encoders. If the encoder senses the change in rotation motion, it is a rotary encoder, whereas the encoders that sense the change in linear movement are known as linear encoders. There are other types of encoders such as an optical encoder, magnetic encoder, and more that are chosen on the requirement of the encoder detection mechanism. An encoder consists

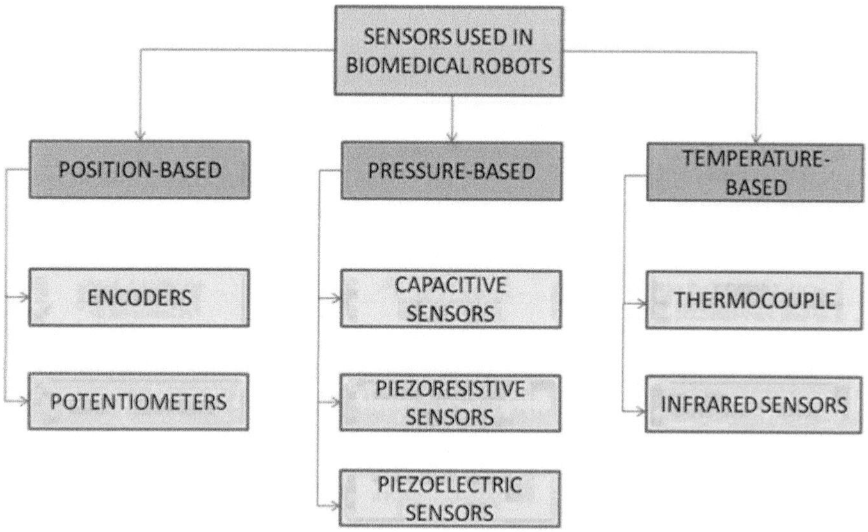

FIGURE 12.6 Classification of sensors used in biomedical robots.

of a disc that rotates along with the joint segment rotation. The light sensor present in the encoder converts these signals into electrical pulses which are used to determine the rate of revolution and exact position of the system [16]. The encoder feedback is fed to the control system which causes movement of the body and provides accurate actions for the surgeon's commands.

B) Potentiometers

The potentiometer relies on the value of change in the resistance. Changes in the length and area of the line can vary the resistance value. In a potentiometer, the change in the resistance is converted into an electrical signal and fed as feedback to the console. A potentiometer in a surgical system consists of a wiper that is attached to the joint segment of the robot. When the joint segment undergoes a movement, the wiper position changes (i.e.) the length of the conductive line that the wiper is in contact with varies, thus varying the resistance. This change in resistance is converted into a voltage output and fed to the control system. This value of voltage is considered as the current position value and compared with the surgeon input value from the console. The variations in the reading are adjusted by the actuators from the control signals.

12.3.3.2 Pressure-Based Sensors

A) Capacitance Sensors

A capacitance sensor relies on the working principle of change in capacitance due to the change in distance between the two plates. The capacitor is an electrical storage unit that stores the electric field to its threshold. The threshold value of the electric field the plates of the capacitor can store is expressed in terms of capacitance. Usually, in a capacitance sensor, one of the plates of the capacitor is kept movable and the other is immovable. When a force is exerted on the movable plate of the capacitance sensor, the distance between the plates is varied which causes a change in the capacitance value [16]. The variation in the capacitance value is processed into voltage signal output. Many capacitance sensors that measure force include oscillators or capacitance bridges to decouple the force from the capacitance. The equations for the force and capacitance calculated are listed below [17],

$$\mathbf{C=\varepsilon A/d}$$

$$\frac{CV^2}{2d} = F$$

where

C=Capacitance
D=Distance between two plates
F=force exerted on the mobile plate
ε=Permittivity of dielectric material.

Recent studies on capacitive sensors have resulted in inclusion of these sensors in the MIS. The distance between the plates of the capacitor was reduced to be very minimal, and the capacitance change was noted. This can be used for very-high resolution systems and these can sense a micro-newton force input.

B) Piezoresistive Sensors

A piezoresistive sensor in a surgical system measures the change in deformation by calculating the change in the resistance value. The commonly used piezoelectric sensor in the field of medical robotics includes a strain gauge with a Wheatstone bridge arrangement. As there is a stress or force exerted by the surgeon on the console, the resistance of the arrangement varies which is calculated in terms of electrical output either in terms of voltage or current. The strain gauge arrangement is usually made of a flexible material called flexure [17]. To make the system more reliable, these materials are now replaced by monolithic metals. The major disadvantage of the strain gauge relies on its hysteresis. When the sensor is subjected to excess load force, the flexure cannot recover to its initial state. The data of the resistance change is passed as a voltage signal and is made to be the same of the same force exerted by the surgeon to the console.

C) Piezoelectric Sensors

Piezoelectric materials are those that generate a voltage difference when exposed to a physical stress or a force. This is due to the accumulation of opposite charges on either side of the material that mimics a capacitor design. The voltage thus generated is taken for readings and the material reformations stop the voltage flow. This is known as piezoelectricity. In a surgical instrument, when the surgeon applies force on the device, which has a piezoelectric sensor, it processes a voltage output. The control system is fed with the voltage input compares it with the force exerted and adjusts the actuation accordingly. The feedback signal is then transferred to the system for further calculations.

12.3.3.3 Temperature-Based Sensors

A) Thermocouple

A thermocouple is made up of two different metals which vary in their temperature coefficient. It usually has two junctions, one being the output port through which the potential difference is calculated. The other end is exposed to the environment, whose temperature has to be noted. In the field of surgery, these thermocouples are used to monitor the temperature of the soft tissues during cryosurgery. When the hot junction end of the thermocouple is exposed to the soft tissue of the patient, there is a flow of electrons due to the heat produced [18]. Since the elements are made of two different materials, the electron flow is not the same in both metals due to the difference in the thermal coefficient. This variation in the flow creates an EMF, and the voltage output is noted. This voltage is proportional to the change in temperature. In the case of ablation techniques, these thermocouples can be used to monitor the temperature rise and provide real-time feedback. Figure 12.7 shows a thermocouple medical sensor with the parts detailed. On one end is a pair of metal wires with different coefficients. On the other end is an end-effector junction exposed to the patient's tissues.

B) Infrared Sensors

Infrared sensors are usually used to avoid obstacles and detect objects on the path. In medical robots, these sensors are used to determine the temperature of a patient with its absorption principle. The sensor has two major components: the transmitter and the receiver. The transmitter transmits the IR radiation to the environment, in

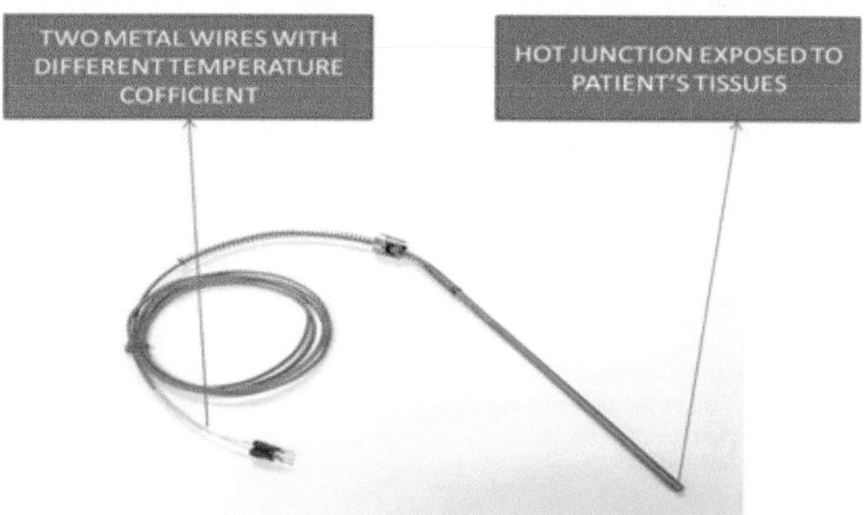

FIGURE 12.7 Thermocouple sensors [19].

this case, the patient's body, and notes the return signals in the receiver end. The change in the intensity of the radiation is calibrated in terms of temperature. These sensors are used in digital thermometers and ensure non-contact temperature detection techniques. This non-contact technique can extend the advantages in terms of the prevention of spread of diseases. Based on the type of material and strategy used for monitoring the temperature of the radiation, these sensors can be divided into pyroelectric sensors and bolometers. The pyroelectric sensors are sensitive materials that sense the change in intensity of the incident infrared radiation. The bolometer measures the small changes in the temperature with high sensitivity. With high resolution, the infrared radiation technique for the determination of temperature is more feasible and widely used in many instruments.

12.4 BROAD CLASSIFICATION OF BIOMEDICAL ROBOTS

12.4.1 Supervisory Robots

Supervisory robots are usually semi-automated, depending on the principle of process control and vehicle control theory. When these robots are used for surgery, the surgeon preplans the surgical steps and loads the mechanism into the robot. The surgery is supervised by human surgeons, hence the name. There are usually two types of approaches to this type of surgery. The first is a fully programmed process in which the programming is preset before the surgery and the surgeon can interrupt the process and make necessary changes whenever needed. The second is a stepwise surgery in which the surgeon programs the robot to complete the particular step in the surgery. As the system passes the feedback, the surgeon programs the robot with the next step. These approaches do not require the surgeon's continuous presence and actions throughout the surgery. The surgeon's work in the surgery relies on the robot programming according to the condition. The proper procedure for the surgery involves three major steps:

1. Planning
2. Registration
3. Navigation

Planning

In this process, the surgeon analyzes the patient's condition and plans the required actions for the surgery. The next step for the surgeon is to analyze the patient's body and go through the vital requirements. The surgeon then designs a 3D mapping of the patient's body part which must undergo the surgery. These data are then fed to the robot, and the robot is programmed to perform the commands from the surgeon. The 3D mapping data of the patient paves the way for the robotic system to identify the location and plan the path for the instruments [20].

Registration

This is the crucial process in the supervisory surgery that marks the success of the surgery. The surgeon places the patient in a particular position that coincides with the 3D mapping model created for the patient. Reference point marking aligns the 3D model and the patient's posture. The reference point marked in the 3D model is compared with the actual patient posture and the alignment of the model and patient position is checked. In some cases, the surgeons make changes in the model to properly align with the patient's posture. In some supervisory robots, the 3D mapping model is replaced with imaging techniques that use ultrasound and fluoroscopy as the principle of operation for the alignment of patient posture and the robot's reference points.

Navigation

In this step, the robot is supervised in the accuracy of movements and proper navigation of the manipulator to the programmed location. There are many navigation techniques. The 3D mapping that has the points of reference can be used for the navigation. The changes in the accuracy can be noted by the sensors or other imaging techniques and the feedback is provided in real time. In the case of discrepancies, the surgeons can change the programming and get the manipulator back to the proper alignment.

Pros and Cons of the Supervisory Robot

The major reason for the usage of the robots is accuracy and precision. The haptic feedback signals can be supervised and can alert the surgeon in case of a change in set point. The manipulator works with very high precision and reduces the recovery time and the chances of Post Traumatic Stress Disorder (PTSD) conditions for the patient. Though the manipulator performs the surgeon's commands, the deviation from the reference point can destroy the entire process. As the surgery is automated, there may be chances of soft tissue damage and other unexpected damage in the patient's body.

12.4.2 Tele Surgical Robots

As mentioned above, the idea of teleoperation for a surgery was raised to treat soldiers injured in combat remotely. The tele surgical robot can also be called a remote surgical robot, or a master-slave surgical system. The main focus of the tele surgery system was to bring a gap between the patient and the surgeon and perform surgeries with communication technologies. A robotic manipulator is in contact with the patient and performs the commands given by the console controlled by the surgeon. In this surgical technique, the manipulator and the console unit are connected via a wireless communication system that is suitable for remote operations. There is a series of technical and technological developments in the system design which marked the reliability of the system for medical surgeries. The tele surgical system consists of two major parts: the console unit and the robotic manipulator. One such system is shown in Figure 12.8. The first telesurgical operation was done in 2001 in France for a patient with cholecystectomy [21]. The surgery took about 54 minutes and the patient recovered without any complications. Telesurgery in the 2000s was over a low grade network when compared to the present 4G and 5G network communications. Figure 12.9 shows the control system loop of the tele surgical system. The technique was tested in China where a single surgeon console controlled about 12 manipulators without latency error and network lag.

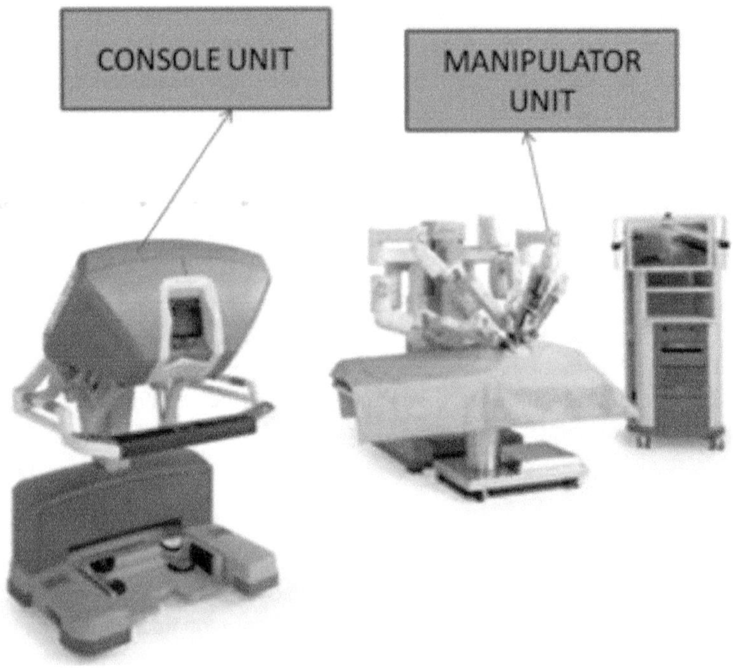

FIGURE 12.8 da Vinci tele surgical system.

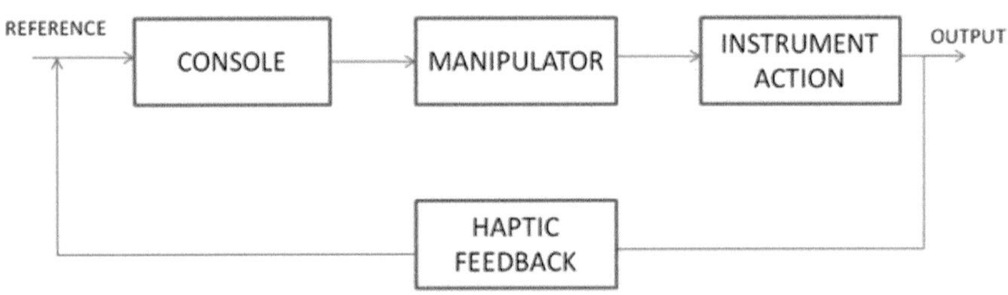

FIGURE 12.9 Control loop for a tele-surgical system.

The da Vinci system has a console unit and a manipulator unit [22]. The console unit has a monitor screen and a controller joystick to direct the manipulator arm motion. On the other side, a manipulator arm is equipped with a robotic arm. The end-effector of the arm includes a medical instrument that is controlled by the surgeon motion command.

The reference input is fed to the console, which is then passed to the manipulator. The error is calculated, and the instrument action is the output. There is haptic feedback that derives data from output instrument action passed to the reference input.

Pros and Cons of the Tele surgical Robots

The idea of remote surgery increased the accessibility of surgical systems into unreachable networks. The distance between the patient and the surgeon could at times prevent the transmission of diseases. Though network technologies have developed, there is always a latent time lag in this system. This value being 100 milliseconds does not cause any serious damage but can produce discrepancies in MIS. Other ethical concerns often limit the tele surgical methods for other surgeries.

12.4.3 Shared-Control Robot

As shown in Figure 12.10, in a shared control robot, the manipulator system assists the surgeon during the surgery. In a shared-control surgical robot, the surgeon does most of the work, unlike in the other two classifications. The manipulator system does not actuate without control signals from the surgeon. In this surgical robot, there is a preprogrammed action or console unit that makes a gap between the patient and the surgeon. The surgeon is in the field of surgery and uses the manipulator system to perform the surgery. Instead of the traditional surgical tools used for surgery, the manipulator has surgical instruments built into it that work on the control signals from the surgeon. The manipulator system manages to control the commands from the surgeon as well as the robot's autonomy and drive the surgical instruments. Watanabe introduced a shared-control robot that does one of the processes, and the surgeon cares for the other process in a surgery [23]. For example, if the patient has a cut and needs a stitch, the surgeon does the cleaning and other work while the manipulator

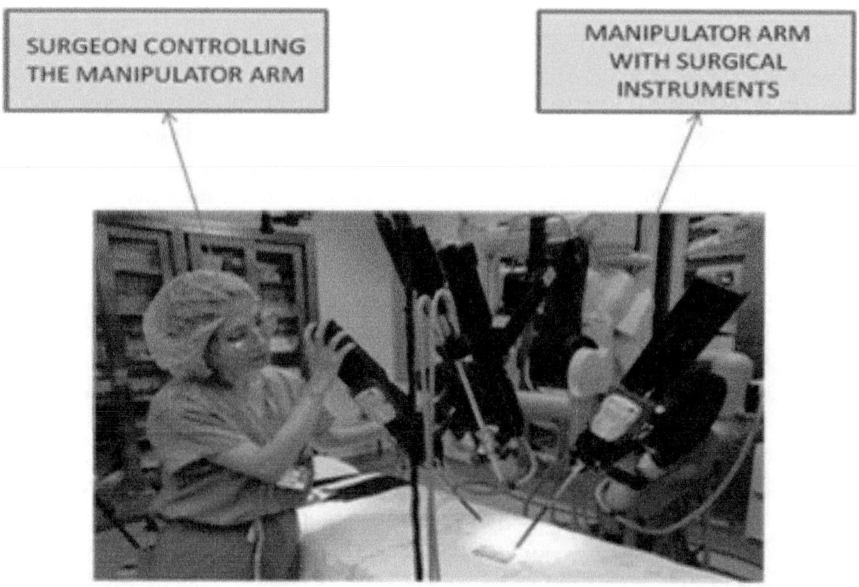

FIGURE 12.10 Shared-control robot [24].

arm does the stitching process. In this process, the surgeon and the manipulator arm do different functions for the same surgery by sharing control.

Pros and Cons of the Shared-Control Robot

The shared-control system involves direct involvement of the surgeon's actions in the field and allows them to directly handle the patient's body. The introduction of haptic feedback in the shared control systems is an added advantage for the surgeon which makes them feel the pressure given by the surgical instrument. Continuous steps can be performed by the manipulator arm automatically without the surgeon's intervention and command. Though the system has a haptic feedback mechanism [24], the commands from both the surgeon and the robot autonomy may direct the manipulator arm in the wrong kinematics. This may reduce the accuracy and reliability of the system.

12.5 FUTURE ADVANCES IN THE FIELD OF BIOMEDICAL ROBOTS

The field of biomedical robots has gained interest from the public. Invention has no boundary to stop them from further attainment and the field of biomedical robots is still an improving technology. For example, the integration of Artificial Intelligence and Machine Learning techniques is a good involvement in the field of medical surgery as it ensures high-end decision-making and understanding of the patient better in emotional aspects as well [25]. Assistant robots are now being introduced to take a stand with patients, converse with them, and become post-surgery companions for patients. The next form of development could be the time lag with the communications systems. In tele surgery systems, the distance between remote locations is still a development, and the introduction of high-speed networks is in progress. This can increase the range of the tele surgical techniques. In the case of data transmission, cyber security plays a vital role. The data from the patient during the surgery should meet the ethical code of conduct and hence have to be secure. Improving cyber security has been a great improvement in the field of robotic surgery. Miniaturization and microbots are the trending biomedical robots that are capsule-like in structure and have a camera module with them. This technology can be used to visualize inner body parts and increases the efficiency in analyzing the patient's condition.

12.6 CONCLUSION

This chapter covers the evolution of biomedical robots to the present day and future extended divisions. Continuous data on the patient can be passed on to the public to determine the current status of the patient. The rapid growth of the stream relies on the day-to-day updates of the technologies involved. The telepresence technology introduced by Dr. Green and his colleagues revolutionized the field of medicine. The communication between the monitor and the manipulator is the major reason for the system's limitations of the robot manipulator. However, modern wireless communication systems go hand-in-hand with this issue and mark the success of such direct-contactless surgery techniques. Integration of various fields such as engineering design, construction, automation, kinematics, etc., has resulted in the introduction of robotics into medical science. Through this chapter, we analyzed the involvement of automation in the field of medicine and reviewed the major components of a robot manipulator used for surgery. We discussed the major classification of sensors and the workings of the sensors. Sensor elements used in the surgery need an increase in resolution, as in the case of supervisory controlled surgery, only the manipulator decides the area of location. A sensor in this case is the major controller along with the reference to decide the area of action for the manipulator. A few suggestions for self-error techniques are appreciable and the major drift in the context is the post-surgery sanitation for the manipulator. There is a need for the biomedical robots to become an inevitable part of the future and MIS requires the integration of biomedical robots to establish the success of surgical technologies.

REFERENCES

[1] Guo, Yingwei, Yingjian Yang, Yang Liu, Qiang Li, Fengqiu Cao, Mengting Feng, Hanhui Wu, Wei Li, and Yan Kan. (2021). "Development Status and Multilevel Classification Strategy of Medical Robots." *Electronics (Switzerland)*, vol. 10, no. 11 pp 3-7.

[2] George, Evalyn I., COL Timothy C. Brand, and Jacques Marescaux. (2018). "Origins of Robotic Surgery: From Skepticism to Standard of Care." *JSLS*, vol. 22, no. 4, p. e2018.00039. https://doi.org/10.4293/JSLS.2018.00039

[3] Chitwood, W. Randolph. "Historical Evolution of Robot-Assisted Cardiac Surgery: A 25-Year Journey." *Annals of Cardiothoracic Surgery*, vol. 11, no. 6, pp. 564–82. https://doi.org/10.21037/acs-2022-rmvs-26 (2022)

[4] Rahman, M., G. J. Murad, and J. Mocco. (2009). "Early History of the Stereotactic Apparatus in Neurosurgery." *Neurosurgical Focus*, vol. 27, no. 3, p. E12. https://doi.org/10.3171/2009.7.FOCUS09118

[5] De Rosa, Michele, Walter Bugiantella, Federica Arteritano, Lorenzo Mariani, Fabio Ermili, and Graziano Ceccarelli. (2024). "The Evolution of Minimally Invasive Robotic Surgery in the Last 20 Years." In *Robotic Surgery of Colon and Rectum*, edited by Graziano Ceccarelli and Alessandro Coratti, p. 1. Updates in Surgery. Cham: Springer. https://doi.org/10.1007/978-3-031-33020-9_1

[6] Marcelissen, Tom, and Guy H.E.J. Vijgen. (2023). "The Endoscope." *British Journal of Surgery*, vol. 110, no. 12, pp. 1641–43. https://doi.org/10.1093/bjs/znad220

[7] Ashrafian, H., O. Clancy, V. Grover, and A. Darzi. (2017). "The Evolution of Robotic Surgery: Surgical and Anaesthetic Aspects." *British Journal of Anaesthesia*, vol. 119, pp. i72–i84. https://doi.org/10.1093/bja/aex383

[8] Ginoya, Tirth, Yaser Maddahi, and Kourosh Zareinia. (2021). "A Historical Review of Medical Robotic Platforms." *Journal of Robotics*. pp. 1-7. https://doi.org/10.1155/2021/6640031

[9] Tung, Tran Thanh, Nguyen Van Tinh, Dinh Thi Phuong Thao, and Tran Vu Minh. (2023). "Development of a Prototype 6 Degree of Freedom Robot Arm." *Results in Engineering*, vol. 18. https://doi.org/10.1016/j.rineng.2023.101049

[10] Zhang, Zhizhou, Zeqing Jin, and Grace X. Gu. (2022). “Efficient Pneumatic Actuation Modeling Using Hybrid Physics-Based and Data-Driven Framework.” *Cell Reports Physical Science*, vol. 3, no. 4, pp 7-9. https://doi.org/10.1016/j.xcrp.2022.100842

[11] Ueda, Yuichiro, So Miyahara, Keita Tokuishi, Hiroyasu Nakajima, Ryuichi Waseda, Takeshi Shiraishi, and Toshihiko Sato. (2023). “Impact of a Pneumatic Surgical Robot with Haptic Feedback Function on Surgical Manipulation.” *Scientific Reports*, vol. 13, no. 1, pp.-2. https://doi.org/10.1038/s41598-023-49876-7

[12] Grochulla, F., Vieweg, U. (2023). “Surgical Motor Systems in Spinal Surgery.” In Heidelberg: Vieweg, U., Grochulla, F. (eds.), *Manual of Spine Surgery*. Berlin, Heidelberg: Springer. https://doi.org/10.1007/978-3-662-64062-3_11

[13] Dinesh, Sharad, Umesh Kumar Sahu, Dameshwari Sahu, Santanu Kumar Dash, and Umesh Kumar Yadav. (2023). “Review on Sensors and Components Used in Robotic Surgery: Recent Advances and New Challenges.” *IEEE Access*, vol. 11, pp. 140722–39. https://doi.org/10.1109/ACCESS.2023.3339555

[14] Gafford, Joshua B., Scott Webster, Neal Dillon, Evan Blum, Richard Hendrick, Fabien Maldonado, Erin A. Gillaspie, Otis B. Rickman, S. Duke Herrell, and Robert J. Webster. (2020). “A Concentric Tube Robot System for Rigid Bronchoscopy: A Feasibility Study on Central Airway Obstruction Removal.” *Annals of Biomedical Engineering*, vol. 48, no. 1, pp. 181–91.

[15] Gilbert, H.B., D.C. Rucker, and R.J. Webster III. (2016). “Concentric Tube Robots: The State of the Art and Future Directions.” In Masayuki Inaba and Peter Corke(eds.), *Robotics Research*, vol. 114. Cham: Springer.

[16] Dibekci, A., and O Bebek. (2018, August). “Improving the Safety of Medical Robotic Systems.” In Sarthak Misra (eds.), *2018 7th IEEE International Conference on Biomedical Robotics and Biomechatronics (Biorob)*, pp. 73–78. IEEE.

[17] Gao, Hongyan, Xiaojie Ai, Zhenglong Sun, Weidong Chen, and Anzhu Gao. (2023). “Progress in Force-Sensing Techniques for Surgical Robots.” *Journal of Shanghai Jiaotong University (Science)*, vol. 28, no. 3, pp. 370–81. https://doi.org/10.1007/s12204-023-2607-x

[18] Hu, J. Y., Y. I. Li, and K. W. Yeung. (2006). In vivo physiological measurements. *Clothing Biosensory Engineering*, pp. 285–300.

[19] *Medical Device Network*. (2021). “Medical Devices: In-Depth Review of Medical-Grade Thermocouples.” *Medical Device Network*. January 22. www.medicaldevice-network.com/sponsored/medical-devices-in-depth-review-medical-grade-thermocouples/

[20] Sumit Suri, Yashpal Singh. (2015). “A Review on Robotics in Surgery.” *International Journal of Engineering Research & Technology (IJERT)*, NCETEMS, vol. 3, no. 10. pp. 1-3.

[21] Abouelseoud, Gehan. (2012). “Biomedical Engineering: A Brief Survey into Current Challenges and a Proposed Research Roadmap.” *International Journal of Healthcare Technology and Management*, vol. 13, no. 1–3, pp. 1–31. https://doi.org/10.1504/IJHTM.2012.048971

[22] McGuinness, L. A., and B. Prasad Rai. (2018). “Robotics in Urology.” *The Annals of The Royal College of Surgeons of England*, vol. 100, no. 6_sup, pp. 45–54.

[23] Xiong, Linfei, Chin Boon Chng, Chee Kong Chui, Peiwu Yu, and Yao Li. (2017). “Shared Control of a Medical Robot with Haptic Guidance.” *International Journal of Computer Assisted Radiology and Surgery*, vol. 12, no. 1, pp. 137–47. https://doi.org/10.1007/s11548-016-1425-0

[24] Kevin Bonsor and Jonathan Strickland. (2000). "How Robotic Surgery Will Work." *HowStuffWorks*, 30 October 2000. https://health.howstuffworks.com/medicine/moderntechnology/robotc-surgery

[25] Reddy, Kavyanjali, Pankaj Gharde, Harshal Tayade, Mihir Patil, Lucky Srivani Reddy, and Dheeraj Surya. (2023). "Advancements in Robotic Surgery: A Comprehensive Overview of Current Utilizations and Upcoming Frontiers." *Cureus*, December. https://doi.org/10.7759/cureus.50415

13 The Digital Technologies in Healthcare

Navigating the Digital Transformation with Security and Operational Efficiencies

R. Sangeetha, M. Premkumar, S.R. Ashokkumar, G Mohanbabu, S. Anupallavi, and Josephine Pon Gloria Jeyaraj

13.1 INTRODUCTION

The evolution of digital health technology is a critical facet in healthcare delivery. Especially in wearables, telemedicine, and e-pharmacies, the health technology sector has boomed over recent years. In addition, considerable work has been conducted in the medicine domain to integrate advanced technologies such as robotics, Artificial Intelligence (AI), blockchain, etc. into healthcare [1]. Market expansion is being driven by the high demand for digital healthcare solutions given current world trends, the increase in public and private sector investments, as well as innovations made within telehealth and telemedicine to provide more safety. Healthcare not only harbors new areas of economic growth and jobs but is essential for maintaining a nation's health.

Technological innovation is enabling healthcare companies to reach the next wave of growth, while investors are increasingly eyeing up the sector as an attractive investment opportunity. Digital health solutions span across mobile healthcare (mHealth). Various forms of healthcare information technology (e-prescriptions, EHRs etc.) are shown in Figure 13.1, e.g. wearable technologies, personalized medicine, telehealth services, AI-assisted diagnostics, and surgical robotics [2].

Technology involving the adaptation of comprehensive health data is quickly progressing throughout the world through a concept known as IoT in the medical industry. This growth has been even more accelerated by the COVID-19 pandemic to make IoT more prominent in health care. The fast-growing innovative methods are influencing the future of IoT in healthcare, but great barriers still exist in the advancement of technologies, healthcare, data privacy, the digital enabling gap, government and stakeholder involvement, and medical practitioners and hospitals [3].

This system of connected devices, sensors, and gadgets can upset industries and optimize almost everything in our lives. Interconnectivity is the basic foundation of the IoT paradigm that needs to occur everywhere for any gadget. This starts from

 DOI: 10.1201/9781003561309-13

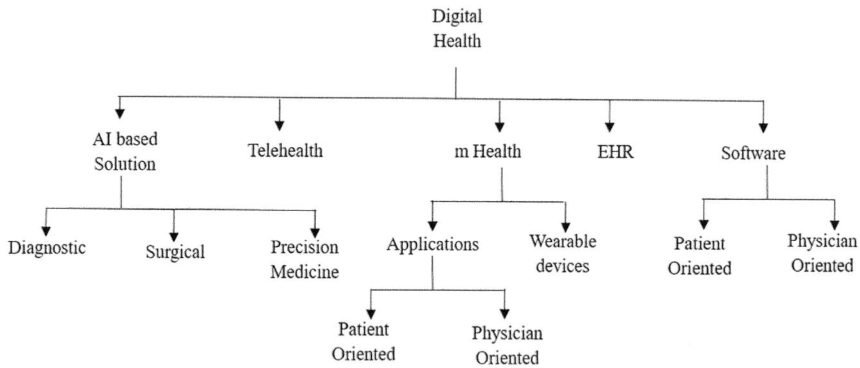

FIGURE 13.1 Components of digital health.

simple domestic appliances like the climate control units and refrigerators to the larger industrial applications and even health-related devices. This is made possible through sensors and actuators placed in these objects to enable IoT to collect data, process the same and even independently make decisions. The one major benefit of IoT is to make environments intelligent, in terms of efficiency in utilization of resources, forecasting when they will require to be replaced or repaired, and to optimize processes based on data analysis [4]. IoT devices like wearable sensors and even implants can relay the patient's vitals in real time to doctors and other healthcare givers. This ensures that health concerns are resolved before they develop to an extent that hospitalization is required, thus leading to healthier patients.

However, healthcare data protection remains one of the biggest hurdles for the fulfilment of IoT concepts. From wearables, remote monitoring tools, and equipment to smart, connected technologies in healthcare, IoT has developed a massive attack surface. These risks include risk of theft or loss, hacking, tampering, and compromise of the patient's records [5]. Medical data are also usually private, and include patient's medical history, prescribed treatment, and additional personal information, which if disclosed even unintentionally pose a severe privacy threat to patients.

Conventional centralized database models are not safe from intrusion and alteration, and this is dangerous when it comes to healthcare. For this reason, the integrity and origin of the records must be unaltered to sustain the consumers' confidence. The implementation of blockchain and machine learning (ML) in infrastructures of healthcare is not an easy thing to achieve. For the implementation of smart contracts based on blockchain technology, problems associated with decentralization and cryptographic features regarding the distribution of storage arise, along with problems of integrating solutions and scaling. Meanwhile, ML algorithms such as SVM, Decision Trees, KNN, Random Forest and Naïve Bayes must overcome challenges related to data confidentiality and stability of models used in healthcare analytics. This review aims to summarize the recent state of digital medical technologies and the opportunities of applying AI, big data, telemedicine, and blockchain in solving the actual problems in healthcare and medical education.

13.2 DIGITAL TECHNOLOGIES IN HEALTHCARE

"Digital health" is the umbrella word for the broad, interdisciplinary field that includes concepts from technology and healthcare. It transforms the healthcare sector by fusing technology, software, and services. Wearable technology, telehealth and telemedicine, mobile health apps, EHRs, EMRs, and medicines are all included in this category and are shown in Figure 13.2.

13.2.1 Telemedicine and Telehealth

Telemedicine—the provision of health services through the use of technology—has continued to experience phenomenal growth in development. Reducing mortality and enhancing the coverage of health services, telemedicine is a viewpoint to respond to the issues of healthcare provision for rural and other undersupplied zones. Telemedicine has emerged as the most prominent force of digital health change throughout the developing nations, especially as more emphasis is placed on digital healthcare service delivery [6].

Telemedicine is a medical practice that can be delivered over various distances, thereby overcoming most associated distances. Health care specialists use telemedicine

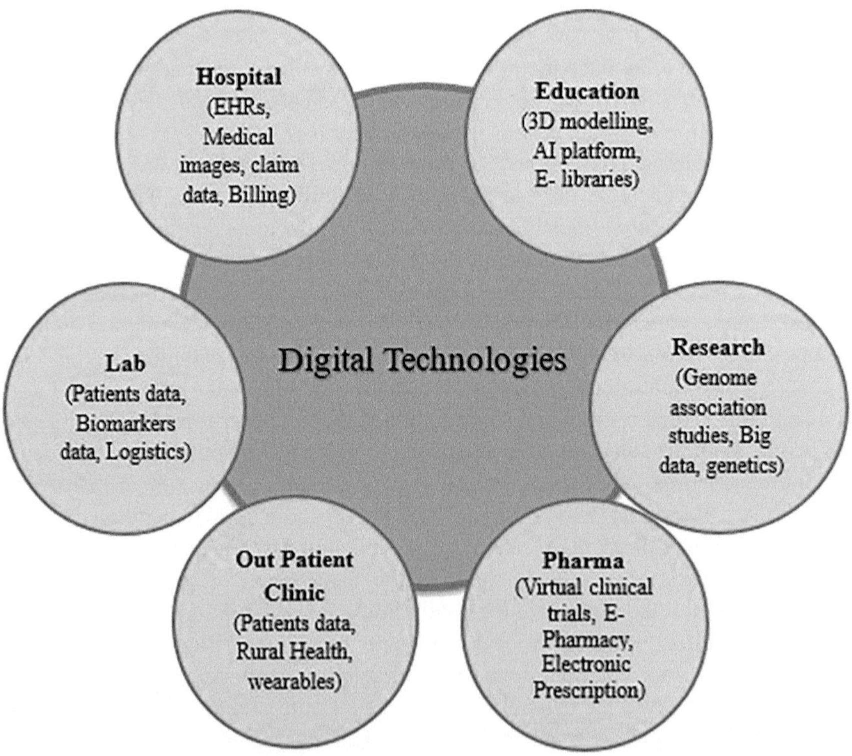

FIGURE 13.2 Digital technology in medical industry.

equipment to offer treatment in areas where geographical separation is a constraining factor. This technology is used by the care givers in the health sector to share information concerning the treatment strategies and analysis and to disseminate knowledge to other people where necessary. Telemedicine encompasses three primary types: store-and-forward, real Â time, and remote monitoring services. By incorporating ICT, telemedicine provides valuable, cheap, and easily accessible information on health care, thus improving on the type of services offered to patients. It is worth emphasizing the following telemedical services: tele dermatology, telehealth, telesurgery, telecardiology, and tele education, all of which enhance the delivery of healthcare in any part of the world. Medical services are important in attending to the health needs of people particularly those in remote areas and this is where ICT proved vital in support. However, the full potential of telemedicine can only be unlocked if it offers the potential of being integrated with other technologies—the second-generation 5G networks, smart wearables, robot, drones among other connected technologies. As clearly depicted in Figure 13.3, these integrated technologies enable an efficient and responsive health care sector to monitor patients from a distance and to take care of the severe cases, including coronavirus-infected patients [7].

Telemedicine technology is discussed, including aspects of video conferencing virtual consultation and electronic health record (EHR). Medical imaging algorithms are explored as an example of how AI is used in diagnostics. Of further interest, factors related to the patient and healthcare provider acceptance are considered based on the literature, namely, patient involvement, handling the technology-facilitated impediments, and the issue of health professions when they engage in the virtual space [8].

The implementation of VR and AR in telemedicine is taking the healthcare industry towards patient-centered care and education approaches. In this case, the

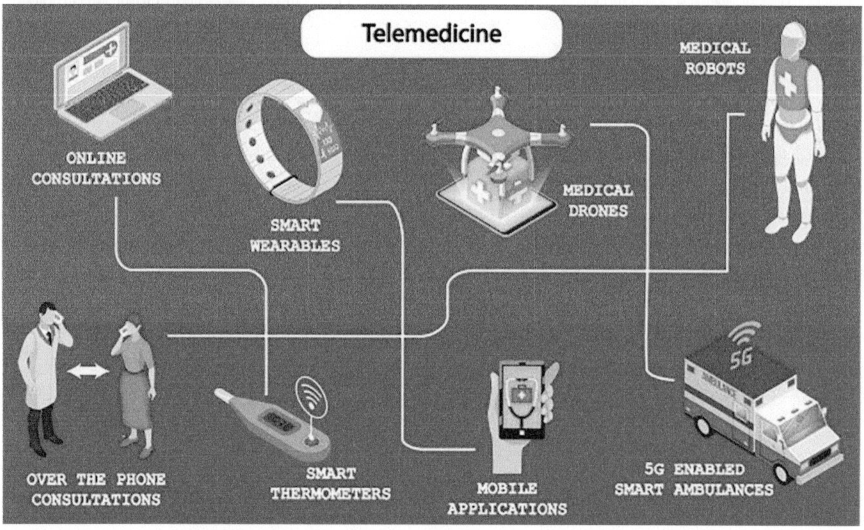

FIGURE 13.3 Different telemedicine enabling technologies [7].

incorporation of AI, the use of RPM, and the incorporation of VR and AR in telemedicine point to the future of health care delivery. These emerging trends do not only increase the effectiveness of the telemedicine but also help in the changing perspective of the healthcare delivery model. It is the delivery of health care services using audio-video and graphical information transfer through telecommunications infrastructure and includes consultative, diagnostic, collaborative and coordinated care. Telemedicine is expected to transform the public health service delivery since it impacts on processes and structures of the health care system.

13.2.2 Electronic Health Records (EHR)

EHRs have brought substantial changes into the practice of healthcare through offering an online solution on patient data storage, processing, and sharing. EHRs shown in Figure 13.4 include a myriad of information, which include medical history, prescribed drugs, known allergies, test results, and a patient's treatment plan.

The use of EHRs in healthcare systems has been observed to have the following benefits: improved patient care, better co-ordination of care, and increased efficiency. EHRs help physicians to view patient's information easily, which helps in diagnosis and forming an action plan with the patient. Also, EHRs reduce the flow of information among clinicians, which results in improved management of care and fewer mistakes [9]. However, there have been some difficulties with the implementation of EHRs such as the problems of exchanging data and information between the systems, and security risks and concerns among the healthcare practitioners. Nonetheless, continued work to address these difficulties and enhance EHR systems should help to continue finalizing the systems' position as key tools for renaissance in healthcare delivery. EHR increases record retrieval by acting as the source of all patient records and information. This centralization makes it convenient for the health care providers where all the data can be retrieved from numerous papers. Also, EHRs can relieve

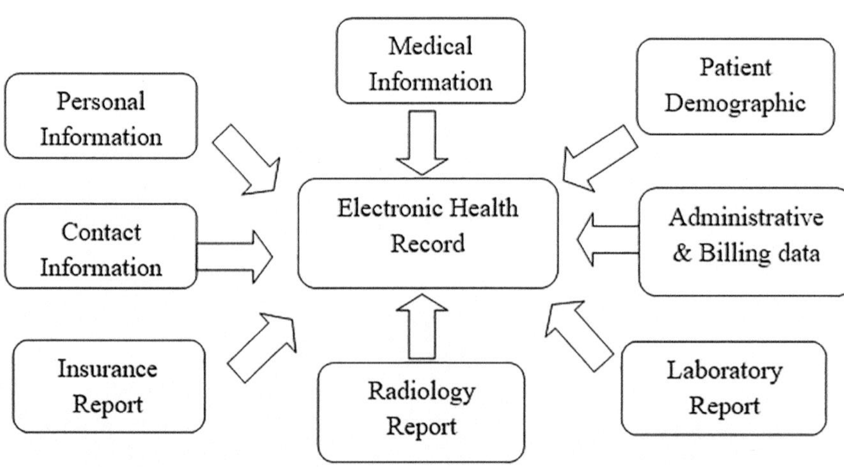

FIGURE 13.4 EHR model.

documentation processes involved in coding and billing, among others, which serves to increase efficiency. EHRs also provide extended patient information, which has contributed to the reduction of medical errors as well as the repetition of tests.

13.2.3 Artificial Intelligence (AI) and Machine Learning (ML)

The healthcare sector has several prominent problems which are rather general, namely the shortage of the workforce and the challenges in treatment of chronic diseases. As a result of population increase and economic development the world market for health human resources is predicted to scale new heights. Similarly, it is established that chronic non-communicable diseases (NCDs) are said to be the major killer in the world today contributing to about 73% of deaths and impacting on millions of people indefinitely [10]. This shortage reflects demographic and epidemiological changes at the current time, and the number of health care workers is already scarce.

This is, however, an area of interest where digital health interventions, especially the ones that incorporate AI, have been deemed to have the prospects of addressing these gaps in health care. Machine learning (ML) is one of the branches of AI that involves using data-trained algorithms for the creation of models that are capable of carrying out tasks.

Digital health interventions range from assisting in clerical work and making evidence-based clinical diagnoses or decisions to analyzing health data quickly, as a means of determining potential treatment. AI in healthcare has been described to elevate the conditions of the patient and overall, well-being of the caregivers. Regulatory authorities are a critical component in the regulation of AI systems since such systems make determinations that have bearings on the health, welfare, and safety of an individual. Thus, regulations are useful in eliminating errors or malfunctions that may pose a danger to the lives of the patient, as well as highlighting the policy on the ethical use of the AI, including on issues such as privacy of the patient, consent to use their information in the program, and the security of the data [11]. Appropriate rules are pertinent to avoid any form of violation, or violation of privacy concerning the individual's health data. These are codes of conduct and regulation that set up rules and policies of AI systems, API that encourage compatibility and integration of various systems, and assurance to clinicians, patients, and the general public. The awareness that the AI systems function according to the set standards has increased the faith in the efficiency and reliability of the systems.

13.2.4 Robotics and Automation

Robotic Process Automation (RPA) aims at automating business processes or segments of them through utilizing software robots to emulate users' actions on GUI. It is an extended form of automating lower-skilled back-office and administrative work that was formally done manually by employees. In 2018, the RPA software market experienced growth of 60% [12]. In this case, organizations strive to employ RPA in the execution of enhancing their efficiency in formulating and providing new products or services in the market fast and as a response to possible opportunities in the market.

The aspects of sustainability in organizations include an organization's social and environmental responsibilities based on changing organizational values and legislations. It has become a trend in today's business society for organizations to take cognizance of their corporate social, environmental, and economic responsibilities.

Technology has more or less changed the arena of diagnosing and treating diseases in the medical field. Technology helps to bring science advances in diagnosis and treatment of diseases as they contribute toward the early detection and control of diseases. Also, together with cost optimization, automation helps to coordinate the personnel, supplies, and financial activities and improve their effectiveness and productivity [13]. The benefits of RPA in healthcare administration can be highlighted through the analysis of elements related to value creation and adoption of RPA in relation to time optimization and possible impact on both employee satisfaction and customers' satisfaction.

Application of medical robotics can significantly change the clinical processes as it can enhance the performance of surgical procedures, avoid different complications, and simplify the existing processes together with the improvement of patients' safety and outcomes. Nevertheless, there are several challenges, which include high costs, training, and ethical issues, which are a hindrance to the general use of the technology. Further development and studies are required to improve robotic platforms as well as to identify new uses and expand robotics in many fields of medicine. Multidisciplinary efforts between engineers, clinicians, and interdisciplinary researchers will be pertinent in developing safe, efficients and enjoyable robotic technologies.

13.2.5 Internet of Medical Things (IoMT) Devices

The IoMT is defined as the connected use of healthcare systems, devices, and technologies through the Internet for enhancing the delivery of efficient health care services. As IoT grows, IoMT has been made more available and cheaper; this is sort of a postmodern way of health care. IoT devices allow monitoring data in real-time through the use of Internet connection to collect, store, and analyze data. This section aims at highlighting IoT devices for health care, the characteristics of the devices and how the introduction of the devices will improve health care systems [14]. Wearable IoT devices include Smart Watches, Fitness Trackers, and Smart clothing which are clipped or worn on the body and sense bodily parameters like the sleep cycle, blood pressure, heart rate, and activity level. Such devices enable real-time health monitoring by interacting with the health care providers. For instance, abnormally high blood pressure rates can be identified by individual wearable devices and call the attention of doctors to a health concern. A few details regarding the IoMT model for smart health control systems are provided in Figure 13.5.

The process starts with the intake of a patient's health parameters and other peculiarities through sensors of wearable devices. Then all the information obtained is transferred to a cloud type server. In an emergency the information is transmitted from the cloud server to a database station that checks and sends the information to

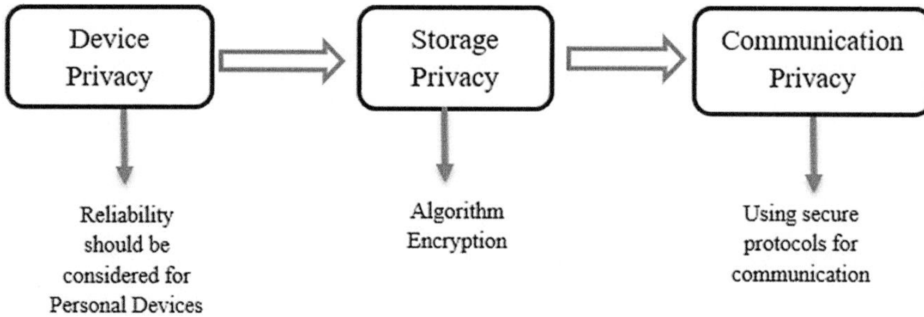

FIGURE 13.5 Privacy issues in IoT and their solutions.

a medical server [15]. The medical server then alerts the hospital so that the patient's health care necessities can be attended to. Furthermore, IoMT optimizes the interoperability of information between and across patients, family/caregivers, clinicians, and insurers. With links between electronic health records and telemedicine tools, as well as HIEs, IoMT helps providers enter and receive the necessary information in an efficient and timely manner and engage in cross-disciplinary cooperation.

Examples of IoMT devices are smartwatches, fitness trackers, heart monitors, glucose monitors, and many more. These wearables continuously monitor vitals and send the information in real time to caregivers. Such devices also enable the healthcare givers to monitor and, thus, reach better conclusions regarding their treatment. However, the generation and collection of large amounts of data is a concern owing to the possible security risks that come with it, which are very likely to infringe on the rights of privacy.

Wearable ECG monitors, smart blood glucose meters, and remote respiratory monitors are some of the examples of the highly developed medical devices that monitor different health conditions like blood sugar levels, oxygen saturation, and body temperature continuously [16]. They play an integral part in real-time communication with the healthcare professional and enhance the quality of treatment and decrease the overall healthcare expenditure, as there is no need for continuous follow-up appointments with the physician. However, these devices have potential problems such as software problems, breakdowns in the devices, and connection problems that may compromise the reliability and safety of the devices.

Medical accessories such as the wearable fitness tracking devices and remote patient monitoring tools including stethoscopes and telecommunication tools enable medical services at patients' homes. These devices enhance live video calls, remote supervision, and mobile health services, hence making an approach that once appeared fairly straightforward was regarded as both simple and efficient [17]. Telecare helps the provider track the patient's condition and the changes in the status hence improving the quality of the health of the patient. However, the technology that is employed in telemedicine and its collection of data is questionable as such gadgets may be susceptible to fraud incidents. Similar to other IoMT devices, connected devices present various security and privacy issues because attackers can easily launch cyber attacks on them. It is very important to enforce the most secure protection on these devices to get best possible utilization in the system of health care.

13.3 SECURITY IN DIGITAL HEALTHCARE

The IoT works on the principle of a heterogeneous network which poses problems in matters to do with protection and security. These privacy concerns and protection mechanisms are depicted in Figure 13.5. There are several weaknesses in IoT, and they arise from the use of smart objects. The data collected by these devices is transferred to monitoring bodies and this process can be another vulnerable area which affects the system's security. In light of this, IoT devices should be endowed with self-diagnostics, which would allow identifying security threats and informing the user of third parties' unauthorized access. There is a need to automate how these threats are detected and addressed.

Data provenance can be defined as the practice of data information and tracking of its history from the time it is created up to the time it is destroyed while recording what has been done with it in the process. This assists in detecting data misuse or forbidden changes within the company. There are different ways to apply data models to track data origin with regard to individual patients. The following are some of the tools, which can be used to develop a secure service model: authentication, access control, confidentiality, enforcement, and mobile protocols to enhance the development of a strong network [18]. As shown in Table 13.1, the security goals are centered on safeguarding patient data, guaranteeing confidentiality and privacy, and preserving the availability of the systems.

13.3.1 Authentication Solution

A3 factor authentication protocol was proposed in [31], that aims at addressing most of the security issues in health IoT. It includes the authentication to verify users' rights and the key distribution for confidentiality. Furthermore, biometrics are used to hide users' identities and to provide a better user experience. Thus, owing to the application of encryption, the respective protocol provides increased protection. Additionally, a comparison with other comparable protocols showed that the presented protocol yields significant performance gains in terms of computation, time, and security.

The security scheme using Blockchain is intended to promise security, devolution, and transparency. The scheme is efficiently protected from several security threats with mutual authentication, untrace ability, and anonymity. Simulation and analytical mathematical verifications were used alongside test bed experimental results that employed cryptographic methods in enforcing its security. The proposed strategic frame was compared with the currently existing schemes to observe the advantage of this approach in terms of computational and communication complexity as well as security considerations.

RAPCHI is a novel approach to optimize privacy concerns of IoMT in health systems [32]. RAPCHI achieves authentication and key agreement among the patients, the cloud server, and the doctors. It was also found that the proposed method

TABLE 13.1
Security Objectives in the Healthcare Industry

Security Objective	Technique	Description	Advantages	Challenges	Ref
Confidentiality	Encryption (e.g., AES, RSA)	Encrypts patient data to prevent unauthorized access.	High data protection; widely adopted standards.	Computationally intensive; requires strong key management.	[19]
	RBAC	Limits data access based on users' roles.	Easy to implement and manage; clear access levels.	Complex role definitions; requires continuous monitoring and updates.	
	Data Masking	Hides sensitive data in non-production environments.	Protects data during training and testing phases.	Can be bypassed if improperly configured.	[20]
Integrity	Digital Signatures	Verifies the authenticity of data and ensures it hasn't been altered.	Strong protection against data tampering.	Requires secure management of keys and certificates.	[21]
	Hashing (e.g., SHA-256)	Generates a unique hash value for data, ensuring that changes are detectable.	Quick verification of data integrity.	Vulnerable to collisions with weaker hash functions.	
Availability	Redundancy and Backup Systems	Ensures data and services remain available through backups and failover systems.	Minimizes downtime and data loss during failures.	Costs associated with storage and infrastructure.	[22]

(continued)

TABLE 13.1 (Continued)
Security Objectives in the Healthcare Industry

Security Objective	Technique	Description	Advantages	Challenges	Ref
	Distributed Denial-of-Service (DDoS) Protection	Defends against DDoS attacks that can overwhelm healthcare systems.	Maintains availability during attacks.	Requires continuous monitoring and evolving defense mechanisms.	[23]
	Cloud Solutions with SLAs	Ensures high uptime and availability through service-level agreements (SLAs).	Reliable availability with cloud-based solutions.	Potential data sovereignty and latency issues.	[24]
Accountability	Audit Logs	Tracks all access and modifications to sensitive data.	Facilitates tracking unauthorized access and creating accountability.	Logs can be voluminous; requires proper analysis tools.	[25]
	MFA	Requires multiple forms of authentication (e.g., password + biometrics).	Strong verification of user identity, reducing fraud.	Increased complexity in user experience.	[26]
Non-repudiation	Blockchain	Provides an immutable ledger for medical transactions and data access records.	High trust and transparency; resistant to tampering.	Energy-intensive and complex to implement at scale.	[27]
	Timestamping	Adds trusted timestamps to records, ensuring the authenticity of when actions occur.	Clear evidence of when specific actions were taken.	Requires a trusted timestamp authority.	[28]

Privacy	Data Anonymization	Removes personally identifiable information (PII) from healthcare data.	Protects patient identities during data sharing and analysis.	May reduce the usability of data for research and analysis.	[29]
	Consent Management Systems	Manages patient consent for data sharing and use.	Ensures compliance with privacy laws and patient preferences.	Requires complex user interface and consistent updates.	[30]

is immune to various types of security threats and meets the need for different security standards. Security formalisms were applied; the AVISPA tool was used to study the protocols' behavior. Another comparative analysis proved that RAPCHI yielded better results compared to other similar protocols, particularly in cases such as pandemics.

13.3.2 RFID Security Solution

RFID has gained popularity in managing medical processes in an effort to improve the pharmaceutical service provision, patient care, and security. It is invaluable in drug management especially through the ability to track the supply of medicine in the system. Some of these drugs are used very rarely but must necessarily be stockpiled in a hospital, for example, antivenom, rabies vaccines, and others. These are usually short shelf-life drugs, with low stock turnover, and are very expensive which calls for constant stock checking on these classified medications. The tracking of these medications, when done manually requires a lot of time and can be cumbersome and can lead to a number of mistakes. To counter this, the pharmaceutical companies have integrated RFID-based medication management systems that put into practice the restocking procedures. These systems act as a timely counter and bring down the error rates as well as improve efficiency of the pharmacies.

An RFID tag is assigned to each tray or container of pharmaceuticals, and it carries certain information. Filled trays are scanned in this system and the scanned values are then compared with expected quantity and medicine. It also produces reports on used drugs, expiring products, and products that are almost expiring thus allowing for appropriate action to be taken. Predicting the quantities of the supplies to be procured in healthcare organizations is quite difficult because the needs of the patients are very unpredictable. This results in misplaced or expired items and wrong inventories The absence of a viable tracking system of inventory items such as consumables, lab items and prescriptions contribute to the accumulation of negative consequences, which include forgotten or expired items and expensive emergency orders. RFID technologies installed in refrigerators and storage cabinets can detect inventory levels on a regular basis and will notify users when inventory drops to certain levels or via expiration dates to order new stock for inventory replenishment for essential supplies required by patients [33].

13.3.3 Blockchain-Based Solution

IoMT ecosystem will benefit from safe authentication and key management thanks to the BAKMP-IoMT smart contract blockchain integrated protocol. Because IoMT uses the internet to connect medical devices and apps with healthcare systems, private health information is susceptible to manipulation. This is resolved by ensuring that keys to IMT are safely managed and only allows access to healthcare data stored on BAKMP-IoMT's blockchain by cloud servers to the implantable medical devices [34]. The protocol has been designed, evaluated, and proved to have better security and communication and computational overhead compared with the existing solutions. This is evident through performance simulations that bring out how the approach impacts key parameters. This system is implemented for low power devices by using lightweight cryptographic methods. The organization of the system is effective; it is not bulky and has the possibility of auditing; the transactions are validated within milliseconds.

13.3.4 Cryptographic-Based Solution

A protocol of what we were examining was analyzed in relation to the patients. To these problems, a new protocol introducing biometrics and ECC was introduced to fortify the secure communication in telemedicine information systems. In this research, the effectiveness of this new protocol was analyzed to measure its capability to withstand different security threats such as insider attack and the theft of mobile devices as well as the aspects of patients' anonymity [35]. This new protocol was revealed to exhibit improved effectiveness as well as security to any of the currently known solutions.

The extension of ICT and its usages in the health sector particularly through IoT were discussed. Application of IoT can enhance the health care with RPM with the help of wearable devices and sensors. Such an RPM system coupled with a smart watch, server, and smartphone app will guarantee the confidentiality of health parameters and can further improve health care delivery and living standards. It was then possible to highlight some of the problems that are bound to be encountered when applying IoT in healthcare, among them high energy consumption and security problems. In order to solve these issues, a scheme was proposed to protect healthcare data by using a homomorphic encryption scheme. The implementation of this system with the help of an E-health sensor shield platform enhanced the quality with a strong security premise.

The generalized privacy-preserving mutual authentication scheme targeting the solution of the security and privacy issue of IoT-based healthcare systems was presented [36]. To address this problem of processing power in IoT devices, this scheme employs useful cryptographic methods like XOR, Concatenation, and Hash Processing. It also creates an encrypted connection between such devices and a gateway besides protecting the healthcare system from unauthorized access. Security and performance analyses showed that this scheme is more effective than current methods of authentication.

13.3.5 Threats to the Healthcare Sector

Security of medical information is a primary concern for the healthcare industry, and this sector has been relatively slow to address the issue in the past. Privacy and security questions are examined in the framework of the healthcare sector, and the necessity of incorporating the safety of sophisticated medical technologies and maintaining the secrecy of the patient's data in the development of cybercrime in today's world is underlined by this study [37]. When it comes to the connection within the healthcare devices, it has enhanced the integration within the health sector's framework with many advantages like better efficiency, remote access, automation, and few errors.

It is through such advancements that the management of serious and chronic disease is being enhanced. The new technology system of interconnected care provides practitioners with a chance to track and manage the implantable devices apart from the medical amenities without necessarily going through operations.

However, healthcare management equipment has a poor security regime, making it a high-risk area compared to other sectors. In 2015 over 110 million patients' data were breached. While experiencing a 300% boost in cyber threats within the last three years, less than half of the US healthcare organizations say they are ready to protect themselves from such intrusions [38]. The healthcare industry has been targeted as a soft target.

Threats to healthcare are mainly for economic or political leverage but a future malicious cyber attack could be intentionally or unintentionally capable of changing a patient's blood group or test reports. Another very grave threat is attacks on medical devices. It should also be noted that, in 2014, more than 300 medical devices were identified that could be potentially unsafe. People who suffer from ineffective or more tangential cyber security with IoT technology might be more likely to hold off their information to the clinicians and researchers which might hamper the precision and quality of their treatment.

One major problem when it comes to identifying cyber-attacks is the fact that many of them occur and are rarely reported. Medical Equipment Management Programs (MEMPs), controlled through hospital biomedical engineering team, are intended for the protection and safety of medical equipment. Yet, as medical devices use data and communication technology in an increasing manner, security risks remain massive internally and externally. In order to combat all these threats adequately, there is a need to classify and prioritize the critical systems. This is because public healthcare organizations have implemented MEMPs in their organizations for over three decades and there is still a need to conduct more research in enhancing these programs to suit the health care organizations finances, safety, and reliability in delivering a quality service of this medical equipment [39].

13.3.6 Developing Specific Regulatory Frameworks

This advancement in technology can very much benefit applications that require computing in real time for functioning and other uses such as in the healthcare profession where patient data are analyzed in real time since proximity of computing to the data results in faster response time. However, the incorporation of fog computing (fog computing refers to a decentralized computing infrastructure in which data, processing, storage, and applications are distributed in the most efficient place between the data source and the cloud, often at the edge of the network) in the delicate health care system presents several issues concerning regulation, privacy and security that warrants further analysis. At this moment, the structure of healthcare data solutions meets the requirements of the HIPAA regulation in the US or GDPR in EU [40].

HIPAA is the leading healthcare data regulation in the US. HIPAA regulates entities and their associates who deal with the PHI and entails the application of physical, administrative, as well as technical controls. Fog computing systems must meet the HIPAA standards regarding data security and privacy, especially on communication of PHI by the fog nodes with other elements. Relatively to HIPAA the HITECH Act raises the penalties for violating the rules and expands the responsibilities to the healthcare provider's affiliates. It supports EHR and improves data security measures; both of which are important in fog computing environments [41]. FDA particularly has the responsibility of overseeing many of the devices employing technologies especially for time-sensitive diagnosis. The FDA has provided guidelines that classify SaMD terms, which also cover software functions in the different layers of fog computing systems. Manufacturers have to make certain that their device conforms to safety and efficacy regulations which means that firms will have to test and validate the fog computing components. Although the current FDA approach to SaMD implies that not all fog components should be validated, components affecting the diagnosis or therapy decision may require specific validation. Together with the FDA efforts are being made to identify areas where the fog computing infrastructure might benefit from a regulatory approach while also preserving innovation. As this sector continues to advance, it is possible for the FDA to produce elaborate guidelines to tackle problems of distributed systems.

GDPR is one of the main instruments ensuring the processing of personal data protection in the EU and greatly influences the processing of health data. GDPR enhances the legal protection of individual privileges on the use of personal data and also provides extra obligations to acting organizations. For the case of fog computing, GDPR set a mandate that protection of data privacy has to be a principle that is considered when designing systems, leading to the enhanced protection of data [42]. The biggest challenge that GDPR imposed on healthcare structures is the consent requirement that requests clear and unambiguous permission for processing patient data; this can be solved by decentralized consent layers like smart contracts on the block chain that can enforce consistent patient consent across nodes as data travels.

One of the most pressing issues under GDPR is data consent which must be obtained in a transparent manner, and this means that consent must be freely given, for a specific purpose, the process must be informed, and the consent must be unequivocal. This may be challenging particularly in fog implementation structures where data processing transcends nodal level, and therefore may be challenging to single handedly manage consent.

Furthermore, GDPR bans data transfer; consequently, the fog nodes situated in the territory of third countries must apply the same level of protection. The compliance may be achieved by using tools such as BCRs or SCCs. The new proposal for regulation that is going to replace the current ePrivacy Directive is the ePrivacy Regulation which will build on the framework of GDPR while dealing with privacy. While this regulation is not yet in force, it will definitely shed more light on dealing with healthcare data that is transmitted through fog computing networks. The comparison of data privacy regulations relevant to fog computing in healthcare is shown in Table 13.2.

TABLE 13.2
Comparison of Data Privacy Regulations Relevant to Fog Computing in Healthcare [43]

Region/Country	Regulation	Key Provisions Impacting Fog Computing	Challenges in Fog Computing Context
United States	HIPAA	Requires secure handling of PHI; mandates physical, administrative, and technical safeguards.	Ensuring PHI security across dispersed fog nodes.
European Union	GDPR	Data protection by design and by default; strict cross-border data transfer regulations.	Managing consent and data integrity across multiple nodes in different jurisdictions.
Japan	APPI	Enhanced protection for personal data; strict cross-border data transfer rules.	Ensuring all nodes comply with stringent data protection standards.
China	Cybersecurity Law & PIPL	Data localization; strong protection for personal and critical data.	Complying with data localization and ensuring protection in multi-node environments.
Brazil	LGPD	Strong emphasis on consent and data subject rights.	Integrating dynamic consent mechanisms across decentralized platforms.
India	Proposed Personal Data Protection Bill	Inspired by GDPR; includes data localization and consent requirements.	Harmonizing fog computing operations with evolving national standards.

13.4 ENHANCING OPERATIONAL EFFICIENCIES

Optimization of the utilization of the available resources in the delivery of healthcare services is a critical area that needs to be addressed in order to cultivate operational efficiencies with an effect of improving the quality of the care delivered at an increased rate and more efficiency at a lower cost. Many organizations, particularly the large ones, embrace use of technology, integrated operations, and rational analysis in accomplishing these objectives.

13.4.1 Big Data Improving Healthcare Management

Over the past few decades, Big Data Analytics (BDA) has become an important factor through which healthcare organizations operate. Today clinical data remains an instrumental component that shapes healthcare by providing the basis for the creation of multiple digital applications in this industry. A new phase in making information more open is being supported by both government and private organizations, after improving the attempts of the previous decade for digitizing the medical records. Federal and native authorities have provided for entry to years of compiled information which in turn help the healthcare sector in coming to wiser decisions. However, with the development of the technology and liberty to share the information, the protection of the patient's identity is rather paramount. It is crucial to guarantee that the organizations' protection is sound when they disclose personal information.

Hence the increase in use of evidence-based medicine that aims at involving the medical decision makers in developing treatment practices based on thoroughly conducted research findings. Big data algorithms consist of large data and therefore offer more substantial proof as compared to the smaller quantitative data. He further acknowledges that organizations that escalate the venture of BDA will experience more positive impacts, so the research shows [44]. This expectation has forced other organizations to embrace analytics, to close the gap that is being created. Apart from increasing the attractiveness of services and growth of premium segments, healthcare providers have to actively pursue value improvement with the help of BDA. This can be done by improving the access and cost of care and/or by dealing with fraud, abuse or waste in the system. Platforms and Tools for Processing, Storing, and Analyzing Huge Health Datasets

Data Storage: It is increasingly significant to efficiently manage large complex health care datasets, and several storage options exist. The HDFS is one of the building blocks of Hadoop that allow unstructured big data to be stored on different clusters. HDFS is widely used in healthcare organizations in processing and storing big data, for instance, medical images and genome data [45]. Moreover, especially for the unstructured healthcare information, there are the NoSQL databases such as MongoDB and Cassandra which are essential as they are capable of providing the flexibility and scalability which is needed owing to the constant change in healthcare information.

Data Processing: Health systems rely on frameworks and the appropriate processing of data for timely input and insights. Apache Spark has been lauded for its computational abilities for memory data processing and it is equipped for iterative calculations which make it good for data of large sizes. Spark is well suited to be used in healthcare as it can be used for streaming real-time data and machine learning. The other important framework is Apache Flink, it is specifically designed for stream processing and best suited for event-driven applications. It therefore is useful where there is a need to get an analytics from the streaming data such as in the healthcare field.

Data Analysis: Business intelligence is critical in healthcare informatics and thus requires analytics tools to make informative analysis of the data. SAS Analytics provides a wide range of capabilities for different aspects of healthcare analytics such as growth modeling, clinical analytics, and scam identity. Popular programming languages like R and python, which have executory libraries, are widely adopted in healthcare sectors for statistical analysis as well as for machine learning purposes. As such these languages assist healthcare professionals and data scientists to undertake the analyses required in the field in order to enable evidence-based decision making in healthcare.

Cloud Platforms: Cloud platforms have become essential for modern healthcare data management, offering scalable infrastructure and services. They provide robust solutions for storing, processing, and analyzing healthcare data. Key tools include AWS S3 for storage, AWS Lambda for serverless computing and Azure Machine Learning for advanced analytics. Utilizing cloud platforms enhances the agility and accessibility of healthcare data, fosters collaboration, and allows organizations to leverage advanced analytics technologies effectively.

Integrating big data technologies into healthcare management represents a dynamic journey filled with both challenges and opportunities. As technology evolves, addressing issues related to data privacy, interoperability, and resource constraints is crucial for healthcare organizations. Successfully leveraging the full potential of big data has the potential to enhance patient care and transform the healthcare landscape, fostering a data-driven, efficient, and patient-centric paradigm.

13.4.2 Supply Chain and Resource Management

Healthcare resource management comprises functions that address issues of budgets and proper utilization of important resources such as drugs, equipment, and employees to meet objectives of healthcare institutions. Optimal resource allocation in epidemic situations has been reviewed in detail [46]. Current modern healthcare systems involve the treatment of large numbers of patients, disease and diagnosis information, availability of hospital resources, machinery, and medical devices. This abundance of information makes it possible for planners or researchers and other experts to produce better ways of tackling the tasks of managing these resources.

While reviewing the literature, we found several publications that utilize accurate data in observational studies, including cohort research, cross-sectional research, and case-control research, to help decision-makers analyze and improve the performance of healthcare centers. A cross-sectional research study aimed to establish the extent to which trauma care was managed adequately in Tanzanian hospitals due to the few resources available in the management of trauma, together with other health services. It also identified potential areas for development and suggested interventions, including enhancing financial support for implementing universal treatment guidelines and centralizing clinical staff training.

COVID-19 challenges the healthcare system; several observational studies have focused on addressing the identified gaps and healthcare resource management. The detailed issues involving planning at a healthcare facility in the Singapore outbreak setting. They also recommended staff redeployment, differential training programs for ward staff, adjustments in staff-to-patient ratios, and the transfer of experienced physiotherapists, dieticians, and pharmacists into the wards. In the same vein, [47] discussed pandemic planning from a single-center healthcare perspective, highlighting the importance of timely actions in respect of spatial layout, human resources, training, and infection control for effective healthcare management planning. To estimate the quantity required to meet demand and maximize the number of discharges, a combined planning, optimization, and simulation model was developed. Similarly, using a multi-period resource allocation model, [48] created a model for a newly forming cholera outbreak. Their optimization methodology addresses disease transmission parameters in real time using a rolling horizon approach and utilizes Ordinary Differential Equations. They also accepted the idea of stochastic programming based on scenarios, which included uncertainty in the dynamic behavior of systems.

Sustainable Supply Chain Management (SSCM) has emerged as a key agenda item for healthcare organizations, driven by concerns for the environment, social responsibility, and prosperity. Suppliers, manufacturers, distributors, and healthcare providers that comprise the medical industry require sustainability, while also delivering quality healthcare to their patients. Implementing this has been a result of increased societal concern regarding responsible and ethical conduct in business [49]. This is due to rising instances of pollution, ethical considerations in sourcing raw materials, and the need to reduce costs amid increasing demand for healthcare services.

This means that the implementation of alternative solutions creates significant chances to boost the sustainability of the medical supply chain. Hence, solutions such as blockchain for supply chain traceability and AI optimization techniques enhance system transparency and increase accountability. Healthcare sustainability is therefore essential because the use of chemicals, toxic materials, and hazardous wastes in the process of delivering health services may be hazardous to the health of clients. Poor disposal of drugs, for instance, results in water pollution and the emergence of powerful bacteria resistant to antibiotics, while exposing patients and healthcare providers to hazardous chemicals from medical devices. In this way, sustainable management of the healthcare supply chain involves the use and disposal of safer substitutes to control environmentally induced diseases.

This is particularly so because, as the healthcare industry continues to grow, it is under pressure to prove its social responsibility and environmental responsibility, and most importantly, it is required to ensure it has high levels of ethics when hiring its workforce, protecting human rights, and having sustainable purchasing practices when sourcing its supplies. Environmentally and socially responsible healthcare firms have begun adopting supplier-buyer management operations to reduce power consumption, waste, and pollution generated by production processes, and to implement cleaner production technologies. Setting up factories and depots can result in the creation of employment opportunities, the investment in and improvement of infrastructure, and the provision of healthcare services to local people.

These effects must be positive and long-lasting; that is why healthcare companies interact with the stakeholders of the community, including community leaders, NGOs, and the government. This involves ensuring that poverty reduction strategies reach all people through participation in community-based activities, provision of timely basic infrastructure, and encouragement of partnerships for sustainable and efficient development.

In this case, compliance with regulatory frameworks is about the need to endorse a sustainable and accountable medical supply chain, with consideration for patient safety [50]. Environmental standards focus on reducing emissions, optimizing resource utilization, and responding to climate change. Social and ethical standards are in place to defend workers, aimed at preventing exploitation and enhancing transparency. Quality and safety regulations also assess the manufacturer's ability to provide high-quality products in the medical field, which improves the health of the people. In this regard, by embracing these regulations, healthcare organizations will be in a position to create sustainable supply chain networks that can deliver high-standard, safe, ethical, and environmentally sensitive medical products.

13.5 CHALLENGES IN DIGITAL HEALTHCARE TRANSFORMATION

Considering the recent advancements in digital technology across the healthcare system, the following changes have occurred. Some of the difficulties that have accompanied digital technology include cybersecurity, which is a primary concern in the Department of Health. The threats born in cyberspace are most expensive and influential. The stated problems are relatively widespread and pose a significant threat to the security of healthcare systems. Furthermore, the increased implementation of the IoMT has escalated threats to data handling systems. Ransomware is a significant problem in the healthcare industry in terms of cybersecurity. According to an FBI report from 2021, the healthcare sector is the most targeted by ransomware attacks compared to other sectors. The FBI reported receiving 148 complaints from the healthcare industry in 2021, surpassing even the financial sector. The techniques used by attackers to execute ransomware in healthcare settings include exploiting software weaknesses, phishing, and RDP attacks. This proves that the cybersecurity threat in this sector is very real and pressing. Personal data and protection are fundamental rights, and the details provided to healthcare organizations contain both personal and medical data, which are at risk of loss in the event of a breach. Bargaining breaches like these contradict the concept of digitization in the context of medicine. This emphasizes the need to apply suitable methods for protecting data in the health industry and highlights the significance of conducting and presenting research and design frameworks on these critical topics. Electronic Health Records (EHRs) are one of the most widespread digital tools that allow patients to view their medical records and provide service providers with the client's Health Information Exchanges (HIEs). However, this process poses a risk to data security and results in an increase in the number of protocol layers within the system. Data in EHRs includes past health history, social security numbers, payment information, and as such, EHRs attract hackers and cybercriminals.

13.6 FUTURE TRENDS

In the healthcare sector, several privacy and security measures are required to safeguard patients' personal information. Encryption is one technology used to protect data in transit and storage, thereby minimizing access by unauthorized personnel. Another is access controls, whereby data is only made available to those with specific clearances or assigned roles. For example, HIPAA and GDPR require particular measures to be taken as guidance for protecting the privacy of patients and their data. Altogether, the healthcare sector employs a technical and policy approach to protect patient data. Studies in this field could therefore concentrate efforts on assessing the impact of privacy and security laws in the industry. In examining the privacy and security concerns of wearable technology, several steps are taken. One is to scan the overall areas of the device or service, including software and hardware, to detect potential points of attack. As penetration testing approaches, it becomes apparent that some of them focus on reproducing real-life attacks to demonstrate vulnerabilities in security layers. The approach of surveying and interviewing wearable technology users would offer insight into the actual issues they have with privacy and security, and where assistance with awareness may be required. It is essential to employ a methodical and fine-tuned approach based on technical methods, testing, and user feedback to address these risks.

Automated diagnosis and recommendations for treatment, which are used in handling patient data, are made possible by natural language processing (NLP), which enables computers to interpret human language. Machine learning approaches, in the form of intelligent chatbots, enhance the flow of pertinent medical data to patients or between patients and doctors. Diagnostic imaging techniques jointly enable doctors and AI-based imaging analysis instruments in the evaluation of images and the determination of health consequences. The use of AI in healthcare provision aims to redefine the delivery of care and enhance patient health outcomes.

Blockchain technology can transform the healthcare sector by providing a secure, transparent, and shared method of handling patient information. In the EMR on blockchain, the sharing of information among healthcare professionals is safe and less complex. Insurance claims and reimbursement are two areas where smart contracts can bring about changes through automation. Thirdly, blockchain can also be applied as an effective tool for supply chain management in the healthcare and pharmaceutical industries to enhance the identity and track record of drugs and medical devices. In general, the application of blockchain technology offers a higher level of optimization and protection for healthcare processes, benefiting both patients and healthcare providers.

13.7 CONCLUSION

To align employment expectations and realities, healthcare operations, regulations, and activities must be digitized. Due to the prospects and challenges of patient safety and the integration of digital technology in the clinical setting, it is valuable to evaluate the digital readiness of clinicians. As such, digital health systems and other health information technologies are emerging as efficient substitutes for the obsolete paper-based systems prevalent within developing economies. Therefore, different digital technologies are being sought to be incorporated into healthcare organizations due to the increasing requirement for efficient processes. The main factors that promoted this trend are cost reduction, improvements in reliable and energy-efficient hardware and software, the spread of the Internet, and the successful implementation of numerous large-scale projects in many countries. These digital innovations are expected to increase efficiency and effectiveness when adopted widely across healthcare organizations, as most healthcare delivery is time-sensitive, while also significantly reducing costs. In poor countries there is an opportunity to harness digital health systems to enhance the achievement of health-related goals within the nation's strategic frameworks. Although the possibilities and advantages of digitalization are apparent, its application in the healthcare sphere is regularly hindered by specific contextual conditions that become the keys to failure. Therefore, healthcare organizations must pay particular attention to creating a high level of workplace organizational culture and an organizational attitude towards digitalization. Digital systems imply practical solutions that need to be implemented in a systematic, managerial, and collaborative manner. Some authors have stated that not all developed digital healthcare systems have met expectations, and more often the expectations promoted with the actual possibilities of enhancement through digitization may not be fully realized.

REFERENCES

[1] Vasanthan, L., Natarajan, S. K., Babu, A., Kamath, M. S., & Kamalakannan, S. (2024). Digital health interventions for improving access to primary care in India: A scoping review. *PLOS Glob Public Health*, 4(5), e0002645. https://doi.org/10.1371/journal.pgph.0002645

[2] Dal Mas, F., Massaro, M., Rippa, P., & Secundo, G. (2023). The challenges of digital transformation in healthcare: An interdisciplinary literature review, framework, and future research agenda. *Technovation*, 123, 102716. https://doi.org/10.1016/j.technovation.2023.102716

[3] Dash, S. P. (2020). The impact of IoT in healthcare: Global technological change & the roadmap to a networked architecture in India. *Journal Indian Institution Sciences*, 100, 773–785. https://doi.org/10.1007/s41745-020-00208-y

[4] Sikandar, H., Abbas, A. F., Khan, N., & Qureshi, M. I. (2022). *Digital technologies in healthcare: A systematic review and bibliometric analysis*.International Journal of Online and Biomedical Engineering (iJOE), 18(08), 34–48. https://doi.org/10.3991/ijoe.v18i08.31961

[5] Tortorella, G. L., Saurin, T. A., Fogliatto, F. S., Rosa, V. M., Tonetto, L. M., & Magrabi, F. (2021). Impacts of Healthcare 4.0 digital technologies on the resilience of hospitals. *Technological Forecasting and Social Change*, 166, 120666. https://doi.org/10.1016/j.techfore.2021.120666

[6] Sharifi Kia, A., Rafizadeh, M., & Shahmoradi, L. (2023). Telemedicine in the emergency department: An overview of systematic reviews. *Journal of Public Health (Berl.)*, 31, 1193–1207. https://doi.org/10.1007/s10389-021-01684-x

[7] Chamola, V., Hassija, V., Gupta, V., & Guizani, M. (2020). A comprehensive review of the COVID-19 pandemic and the role of IoT, drones, AI, blockchain, and 5G in managing its impact. *IEEE Access*, 8, 90225–90265. https://doi.org/10.1109/ACCESS.2020.2992341

[8] Adeghe, E. P., Okolo, C. A., & Ojeyinka, O. T. (2024). A review of emerging trends in telemedicine: Healthcare delivery transformations. *International Journal of Life Science Research Archive*, 6(1), 137–147. https://doi.org/10.53771/ijlsra.2024.6.1.0040

[9] Gill, E., Dykes, P. C., Rudin, R. S., Storm, M., McGrath, K., & Bates, D. W. (2020). Technology-facilitated care coordination in rural areas: What is needed? *International Journal of Medical Informatics*, 137, 104102. https://doi.org/10.1016/j.ijmedinf.2020.104102

[10] Howse, E., Rychetnik, L., Marks, L., & Wilson, A. (2020). What does the future hold for chronic disease prevention research?. Australian and New Zealand Journal of Public Health, 44(5), 336–340. https://doi.org/10.1111/1753-6405.13028

[11] Meskó, B., & Topol, E. J. (2023). The imperative for regulatory oversight of large language models (or generative AI) in healthcare. *npj Digital Medical*, 6, 120. https://doi.org/10.1038/s41746-023-00873-0

[12] Patrício, L., Costa, C. R. de S., Varela, L., & Cruz-Cunha, M. M. (2024). Literature review on the sustainable implementation of robotic process automation (RPA) in medical and healthcare administrative services. *Procedia Computer Science*, 239, 166–176. https://doi.org/10.1016/j.procs.2024.06.159

[13] Sangeetha, R., & Mohanbabu, G. (2024). A novel circularly polarized antenna array methodology for early identification of kidney tumors. *Journal of Microwave Power and Electromagnetic Energy*, 58(4), 318–341. https://doi.org/10.1080/08327823.2024.2414710

[14] Mathkor, D. M., Mathkor, N., Bassfar, Z., Bantun, F., Slama, P., Ahmad, F., & Haque, S. (2024). Multirole of the Internet of Medical Things (IoMT) in biomedical systems for managing smart healthcare systems: An overview of current and future innovative trends. *Journal of Infection and Public Health*, 17(4), 559–572. https://doi.org/10.1016/j.jiph.2024.01.013

[15] Ahmed, S. F., Alam, M. S. B., Afrin, S., Rafa, S. J., Rafa, N., & Gandomi, A. H. (2024). Insights into Internet of Medical Things (IoMT): Data fusion, security issues, and potential solutions. *Information Fusion*, 102, Article 102060. https://doi.org/10.1016/j.inffus.2023.102060

[16] S. R., A., M., P., P., D., Manikandan, P., P., N., & Saravanan, M. (2022). Application of multi-domain feature for automated seizure detection from EEG signal. In Proceedings of the *2022 3rd International Conference on Smart Electronics and Communication (ICOSEC), Trichy, India* Institute of Electrical and Electronics Engineers (IEEE). (pp. 280–285). https://doi.org/10.1109/ICOSEC54921.2022.9952003

[17] Solanki, V., Sharma, B., Saluja, K., Gupta, S., & Jeon, G. (2024). Importance and need of IoMT and big data to revolutionizing healthcare industry.

[18] Parihar, A., Prajapati, J. B., Prajapati, B. G., Trambadiya, B., Thakkar, A., & Engineer, P. (2024). Role of IoT in healthcare: Applications, security & privacy concerns. *Intelligent Pharmacy*, 2(5), 707–714. https://doi.org/10.1016/j.ipha.2024.01.003

[19] Marquis, Y. A. (2024). From theory to practice: Implementing effective role-based access control strategies to mitigate insider risks in diverse organizational contexts. *Journal of Engineering Research and Reports*, 26(5), 138–154. https://doi.org/10.9734/jerr/2024/v26i51141

[20] Reddi, S., Rao, P. M., Saraswathi, P., Jangirala, S., Das, A. K., Jamal, S. S., & Park, Y. (2024). Privacy-preserving electronic medical record sharing for IoT-enabled healthcare system using fully homomorphic encryption, IOTA, and masked authenticated messaging. *IEEE Transactions on Industrial Informatics*, 20(9), 10802–10813. https://doi.org/10.1109/TII.2024.3397343

[21] Verma, P., Tripathi, V., & Pant, B. (2024). Secure Hashgraph for Healthcare: Strengthening privacy and data security in patient records. *IEEE Transactions on Consumer Electronics*, 70(1), 1205–1213. https://doi.org/10.1109/TCE.2024.3370737

[22] Pradhan, D., Behera, M., & Gheisari, M. (2024). Dynamic data placement strategy with network security issues in distributed cloud environment for medical issues: An overview. *Recent Advances in Computer Science and Communications,* 17(6), 25–38. https://doi.org/10.2174/0126662558285372240109113226

[23] Bala, I., Pindoo, I., Mijwil, M. M., Abotaleb, M., & Yundong, W. (2024). Ensuring security and privacy in healthcare systems: A review exploring challenges, solutions, future trends, and the practical applications of artificial intelligence. *Jordan Medical Journal*, 58(3) https://jjournals.ju.edu.jo/index.php/JMJ/article/view/2527

[24] Qazi, F., Kwak, D., Khan, F. G., Ali, F., & Khan, S. U. (2024). Service Level Agreement in cloud computing: Taxonomy, prospects, and challenges. *Internet of Things*, 25, Article 101126. https://doi.org/10.1016/j.iot.2024.101126

[25] Akinyele, K., Baudot, L., Koreff, J., & Sutton, S. (2024). Regulatory innovation and (de)legitimisation: Accountability challenges in the healthcare field. *Accounting Forum*, 49(3), 668–696. https://doi.org/10.1080/01559982.2023.2295161

[26] Haapaniemi, H. (2024). Exploring perceptions and coping behaviors regarding imposed multifactor authentication usage: A University case study (Master's thesis, University of Jyväskylä, Finland). Jyväskylä Studies in Information Systems Science and Information Management. Retrieved from https://jyx.jyu.fi/handle/123456789/94575.

[27] Tariq, M. U. (2024). Revolutionizing health data management with blockchain technology: Enhancing security and efficiency in a digital era. In Manuel B. Garcia and Rui Pedro Pereira de Almeida (eds.), *Emerging Technologies for Health Literacy and Medical Practice* (pp. 153–175). IGI Global. https://doi.org/10.4018/979-8-3693-1214-8.ch008

[28] Ramniklal, R. J. (2024). Database security and integrity: Ensuring reliable and secure data management. *Mosaic of Ideas: Multidisciplinary Reflections*, 73.

[29] Al Zaabi, M., & Alhashmi, S. M. (2024). Big data security and privacy in healthcare: A systematic review and future research directions. *Information Development*, 02666669241247781.

[30] Rahman, M., Hasan, M., Rahman, M., & Momotaj, M. (2024). A framework for patient-centric consent management using blockchain smart contracts in predictive analysis for healthcare industry. *International Journal of Health Systems and Medical Sciences*, 3(3), 45–59.

[31] Premkumar, M., & Sundararajan, T. V. P. (2021). Defense countermeasures for DoS attacks in WSNs using deep radial basis networks. *Wireless Personal Communications*, 120(4), 2545–2560.

[32] Sarkar, A., & Jhamb, M. (2024). Secure and portable health monitoring system for cyber physical systems in internet of things. *Engineering Research Express*, 6(2), Article 025357. https://doi.org/10.1088/2631-8695/ad5269

[33] Sangwan, R. S., Qiu, R. G., & Jessen, D. (2005). Using RFID tags for tracking patients, charts, and medical equipment within an integrated health delivery network. In *Proceedings of the 2005 IEEE Networking, Sensing and Control, Tucson, AZ, USA* (pp. 1070–1074). Institute of Electrical and Electronics Engineers (IEEE). https://doi.org/10.1109/ICNSC.2005.1461346

[34] Lin, Q., Li, X., Cai, K., Prakash, M., & Paulraj, D. (2024). Secure Internet of Medical Things (IoMT) based on ECMQV-MAC authentication protocol and EKMC-SCP blockchain networking. *Information Sciences*, 654, Article 119783. https://doi.org/10.1016/j.ins.2023.119783

[35] Marandi, S., Moazami, F., & Malekinezhad, A. (2024). A lightweight and anonymous mutual authentication and key agreement scheme for WBAN. *Peer-to-Peer Networking and Applications*, 17, 2555–2571. https://doi.org/10.1007/s12083-024-01686-y

[36] Premkumar, M., Ashokkumar, S. R., Mohanbabu, G., Jeevanantham, V., & Jayakumar, S. (2022). Security behavior analysis in web of things smart environments using deep belief networks. *International Journal of Intelligent Networks*, 3, 181–187. https://doi.org/10.1016/j.ijin.2022.10.003

[37] George, A. S., Baskar, T., & Srikaanth, P. B. (2024). Cyber threats to critical infrastructure: Assessing vulnerabilities across key sectors. *Partners Universal International Innovation Journal*, 2(1), 51–75. https://doi.org/10.5281/zenodo.10639463
[38] Zhang, X., Tang, Z., Zhang, Y., et al. (2024). Knowledge, attitudes, and practices of primary healthcare practitioners regarding pharmacist clinics: A cross-sectional study in Shanghai. *BMC Health Services Research*, 24, 677. https://doi.org/10.1186/s12913-024-11136-3
[39] Murotova, N. X. (2024). The importance of regularly organizing training for the current medical equipment management to ensure that medical and technical employees can consciously carry out the maintenance of medical equipment. *World Bulletin of Public Health*, 31, 68–70. www.scholarexpress.net/index.php/wbph/article/view/3786
[40] Bakare, S. S., Adeniyi, A. O., Akpuokwe, C. U., & Eneh, N. E. (2024). Data privacy laws and compliance: A comparative review of the EU GDPR and USA regulations. *Computer Science & IT Research Journal*, 5(3), 528–543. https://doi.org/10.51594/csitrj.v5i3.859
[41] Atadoga, A., Farayola, O. A., Ayinla, B. S., Amoo, O. O., Abrahams, T. O., & Osasona, F. (2024). A comparative review of data encryption methods in the USA and Europe. *Computer Science & IT Research Journal*, 5(2), 447–460.
[42] Demirer, M., Jiménez Hernández, D. J., Li, D., & Peng, S. (2024). Data, privacy laws and firm production: Evidence from the GDPR (Working Paper No. 32146). National Bureau of Economic Research. https://doi.org/10.3386/w32146
[43] Jeyaraman, N., Ramasubramanian, S., Yadav, S., Balaji, S., Muthu, S., & Jeyaraman, M. (2024). Regulatory challenges and frameworks for fog computing in healthcare. *Cureus*, 16(8), e66779. https://doi.org/10.7759/cureus.66779
[44] Chowdhury, R. H. (2024). Big data analytics in the field of multifaceted analyses: A study on 'Health care management'. *World Journal of Advanced Research and Reviews*, 22(3), 2165–2172. https://doi.org/10.30574/wjarr.2024.22.3.1995
[45] Goyal, M., Garg, N., Oberoi, N., & Mehta, V. (2024). Resource management in Hadoop clusters at the storing level of hadoop distributed file system. In: Vimal, V., Perikos, I., Mukherjee, A., & Piuri, V. (eds.), *Multi-Strategy Learning Environment. ICMSLE 2024*. Algorithms for Intelligent Systems. Springer, Singapore. https://doi.org/10.1007/978-981-97-1488-9_39
[46] Eriskin, L., Karatas, M., & Zheng, Y. J. (2024). A robust multi-objective model for healthcare resource management and location planning during pandemics. *Annals of Operations Research*, 335, 1471–1518. https://doi.org/10.1007/s10479-022-04760-x
[47] Mehralian, G., Ghaleh, H. H., Wang, P., & Moradi, M. (2024). Expanding capacity for learning and transformation: A new look from human resource configurations towards product innovation in the Healthcare Industry. *British Journal of Management*, 35, 1247–1261. https://doi.org/10.1111/1467-8551.12756
[48] Zhang, J., Tutun, S., Anvaryazdi, S. F., et al. (2024). Management of resource sharing in emergency response using data-driven analytics. *Annals of Operations Research*, 339, 663–692. https://doi.org/10.1007/s10479-023-05702-x
[49] Abaku, E. A., & Odimarha, A. C. (2024). Sustainable supply chain management in the medical industry: A theoretical and practical examination. *International Medical Science Research Journal*, 4(3), 319–340. https://doi.org/10.51594/imsrj.v4i3.931
[50] Dion, H., & Evans, M. (2024). Strategic frameworks for sustainability and corporate governance in healthcare facilities; approaches to energy-efficient hospital management. *Benchmarking: An International Journal*, 31(2), 353–390. https://doi.org/10.1108/BIJ-04-2022-0219

14 Design of Computer Vision-Based Autonomous Wheelchair for Spatially Abled Patients

Rituraj Bhattacharjee and Subhradip Mukherjee

14.1 INTRODUCTION

Since the late 20th century, computer vision has influenced the world's transition to innovative societies. With the adoption of newer, improved, sophisticated, and focused technology, computer vision continues to evolve. Computer vision tools are becoming a basic necessity for all human beings and their daily lives. To obtain solutions tailored to their specific needs, the majority of sectors, including socioeconomic, political, educational, medical, and healthcare, are incorporating cutting-edge computer vision tools developed by the industry into their systems and procedures. A patient with a disability has increased, maintained, or improved their functional capabilities as a result of integrating wireless and sensor technology. An autonomous wheelchair is a form of assistive technology that allows individuals with motor limitations to move independently.

Worldwide, an estimated 65 million individuals are expected to require a wheelchair [1], and over 22% more people are anticipated to require one within the next ten years [2]. The elderly have a high need for wheelchair services, which is challenging to meet. In the early 1980s, research on wheelchairs began. One could move around an office building with the prototype wheelchair [3]. To provide consumers with indoor mobility, other EPWs have been developed and introduced to the market, including TinMan [4], NavChair [5], Maid [6], and SPAM [7]. However, patients with complex disabilities and mobility impairments brought on by cerebral palsy, cognitive decline, and fatigue found it challenging to operate the joystick-controlled classic form of wheelchair [8]. For instance, due to perceptual abnormalities, patients with Parkinson's disease frequently lack the cognitive and motor skills necessary to navigate the EPW. According to research involving 65 doctors, between 10 and 40 percent of their patients had mental problems, limited mobility, or sensory impairments that prevented them from receiving a wheelchair. With the current control features, it was challenging to securely use a wheelchair due to these impairments [9].

 DOI: 10.1201/9781003561309-14

Therefore, persons who are unable to safely and independently operate a wheelchair must be seated in a manual wheelchair and pushed by a caregiver. To address these issues, researchers implemented three primary design improvements to the wheelchair: enhancements to the physical interface, shared power control between the wheelchair and the user, and modifications to the mechanics of assistive technology [10, 11]. Hospitals and airports have tested the smart autonomous wheelchairs. The work on computer vision for obstacle detection as it relates to autonomous wheelchair operation is discussed in a research paper [12]. Researchers developed a voice-activated, intelligent wheelchair navigation system that would enable a deliberate transfer of control between the wheelchair and its user [13]. The concept of the Brain-Computer Interface serves as the basis for the following article, which describes how individuals with disabilities can control the movements of their wheelchairs by blinking their eyes. This is achieved by using an Arduino microcontroller connected to a Bluetooth device [14].

After reviewing the literature, we focused on medical imaging, medical video, and a clinical implementation study. We review the essential algorithmic skills that made these possibilities possible and explore the numerous recent successes. Numerous categories, including screening, diagnosis, condition detection, prognostication, organ-to-cell pathology segmentation, illness monitoring, and clinical research, can benefit from the clinical duties. We consider the technology's potential for growth, as well as its impact on healthcare and medicine.

The goal of this research is to develop a real-time human gesture recognition system that utilizes Mediapipe and OpenCV to track and identify body motions, subsequently sending the gestures to an Arduino for further processing. This study shows how hardware control based on body motions can be integrated with computer vision for gesture recognition. The camera is capable of capturing frames and determining the location of individuals within a specific area marked by wheelchair landmarks by utilizing image processing techniques to identify and evaluate human body landmarks. Serial communication is used to send the digital representations of the resulting states of the human body to an Arduino board. We have developed a 3D model of a wheelchair in a V-REP simulation environment and simulated it using MATLAB code interfacing. The results are efficient enough to compare the real-time results.

14.2 METHODOLOGY

Wheelchairs enable individuals with various disabilities to move freely through the use of an easy-to-use interface, thereby improving their quality of life. With the use of a microcontroller and the development of computer vision technology, the research work provides controls that enable simultaneous control of the chair's speed and direction. Figure 14.1 shows the comprehensive process flow of autonomous roving.

The wheelchair prototype was enhanced and modified from a wheelchair driven by a camera module, and it was integrated with motor controllers to enable both manual and autonomous wheelchair manipulation. The primary component of this research

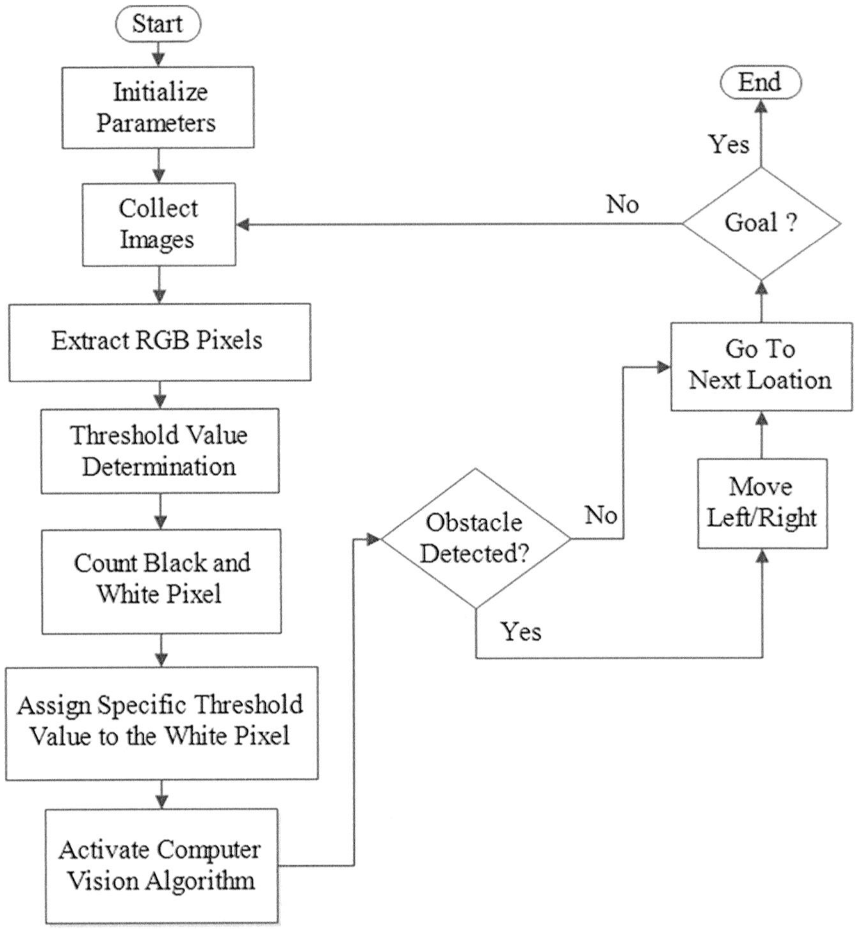

FIGURE 14.1 Process flow diagram for autonomous roving of wheelchair.

work is the image processing method, which is used to process the image and generate the output. Picture customization, picture capture, and image recognition are its three stages. The process of matching the required output signal to the desired image that was gathered is known as image customization. The process of matching the signal of the output to the desired image is known as image customization. The process of capturing the desired person's image and saving it according to the customization setup is known as image capture. The RGB (Red, Green, and Blue) images are then extracted, and the pixel threshold value is established. The RGB images are then masked using the binary masking technique, which turns the masked RGB images into black and white. To determine the desired object, the white pixel values are compared to the threshold value. The last stage is image recognition, and at this point, the camera module sends a specific signal to the microcontroller, allowing it to perform the required action.

14.2.1 Computer Vision Algorithm

It is possible to build deep learning architectures that can learn from non-image data using conventional deep networks and picture data using convolutional networks. Clinical forecasts, prognoses, diagnoses, and combinations of generative models are examples of learned annotations. One can train convolutional neural networks to produce images. Image-to-image regression, super-resolution picture augmentation, creating new images, and other tasks are among them. Deep learning is a subset of machine learning that allows modern computers to define and classify objects. Convolutional neural networks are a specific kind of deep learning algorithm that data scientists mostly use in computer vision. Convolutional neural networks (CNNs) were designed with a multi-layer architecture that minimizes preprocessing while extracting visual features from pixel images. Even though a very deep network could include more than 100 layers, they nonetheless belong to three categories that are essential to every CNN. As shown in Figure 14.2, the primary component of the CNN consists of convolutional (conv) layers. Here, a variety of filters referred to as convolutional kernels move pixel by pixel over an input image to recognize various patterns. Early convolutional layers often extract the fundamental shapes, such as lung edges. Subsequent layers identify more intricate ideas, such as nodes or other anomalous structures. Feature maps are the multiple output images produced by the kernels. To reduce the amount of CPU resources required to process the image, pooling layers are placed before and after convolutional layers to compress the feature maps. The ultimate output (classification) is created by fully connected (FC) layers, which combine the data from earlier layers. All things considered, even the most intricate CNN models can be understood as two-component systems composed of blocks for feature extraction and classification. The pooling and conv layers detect features. The likelihood that an input image belongs to a particular class is determined through fully connected (FC) layers.

14.2.2 Model Description

A wheelchair with two front castor wheels and two rear wheels is a disk with radius r_1 that is centered at (x, y). The system is described in the given equation

$$V = \left\{ \left(z_1, z_2\right) \in R^2 : \left(z_1 - x\right)^2 + \left(z_2 - y\right)^2 \le r_1^2 \right\} \tag{14.1}$$

Figure 14.3 depicts a wheelchair with two front castor wheels and two rear wheels. On opposite ends of a wheelbase of length 1_1 are the two rear drive wheels with radius r_2. The wheelchair's orientational angle with respect to the z1-axis of the z1z2 Cartesian plane is represented by the angle α. The wheelchair's center is located at (x, y), which is μ from the centers of the two opposing rear wheels at an orientational angle of α. The left and right rear wheels have the following angular velocities,

$$\theta_r = s_r \tag{14.2}$$

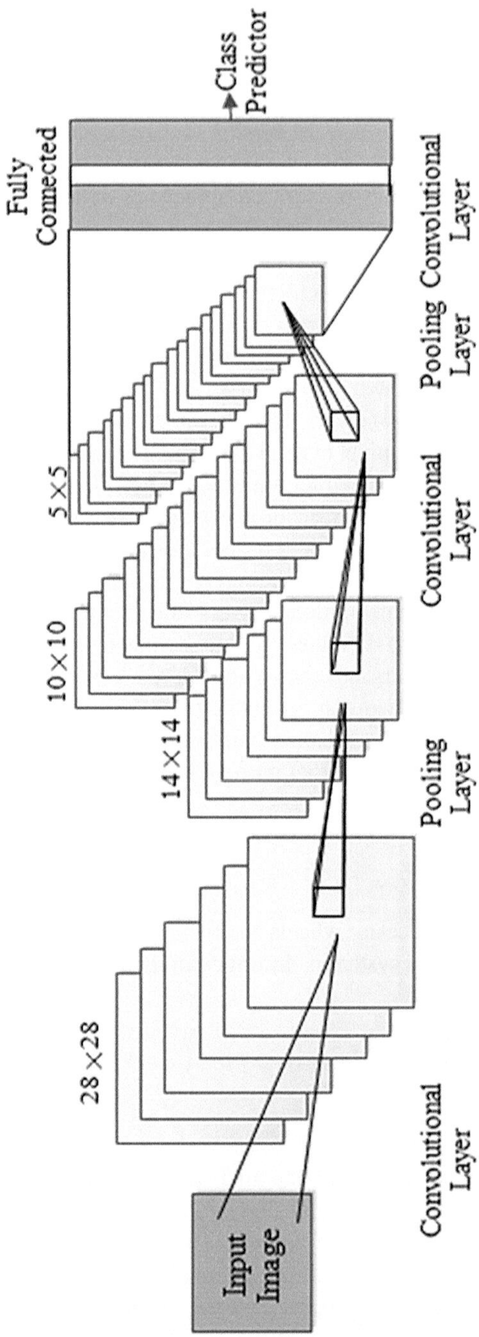

FIGURE 14.2 Basic CNN structure.

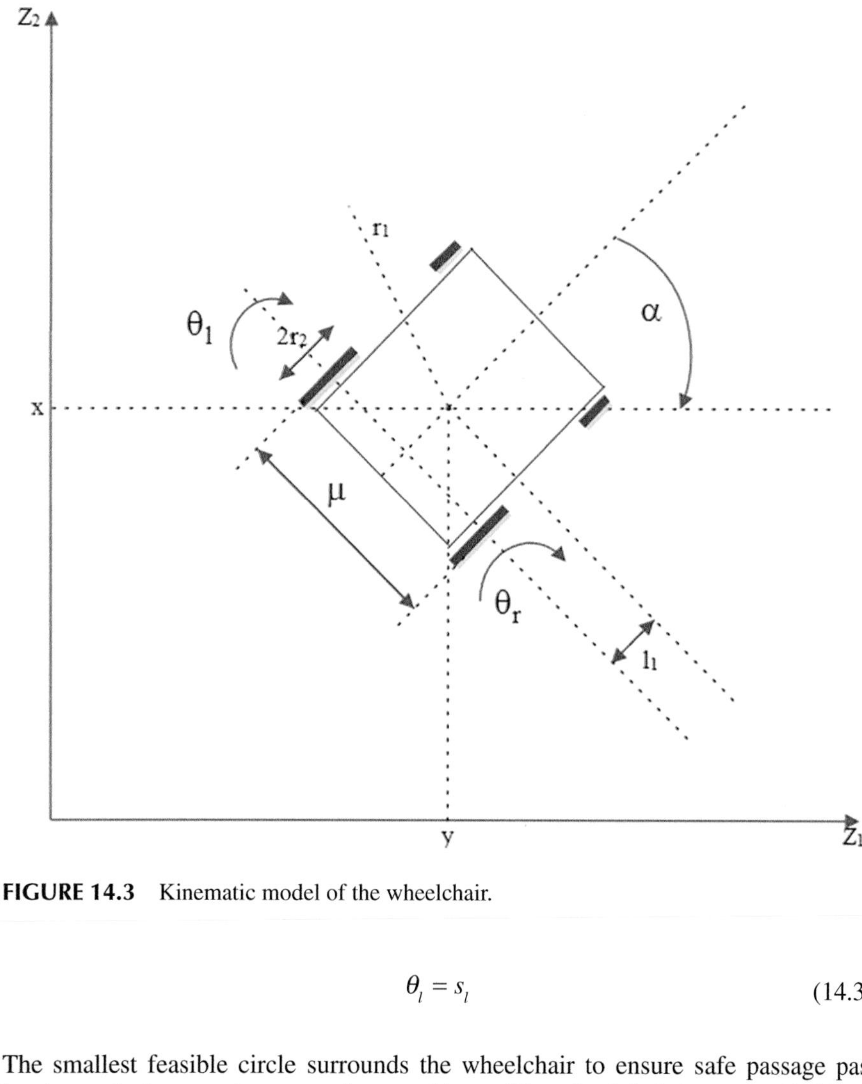

FIGURE 14.3 Kinematic model of the wheelchair.

$$\theta_l = s_l \tag{14.3}$$

The smallest feasible circle surrounds the wheelchair to ensure safe passage past barriers, whether moving or stationary objects. The wheelchair is surrounded by a protected circular zone with a radius r1, centered at (x, y), as illustrated in Figure 14.3.

$$r_1 = \sqrt{\left(\frac{l_1}{2}\right)^2 + \left(\mu + r_2\right)^2} \tag{14.4}$$

The kinematic parameters, namely the wheelbase and wheel radius, are presumed to be free of uncertainty. Additionally, with respect to (x, y), the following limitations are calculated under the assumption that the two back wheels are only rolling and not experiencing any lateral slippage:

$$\dot{y}\, cos\, cos\, \alpha - \dot{x}\, sin\, sin\, \alpha - \dot{\alpha}_{\mu} = 0 \tag{14.5}$$

$$\dot{x}\, cos\, cos\, \alpha + \dot{y}\, sin\, sin\, \alpha + \frac{l_1}{2}\dot{\alpha} - r_2\dot{\theta}_r = 0 \tag{14.6}$$

$$\dot{x}\, cos\, cos\, \alpha + \dot{y}\, sin\, sin\, \alpha + \frac{l_1}{2}\dot{\alpha} - r_2\dot{\theta}_l = 0 \tag{14.7}$$

The robot's kinematic model is generated as follows with respect to its center $(x, y) \in R^2$,

$$\dot{x} = \frac{r_2}{\mu}\left(s_r\left(\frac{l_1}{2} cos\, cos\, \alpha - \mu\, sin\, sin\, \alpha\right) + s_l\left(\frac{l_1}{2} cos\, cos\, \alpha + \mu\, sin\, sin\, \alpha\right)\right) \tag{14.8}$$

$$\dot{y} = \frac{r_2}{\mu}\left(s_r\left(\frac{l_1}{2} sin\, sin\, \alpha + \mu\, cos\, cos\, \alpha\right) + s_l\left(\frac{l_1}{2} sin\, sin\, \alpha - \mu\, cos\, cos\, \alpha\right)\right) \tag{14.9}$$

$$\dot{\alpha} = \frac{r_2}{\mu}\left(s_r - s_l\right) \tag{14.10}$$

$$\dot{\theta}_r = s_r \tag{14.11}$$

$$\dot{\theta}_l = s_l \tag{14.12}$$

The wheelchair has a maximum length of 500 mm, a maximum width of 250 mm, and a minimum turning radius of 200 mm. The hardware architecture of the wheel chair comprises a 5-megapixel infrared camera with an OV5647 sensor, including an adjustable 8 mm focal length, 1.2 Aperture (F), a 1/4-inch CCD size, a 40-degree field of vision, 6.8 Ah rechargeable lithium-ion battery with an input voltage of 12.6 volts and an output voltage of 10.8 to 12.6 volts and 1080-pixel resolution, L298N motor driver module, 12V DC motors with a torque of 43 N cm and a speed of 487 RPM, and an embedded system built on an Arduino Uno board. Using real-time visuals, the camera module offers a medium for communication between the user and the system. The image is transformed into an array of strings, which are then sent to the Arduino Uno that is attached to it. After the camera

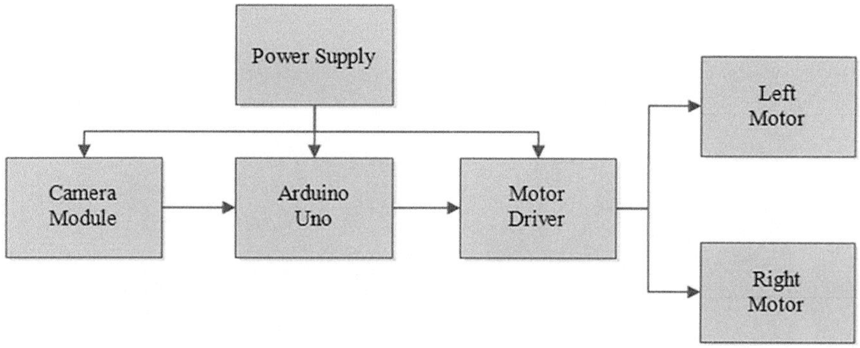

FIGURE 14.4 Basic hardware architecture.

module receives the image, it is extracted and processed by the microcontroller that is attached to it. The motors will then operate by the image that is provided to the motor driver. The wheelchair will be controlled and understood by the system. While the circuit is on, the camera module checks that the path is clear of obstacles and alerts the Arduino if an obstacle is detected. It then halts the wheelchair until the user gives another order. The basic hardware architecture of the wheelchair is shown in Figure 14.4.

14.2.3 V REP Model

Any robot or robotic system can be modeled, edited, programmed, and simulated using the 3D robot simulation application V-REP (Virtual Robot Experimentation Platform), which also features an integrated development environment. A wheelchair simulation model in VREP is displayed in Figure 14.5.

The model comprises a rotating joint, a body or casing, and an infrared camera sensor mounted to the joint. The sensor casing has a non-threaded child script attached to it. Its tasks include reading the sensor, moving the joint by a specified angle, creating a line primitive in the scene (as well as an auxiliary point primitive where a detection happened), and moving on to the next angular position. The child script must handle the number of joint angle positions that the joint would shift in a single simulation phase, as it is not threaded. The model is ready for use during simulation and can be dragged and dropped into an environment. The entire model is contained in a single file that is directly usable on various platforms and compatible with both the most recent and next versions of V-REP. The control code of the model can be modified at any time and copied as often as needed. The MATLAB interface uses v-REP remote APIs. An interface through which commands can be sent to or received from V-REP. The synchronization of V-REP and MATLAB timings is automatic. To start and end V-REP simulations, use MATLAB instructions.

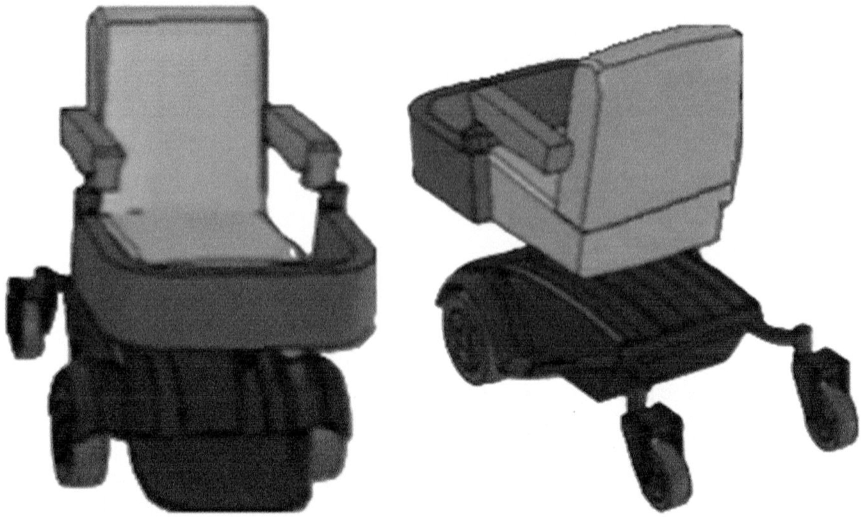

FIGURE 14.5 Design of wheelchair model in V REP.

14.3 RESULTS AND DISCUSSIONS

All the tests required for the system's validation were completed in the MATLAB and VREP simulation because it was not feasible to implement the system in the hospital's facilities.

The computer vision algorithm is simulated in MATLAB in the first step and contrasted with other algorithms. The VREP simulation is used to create and simulate the wheelchair prototype. We present here the results of simulations using the recommended approach. The proposed controller's advantages are demonstrated in various scenarios following several challenging experiments. The laboratory environment's facilities were used for the real-time experiments in the second step.

The following theories have been put out as we simulated the computer vision algorithm in the given scenarios:

i. The wheelchair has a minimum speed and a minimum distance to avoid obstacles in the simulated scenarios.
ii. Every position in the simulation world is known to the wheelchair.
iii. The wheelchair is unable to locate obstructions.
iv. The wheelchair pauses if there is no clear path connecting two locations.
v. All types of slippage and skidding errors are ignored.

14.3.1 MATLAB Results

MATLAB simulation is used in conjunction with multiple tests conducted under various conditions to assess the efficacy of the proposed method. A 100 × 100 cm^2 arena with the obstacles shown in the figures below is used for analysis. To determine the optimal course, ten simulations are conducted, with one agent and multiple agents. Table 14.1 outlines the conditions considered when evaluating the algorithm. The algorithm doesn't increase the iteration number excessively to minimize the time gap. The wheelchair's starting speed was limited to less than 5 meters per second. We test the method in four distinct settings. The wheelchair's threshold distance from an obstacle is adjusted based on its movements. Table 14.2 displays the starting values of the computer vision algorithm's parameters. Figure 14.6 shows the traced paths of the computer vision algorithm under different simulated conditions.

Several iterations are made in each setting until the best outcomes are selected. The algorithm generates its best values after a successful iteration. In general, we have compared the computer vision algorithm's output with previously published methods [6, 11, 12]. Table 14.3 displays the comparative research conducted in various environments.

Ninety percent of iterations ultimately result in success. More than 90% of the time, the accuracy rate across all environments is high. In every situation, a percentage deviation of the computer vision is computed with respect to path length and journey duration. First, time and distance are measured consistently and without any hindrance. After that, the measured values in each example are used to calculate the percentage deviation. Figure 14.7 illustrates one deviation percentage in terms of journey time and another deviation percentage in terms of path length.

Comparing the computer vision algorithm to other methods [6][11][12], the results indicate that it has 32.62%, 21.55%, and 19.23% lower variation in trip time and 30.53%, 20.39%, and 19.33% lower variance in path length. Figure 14.7 presents a comparison of several algorithms based on average percent deviation. Based on the

TABLE 14.1
Different Simulation Environments

Environment	Start (Units)	Goal (Units)	Obstacle
1	(5, 50)	(95, 50)	3
2	(5, 5)	(95, 95)	2
3	(5, 95)	(95, 5)	2
4	(5, 50)	(95, 50)	2

TABLE 14.2
Parameter Values for Computer Vision Algorithm

Parameter	Value
No. of Iteration	100
Wheelchair Speed	0–5 km/hour
Threshold Distance	2 meters
Turning Angle	60^0

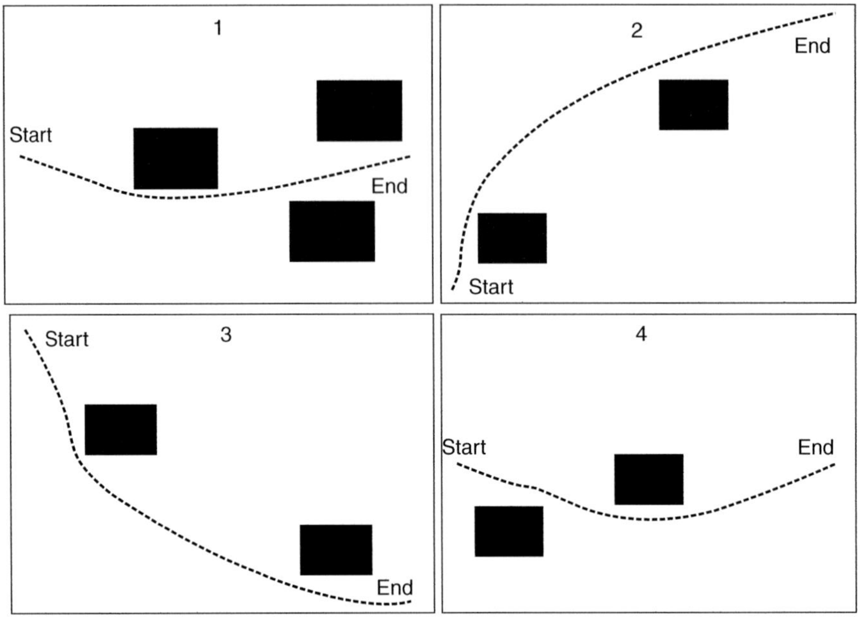

FIGURE 14.6 Path trajectories of wheelchair with computer vision in multiple environments

TABLE 14.3
Comparative Results of Different Approaches

Environment	Method	Path (Unit)	Time (Second)
1	Computer Vision	92.8	71.26
	Approach [6]	95.2	78.54
	Approach [11]	94.7	76.33
	Approach [12]	94.5	76.14
2	Computer Vision	130.2	98.44
	Approach [6]	131.4	99.22
	Approach [11]	130.8	98.75
	Approach [12]	130.4	98.47
3	Computer Vision	129.9	98.32
	Approach [6]	132.2	99.60
	Approach [11]	130.8	98.75
	Approach [12]	130.5	98.46
4	Computer Vision	93.6	71.41
	Approach [6]	95.3	78.52
	Approach [11]	94.6	76.33
	Approach [12]	94.1	75.82

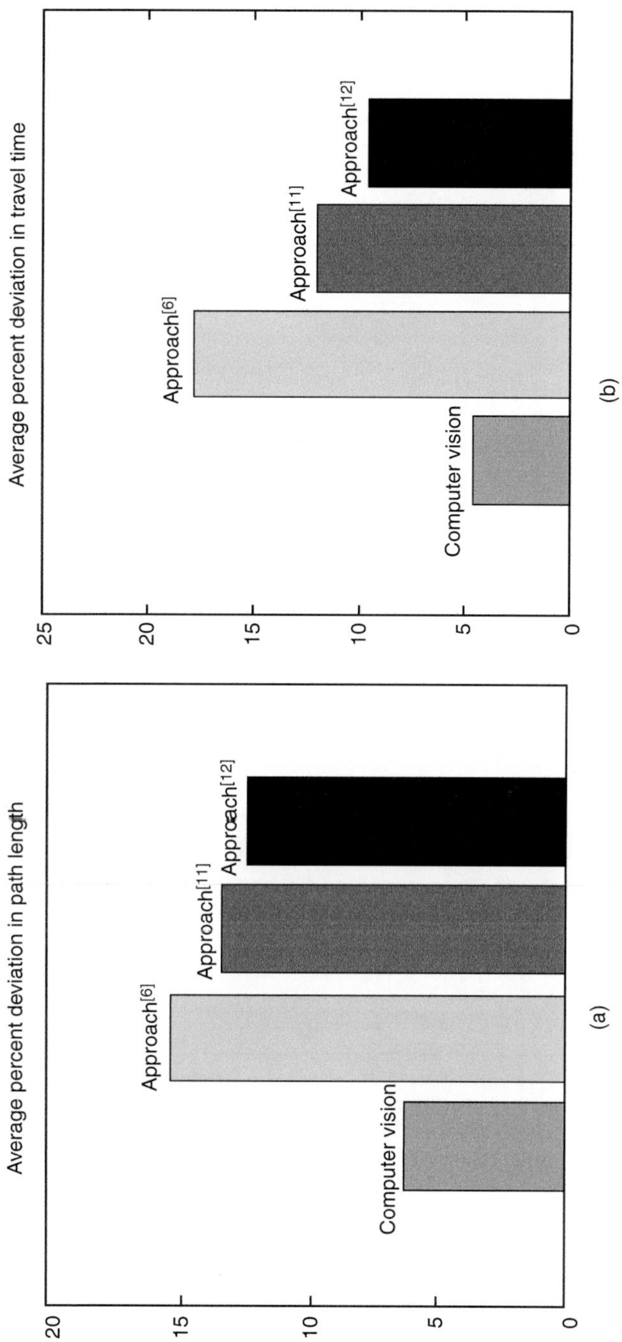

FIGURE 14.7 Comparative percentage deviation in terms of **(a)** travel time and **(b)** path length.

simulation findings, it is evident that the computer vision algorithm performed satisfactorily and accurately in each scenario tested.

14.3.2 V REP Results

A 300 cm by 300 cm simulation platform is shown in Figures 14.8 and 14.9. A red circle represents the start location, a green circle marks the target position, and light

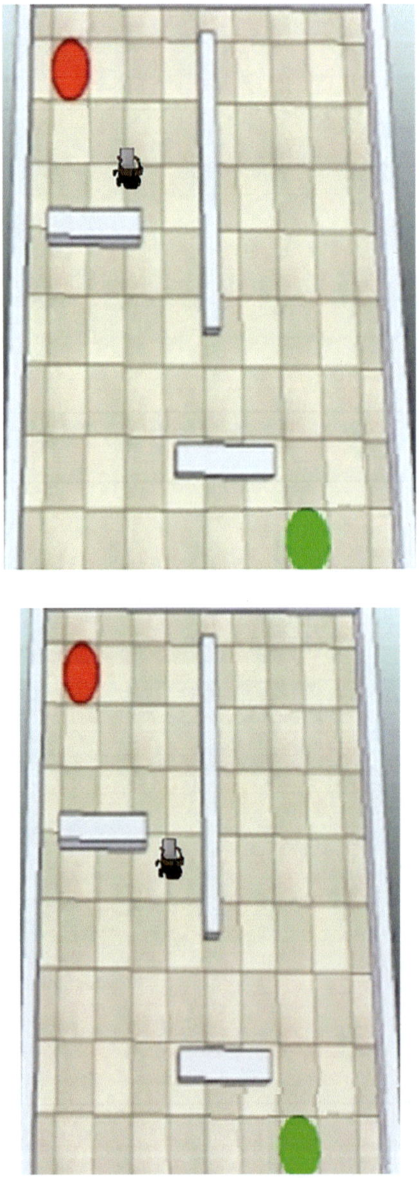

FIGURE 14.8 Performance of wheelchair in V REP Environment-1.

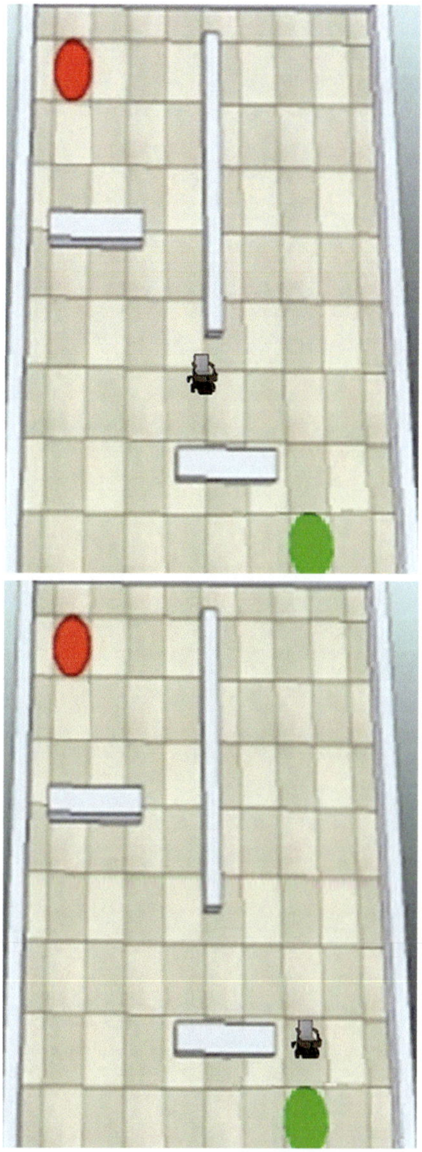

FIGURE 14.8 (Continued)

blue cubic bodies in these surroundings represent the barriers. This configuration aligns with the setup of environment-1 in the VREP platform (see Figure 14.8).

Figure 14.8 illustrates the wheelchair's ability to navigate a course and avoid obstacles in the current setting. The environment has been set up with the same number of obstacles, the same goal, and the same start positions in the exact same locations. In comparison to the 2D simulation, the wheelchair has required more time

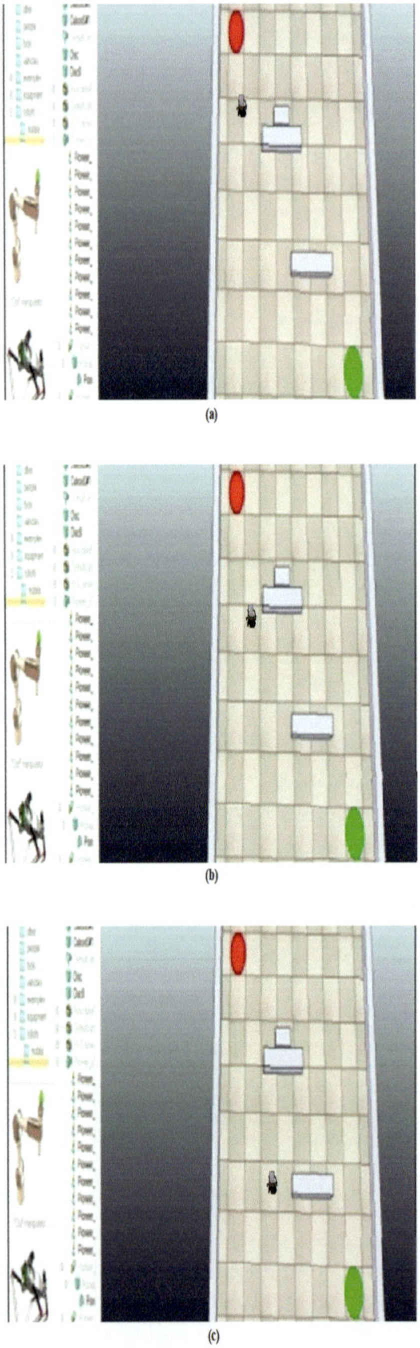

FIGURE 14.9 Performance of wheelchair in V-REP Environment-2.

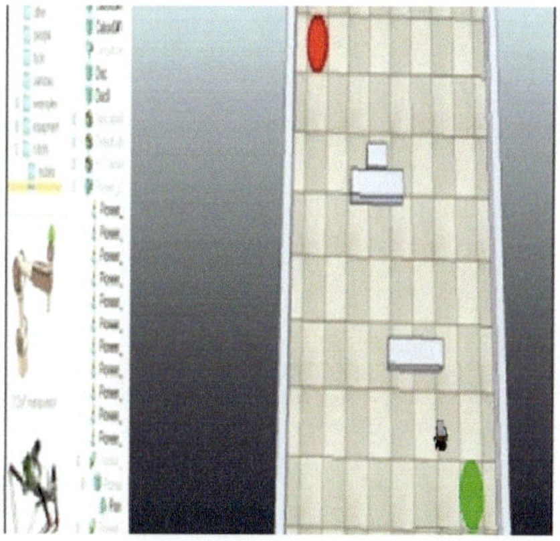
(d)

FIGURE 14.9 (Continued)

TABLE 14.4
Performance of the Wheelchair in the V REP Simulator

Figure No.	*Path Coverage (cm)*	*Travel Time* (seconds)
7	362.6	68
8	351.4	62

on the VREP platform. Furthermore, no severe bends have been made by the wheelchair on this platform. Similarly environments-2 are arranged in Figure 14.9.

In the V-REP environment-2, the wheelchair has performed satisfactorily, as it did in the previous environment. Simulation results demonstrate the effectiveness of the wheelchair in various V-REP environments. A modified obstacle avoidance technique has been developed in this research, and its stability is shown through a 3D simulation. The performance of the wheelchair in the V-REP simulator is given in Table 14.4.

14.3.3 Real-Time Results

The wheelchair's computer vision has been tested in a real-time laboratory setting. The autonomous wheelchair has successfully navigated obstacles in laboratory experiments. Figure 14.10 displays the wheelchair's path navigation in the real-time given environment.

The wheelchair demonstrates its effectiveness through several real-time experiments, with a success rate of 95%. The multiple observations have yielded the best results. The experiment yielded good success rates and lower percent deviations. During the experiment, slippage, skidding mistakes, and other malfunctions are prevented. The experimental test results are presented in terms of travel distance and navigation time, as shown in Table 14.5.

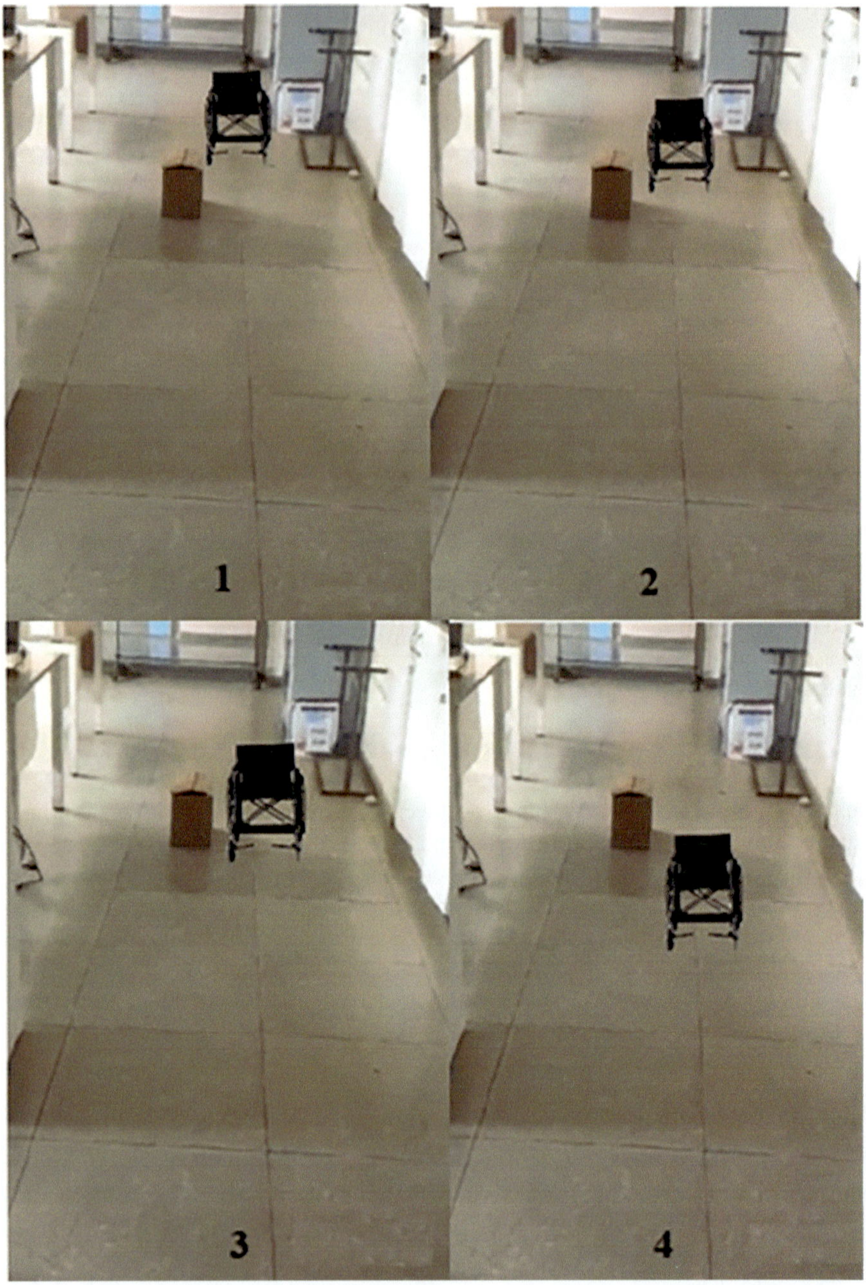

FIGURE 14.10 Real-time path navigation of wheelchair.

TABLE 14.5
Real-time Results of the Wheelchair

Observation	Travel distance (cm)	Navigation time (seconds)
1.	327	1096
2.	335	1230
3.	347	1349
4.	358	1453
5.	367	1678

14.4 CONCLUSION

An installation of the prototype system demonstrates how well the proposed system integrates with the living space. Thus, while some labour is done by hand, our process is entirely automated and distinct. With the help of the proposed algorithm, the wheelchair, which was controlled by its kinematic equations, was able to navigate through an obstacle-filled environment and reach its destination while adhering to the system's constraints and limitations. The wheelchair equipped with computer vision is easily implemented in hospitals, clinics, and healthcare settings. The results demonstrate that the wheelchair achieves greater than 95% accuracy in both simulation and real-time applications. The development of reasonably priced assistive technologies has the potential to accelerate social and economic inclusion.

To create a hybrid system, future research will examine the fusion of the existing algorithm with acceleration controllers using one of the heuristic-based methodologies. The wheelchair user will feel more comfortable with the acceleration controllers. Moreover, the formation control and motion planning of several nonholonomic wheelchairs for realistic applications will be considered.

Acknowledgements: The authors would like to thank all staff in the Robotics and Autonomous Systems Laboratory of the Electronics and Communication Engineering Department, MVJ College of Engineering, Bangalore, India, for their continuous support and encouragement throughout this research work.

REFERENCES

[1] D. Labbé, W. B. Mortenson, P. W. Rushton, L. Demers, and W. C. Miller, "Mobility and participation among ageing powered wheelchair users: Using a lifecourse approach," *Ageing and Society*, vol. 40, no. 3, pp. 626–642, 2020, doi:10.1017/S0144686X18001228.

[2] H. S. Kaye, T. Kang, and M. P. LaPlante, "Mobility device use in the United States," *Disability Statistics Report*, vol. 14, pp. 1–10, 2000.

[3] R. Madarasz, L. Heiny, R. Cromp, and N. Mazur, "The design of an autonomous vehicle for the disabled," *IEEE Journal on Robotics and Automation*, vol. 2, no. 3, pp. 117–126, 1986, doi: 10.1109/JRA.1986.1087052.

[4] D. P. Miller and M. G. Slack, "Design and testing of a low-cost robotic wheelchair prototype," *Autonomous Robots*, vol. 2, pp. 77-88, 1995, doi:10.1007/BF00735440.

[5] S. P. Levine et al., "The NavChair assistive wheelchair navigation system," *IEEE Transactions on Rehabilitation Engineering*, vol. 7. no. 4, pp. 443-451, 1999, doi:10.1109/86.808948.

[6] R. Simpson et al., "A prototype power-assist wheelchair that provides for obstacle detection and avoidance for those with visual impairments," *Journal of NeuroEngineering and Rehabilitation*, vol. 2, no. 30, 2005, doi:10.1186/1743-0003-2-30.

[7] R. C. Simpson, E. F. LoPresti, and R. A. Cooper, "How many people would benefit from a smart wheelchair?" *Journal of Rehabilitation Research and Development*, vol. 45, no. 1, pp. 53-71, 2008, doi:10.1682/JRRD.2007.01.0015.

[8] L. Fehr, W. E. Langbein, and S. B. Skaar, "Adequacy of power wheelchair control interfaces for persons with severe disabilities: A clinical survey," *Journal of Rehabilitation Research and Development*, vol. 37, no. 3, pp. 353-360, 2000.

[9] R. C. Simpson, "Smart wheelchairs: A literature review," *Journal of Rehabilitation Research and Development*, vol. 42, no. 4, pp. 423-436, 2005, doi:10.1682/JRRD.2004.08.0101.

[10] M. R. M. Tomari, Y. Kobayashi, and Y. Kuno, "Development of smart wheelchair system for a user with severe motor impairment," *Procedia Engineering*, vol. 41, pp. 539-546, 2012, doi:10.1016/j.proeng.2012.07.209.

[11] D. Kumar, R. Malhotra, and S. Sharma, "Design and construction of a smart wheelchair," *Procedia Computer Science*, vol. 172, pp. 302–307, 2020, doi:10.1016/j.procs.2020.05.048.

[12] N. Farheen, G. G. Jaman, and M. P. Schoen, "Object detection and navigation strategy for obstacle avoidance applied to autonomous wheelchair driving," in *2022 Intermountain Engineering, Technology and Computing (IETC)*, pp. 1-5, IEEE, Orem, Utah, 2022, doi:10.1109/ietc54973.2022.9796979.

[13] H. M. R. T. Bandara, K. S. Priyanayana, D. P. Chandima, and A. G. B. P. Jayasekara, "Hybrid navigation decision control mechanism for intelligent wheelchair," *IEEE Access*, vol. 11, pp. 118558–118576, 2023, doi:10.1109/access.2023.3318477.

[14] Gupta, P. Sahimkhan, P. Sarmal, and O. Rastogi, "Brain-computer interface (BCI)-inspired Arduino-based wheelchair controller," in *2023 International Conference on Advanced Computing & Communication Technologies (ICACCTech)*, 2023, doi:10.1109/icacctech61146.2023.00052.

15 Privacy-Preserving Machine Learning in Healthcare

Lokesh Ramachandrappa, Krutthika Hirebasur Krishnappa, Aliaa Salim, Ratana Warren, Madhura R, and Manasa R

15.1 INTRODUCTION

PPML is a specialized and rapidly evolving subdomain of ML. The goal of PPML is to ensure that data confidentiality, integrity, and privacy are preserved during the ML lifecycle. The increase in the complexity of ML models is accompanied by an increase in their performance when exposed to larger and more complex datasets. The majority of the documents contain confidential information, particularly those related to critical areas such as health, finance, or law. PPML, therefore, addresses the dual challenge of inferring valuable information from datasets while adhering to the privacy standards imposed to prevent possible exposures or misuse of personal data.

15.1.1 Overview of PPML in Healthcare

Health systems generate and manage immense amounts of data, including electronic health records, medical imaging, genomic sequences, and real-time patient monitoring. This information can potentially be an asset in advancing diagnostic precision, treatment methods, and personalization of care. However, the sensitive data in healthcare requires the application of ML methods that will protect patients' privacy.

PPML makes various techniques available that can help derive insights from data while reducing the risk associated with unauthorized access, data breaches, and misuse. Consequently, PPML will strike a balance between innovation and privacy for healthcare providers, ensuring they remain compliant with regulatory requirements such as the Health Insurance Portability and Accountability Act (HIPAA) in the US and the General Data Protection Regulation (GDPR) in Europe.

15.1.2 Motivation for PPML in Healthcare

The motivation for PPML stems from the critical need to protect sensitive patient information while leveraging the benefits of modern analytics to improve healthcare outcomes. More specifically, serious privacy threats include data breaches, identity inference attacks, model inversion attacks, membership inference attacks, and

DOI: 10.1201/9781003561309-15

adversarial attacks, all of which require effective privacy protection mechanisms tailored to healthcare systems.

Federated learning allows for collaborative model development without the need to exchange data by employing Federated Averaging-based algorithms. Homomorphic encryption enables computation over encrypted data while maintaining confidentiality; it utilizes libraries such as Brakerski-Gentry-Vaikuntanathan (BGV) and Cheon-Kim-Kim-Song (CKKS). Secure Multi-Party Computation (SMPC) enables shared computations with specific assurances of maintaining input data privacy through Yao's Garbled Circuit approach. Blockchain ensures transparency and accountability, as it serves as an immutable log for all interactions and data manipulations. The incorporation of these strategies reduces privacy-related threats, fosters patient confidence, and facilitates smooth transitions among approaches to achieve comprehensive data privacy within healthcare systems.

15.1.3 Literature Review

This literature review will build a strong foundation for understanding the recent developments and challenges that address the existing research and methodologies relevant to PPML in healthcare.

Manoj Ram Tammina [1] elaborated on the application of Differential Privacy in the integration of patient data in the health sector. They have highlighted the challenges in securing data while ensuring privacy and the failure of existing anonymization methods. They have also discussed federated learning for enhancing data usability while preserving patient privacy. The trade-off between data sensitivity and privacy protection, which underlies the requirement for strong privacy-preserving methods in the healthcare sector, is also presented. Amol Khanna [2] adopted Federated Learning with Differential Privacy to develop disease-prediction models that do not expose the private information of individual patients. The challenges of maintaining model accuracy on decentralized data are also discussed. The computational aspects of the study are also presented, along with potential trade-offs in model accuracy resulting from privacy considerations.

Gayathri Hegde [3] compared Neural Networks with traditional approaches in machine learning (ML) in the context of privacy-preserving federated learning for healthcare applications. It demonstrates the effectiveness of neural networks in handling complex data patterns while maintaining strict privacy preservation. The study also addresses the limitations related to computational complexity and the trade-offs between model accuracy and confidentiality. Ahmad Neyaz Khan [4] utilized Homomorphic Encryption for privacy-preserving machine learning in cloud computing, investigating the capabilities of supervised and unsupervised learning tasks through neural networks over encrypted data. The study also addresses the challenges, including sizable computational overhead and complexity in practical implementation. Dominique Mercier [5] evaluated the different approaches to privacy preservation in time-series classification of critical infrastructures, underlining the ineffectiveness of encryption in deep learning, the strong dependence on the dataset of differential privacy, and the general applicability of federated methods. The research further explains the challenges of ensuring data privacy and also of maintaining model performance efficiently. Zahir Alsulaimawi [6] explored privacy-preserving techniques on image data, focused on grayscale images with a single sensitive feature and color images with multiple features. They proposed a new approach that combines adversarial training with modified loss functions to balance privacy and utility appropriately, addressing other critical issues in this study, such as maintaining data utility while ensuring confidentiality, as well as the high computational complexity of the proposed methods.

15.1.4 Key Methods in PPML

Various advanced techniques are followed in PPML, each with its relative strengths and challenges. The most remarkable of them all are:

15.1.4.1 Federated Learning (FL)

FL represents a decentralized methodology, where the various institutions engage in collaborative efforts to develop an ML model without the necessity of exchanging their raw datasets [7]. The local data is managed by each participating institution individually before sending model parameters to a central host. The FL may be utilized in healthcare environments where hospitals develop models using distributed electronic health records. Each user then creates a model based on their segment of the data and sends the model updates to the central server. The central server then aggregates these updates into one global model [8]. In this way, patients' data can be secured and consequently it reduces any chance of leakage. Figure 15.1 shows a healthcare FL setup.

Figure 15.1 depicts the three hospitals participating in FL. Each one of these hospitals will train the model on its own local data and send the updated model parameters to the central server. The server then calculates the average of these parameters to update the global model. This iterative process continues until the model converges. This enables efficient model training while ensuring data privacy [9].

The next aspect of enhancing privacy is through the implementation of secure aggregation methods. A secure aggregation application allows the central server to receive only aggregated results, without updates from participants or users. Specific variant cryptographic solutions for this include SMPC. Consider the case of a FL setup across different hospitals; each party will independently encrypt its model updates before sending them to the central server. It encrypts these updates, decodes the output for the final update, and keeps every single update secret. This provides an additional layer of privacy, thereby enhancing the security of FL when deployed in sensitive fields such as healthcare [10].

15.1.4.2 Differential Privacy (DP)

DP is a mathematically defined set of protocols designed to limit and quantify the possible loss of privacy in data analysis. It works by cautiously adding the measured noise to reduce the possibility of identifying an individual in the dataset through either adjustment made to the dataset or by changing the results of analysis queries.

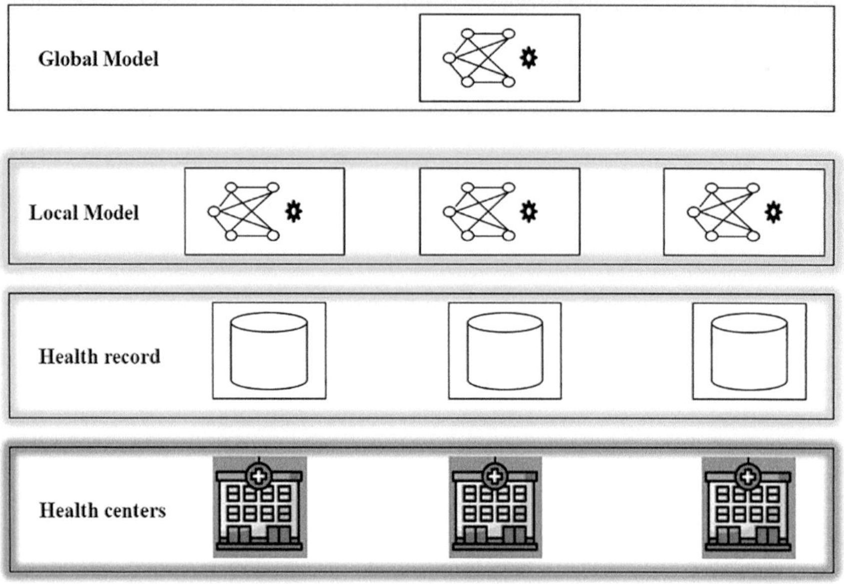

FIGURE 15.1 Diagram of FL in healthcare.

This ensures that adding or removing a single data point will have only a minuscule effect on the analysis result.

Privacy is usually parameterized with a value ε; smaller values of ε imply stronger assurances of confidentiality. For instance, using DP, a dataset of medical records would ensure that the outcome of any analysis conducted on the data remains unchanged, regardless of whether the patients' information is present in the dataset. In such a way, it will be able to protect individual privacy [11].

DP applications include several mechanisms, each personalized to fit different types of data and queries. The Laplace mechanism is one of the most common mechanisms applied to numerical outputs. This mechanism adds noise sampled from a Laplace distribution to query results to ensure the added noise is appropriately scaled with query sensitivity. For example, suppose a hospital wants to publish the average age of patients affected by a specific disease, it would add noise to the average to protect privacy of the patients. Another important usage of the exponential mechanism is choosing one out of various output choices. It assigns a probability to various outcomes based on a utility function and then randomizes the probabilities while keeping the selection process private. Such a mechanism is helpful in several applications, like determining model parameters in ML.

Another application in the analysis of genomic data, where the DP will ensure through genetic studies, no specific participant's information is disclosed. By applying techniques in DP, the researchers may share findings and collaborate on large-scale studies without putting at risk the privacy of individuals as shown in Figure 15.2.

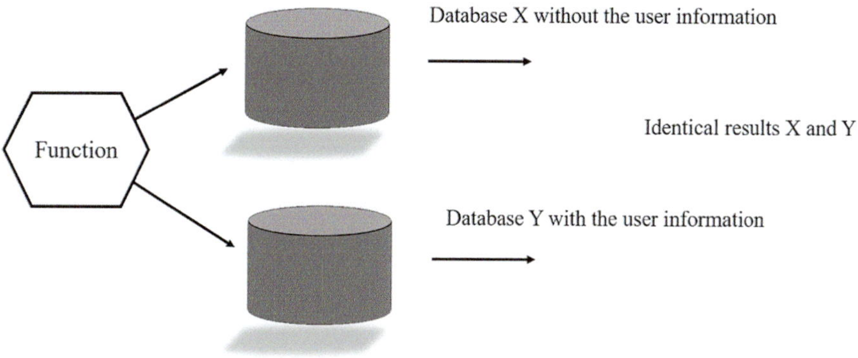

FIGURE 15.2 Differential Privacy in healthcare.

Figure 15.2 shows the process of DP in the healthcare sector.

- Original Data: The raw data contains sensitive data about the individual.
- Query: The query can be used to extract information from data that can be used.
- Noise Addition: Noise is added to the query result, thereby ensuring privacy
- Noisy Output: The final output is a noisy version of the query result that is useful while protecting individual privacy.

This process ensures that any given individual cannot be easily identified within the dataset, thereby providing strong privacy guarantees.

The Laplace mechanism adds noise drawn from a Laplace distribution to the query result to ensure DP. The noise is calibrated based on the sensitivity of the query and the desired privacy level ε.

$$Lap(b) = \frac{1}{2b} exp\, exp\left(\frac{-|x|}{b}\right) \tag{15.1}$$

where:

b is the scale parameter, determined by the sensitivity Δf of the query and the privacy parameter ε. The b is defined as:

$$b = \frac{\Delta f}{\varepsilon} \tag{15.2}$$

where:

Δf : sensitivity of the query
ε : privacy parameter

The exponential mechanism is used for selecting outputs from a range of possibilities [12]. The Equation 15.3 represents the probabilities for various outputs that are assigned based on the utility function $u(x,r)$, where these probabilities are supplemented by noise:

$$P[r] \propto exp\,exp\left(\frac{\varepsilon u(x,r)}{2\Delta u}\right) \tag{15.3}$$

where:

$u(x,r)$: *utility function*
Δu : sensitivity of the utility function
ε : privacy parameter

15.1.4.3 Secure Multi-Party Computation (SMPC)

SMPC is a cryptographic technique that enables multiple parties to jointly compute a function over their inputs while preserving the privacy of the inputs. More precisely, the confidentiality of each party's data is preserved, while external observers gain no additional information about other party's inputs apart from the computed output. The consequences of SMPC become even more critical for secret information; for example, joint research or analytical studies in the field of medicine [12].

SMPC depends on cryptographic methodologies that guarantee both privacy and security. In the context of ML, the Secret Sharing Scheme is employed to collect sensitive data in collaborative model training. Vertical or horizontal FL could be a concrete example, where several parties from different hospitals or different banks jointly train an ML model without data leakage from each party. Using secret sharing, every party divides its input data into shares and distributes these among other parties, where subsequent computations, such as gradient updates, are applied on the shares. After computation, the results are combined to update the model without revealing respective data points and thus, data privacy and collaborative learning are achieved. The secret sharing is one of the solid tools for privacy-preserving ML applications as shown in Figure 15.3 [13].

Figure 15.3 illustrates the following blocks:

- Input Sharing: The parties split their input into shares and send it to other parties.
- Computation on Shares: The parties perform computation on the shares received.
- Result Reconstruction: Computed shares are combined to recreate the result without disclosing individual inputs.

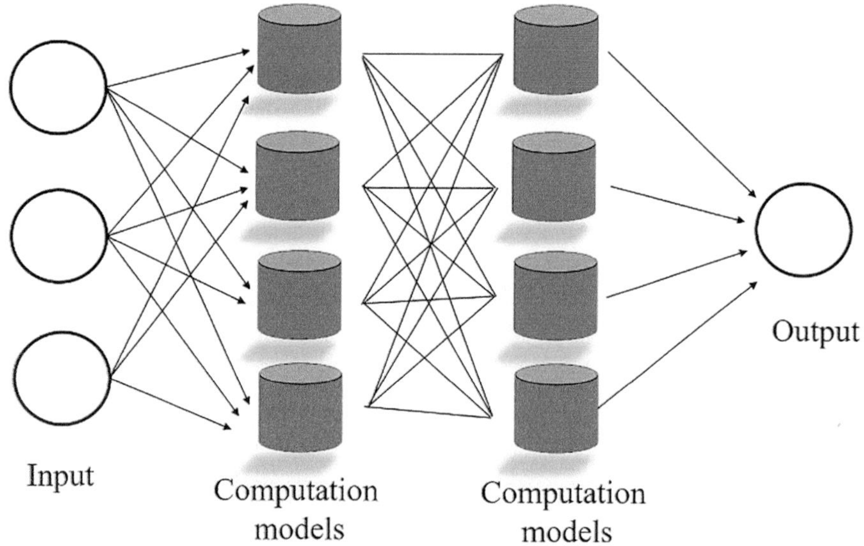

FIGURE 15.3 Secure multi-party computation (SMPC).

15.1.5 Applications of SMPC in Healthcare

1. **Collaborative Genomic Research:** SMPC enables comparative research in genomics, allowing different institutions to jointly analyze genetic information without disclosing the raw datasets. For instance, researchers based at other hospitals can use SMPC to identify genetic markers associated with diseases. Every institution encrypts its genomic data and shares these encrypted inputs with partner institutions. Advanced computations are performed on these encrypted inputs, and the final results are decrypted to reveal integrated data. This approach will ensure that sensitive genetic information remains confidential, thereby enabling the possibility of large-scale collaborative studies [14].
2. **Privacy-Preserving Clinical Trials:** SMPC will enable patient's data to be analyzed securely across different sites for clinical trials. Various pharmaceutical companies and research institutions will use it to compute statistics on trial data without disclosing individual patient information across different sites. For example, SMPC will compute the efficacy of a new drug by collating data from various trial sites. This ensures sensitive patient's information remains private while comprehensive data analysis may occur to determine a new drug's efficacy and safety.
3. **FL for Predictive Modeling:** SMPC enables FL, where numerous health institutions collaboratively train ML models without necessarily sharing raw data. Each institution will train a local model using patient's data and encrypt the model updates before sharing. The central server performs such encrypted update aggregations and final model decryption. This ensures that sensitive

patient information is not disclosed, allowing for the development of a highly predictive model regarding disease diagnosis and treatment.

4. **Secure Health Data Sharing:** SMPC enables clinicians, researchers, and policy analysts to securely share health-related data, allowing hospitals to exchange patient data with public health authorities while maintaining patient confidentiality [15].
5. **Fraud Detection in Health Insurance:** SMPC can be utilized by health insurance companies to identify and assess fraudulent claims. The transaction patterns across different insurers can be effectively analyzed. Each insurer encrypts its transaction data and sends the encrypted input to other insurers. Later, encrypted inputs are analyzed for patterns indicating fraud. This ensures better fraud detection without necessarily revealing sensitive information about individual transactions.
6. **Personalized Medicine:** SMPC enables the creation of personalized treatment plans for patients by securely analyzing information from multiple sources. For example, hospitals will be able to utilize the SMPC concept to combine patient information from various departments and generate a customized treatment program for chronic diseases. Since the data is encrypted and operations are performed on the encrypted datasets, healthcare professionals can develop customized treatment programs without compromising patient privacy.

These applications demonstrate the scope and effectiveness of SMPC in the healthcare industry by ensuring compliance with privacy requirements, facilitating data analysis and collaboration, and providing security.

15.1.6 Challenges and Future Directions

1. **Computational Efficiency:** The significant challenge with PPML is that many of these techniques are computationally expensive. Homomorphic encryption and SMPC techniques can be highly challenging in terms of processing power and time. There is a need to develop algorithms and hardware accelerators of higher efficiency on a large scale in healthcare applications to make it more feasible. For example, optimizing the homomorphic encryption and decryption process can reduce the computational load, making it possible for real-time applications.
2. **Scalability:** Healthcare data is often high-dimensional and voluminous, posing challenges to the scalability of PPML techniques. Ensuring these methods can scale to large datasets is essential for the widespread adoption of PPML. For example, FL must support institutions irrespective of the data volume. Methods like hierarchical federated learning (FL) improve scalability by grouping institutions into clusters, reducing communication overhead, and enhancing efficiency in education.

3. **Interoperability:** A significant challenge to interoperability in PPML arises from standard protocols and data formats, particularly when integrating PPML methods into existing healthcare IT infrastructures. Interoperability ensures that various systems can work together efficiently without issues and facilitate secure data exchange. Standard application programming interfaces and data formats provide the opportunity for different healthcare providers to participate in FL compatibility issues that have previously been addressed.
4. **Verification and Validation:** PPML methodologies need to be validated for their accuracy and reliability to ensure they yield clinically significant results. Testing mechanisms, such as DP, are crucial to ensure that added noise does not compromise the utility of the data. Likewise, FL models must be validated to confirm consistent performance across heterogeneous datasets from various institutions.

15.2 FEDERATED LEARNING (FL) IN HEALTHCARE

15.2.1 FL Technique Overview and its Benefits

FL is a decentralized ML approach that enables collaborative model training across different institutions while maintaining the confidentiality of their raw data. Rather than sharing original datasets, each institution processes its data and sends only the model parameters to the center, which then involves model updates through specific algorithms, such as Federated Averaging, to build a global model. This ensures that sensitive information is still maintained on each institutional local server, thereby reducing the chances of data breaches [16].

Federated Averaging is a crucial algorithm in Federated Learning (FL), enabling different organizations to collectively train a model without sharing any raw data. It can be mathematically represented as:

$$\theta_{t+1} = \sum_{k=1}^{K} \frac{n_k}{n} \theta_{t+1}^{k} \tag{15.4}$$

where:

θ_{t+1} : *updated global model*

K : *number of participating institutions*

n_k : *data points at institution k*

n : *total data points across all institutions*

θ_{t+1}^{k} : *model update from institution k*

15.2.2 Novel Contributions in Federated Learning for Healthcare

FL is well-suited for healthcare, as it allows for collaborative model training without the direct sharing of data between institutions. Nonetheless, this domain faces challenges regarding the efficient scalability of techniques and the protection of privacy. This section introduces hierarchical federated learning (HFL) and secure aggregation methods, which are explicitly designed for multi-hospital collaborations to address these challenges at scale.

1. In standard Federated Learning (FL), each participating entity, such as a hospital, performs local fine-tuning of a global model using local data and then aggregates the results on a central server. However, as the number of institutions increases, network latency and communication overhead become significant issues. HFL implements a dual-tier aggregation framework, categorizing organizations into clusters based on geographical proximity or specific areas of expertise, such as cancer research facilities or rural healthcare coalitions. Within each cluster, a local model is developed, which is subsequently aggregated at the central level, thereby minimizing communication overhead and enhancing the rates of model convergence. The mathematical representation of HFL can be articulated through the hierarchical averaging function:

$$\omega_{global} = \sum_{c=1}^{C} \alpha_c \sum_{i=1}^{N_c} \beta_{i,c}\, \omega_{i,c} \tag{15.5}$$

   where:

   α_c represents the weight assigned to each cluster c

   N_c Is the number of institutions in the cluster c

   $\beta_{i,c}$ denotes the contribution of each institution i In that specific cluster.

   Such a hierarchical structure allows for the flexible utilization of network resources and enhances communication patterns; therefore, FL is achievable even in resource-constrained healthcare settings.

2. Federated learning on a centralized server involves collecting model updates that can pose severe threats to data confidentiality in cases where the server may be compromised. To reduce this risk, an adaptive secure aggregation methodology can be adopted that integrates multi-party computation with differential noise injection techniques. Each participating institution will encrypt its model updates securely and apply a noise factor that adapts to the sensitivity of the data involved. The aggregated update, after MPC processing, still maintains differential privacy, which guarantees the masking of individual updates. The noise factor, calibrated through the privacy budget parameter ε, is applied based on the model update sensitivity:

$$Noise \sim Laplace\frac{\Delta f}{\varepsilon} \tag{15.6}$$

where:

Δf is the sensitivity of the function to individual data points?

This approach enables the secure aggregation of health data, providing reassurance of patient privacy and security, especially in sensitive domains such as genomic or imaging data.

15.2.3 FL Applications and Case Studies

Applications:

1. **Privacy-Preserving Predictive Modeling in Genomic Research:** Privacy-preserving genomic research can be realized by adapting privacy-preserving techniques, especially Secure Data Processing (SDP) and Multiparty Computation (MPC), which identify genetic markers while preserving participant privacy. Such applications are critically significant for the research of rare diseases, where data sharing among organizations is crucial but highly sensitive.
2. **Real-Time Patient Monitoring Using Edge-Based Privacy Techniques:** By integrating privacy-preserving machine learning (ML) at the edge for wearable devices to monitor chronic patients. These devices, along with FL and mechanisms for DP, can facilitate local analyses of health metrics and deliver exclusively encrypted information to healthcare providers, enabling real-time surveillance.
3. **Homomorphic Encryption for Collaborative Diagnostics in Radiology:** Homomorphic encryption allows secure computation over encrypted medical images from different institutions. This permits radiologists to collaboratively examine the encrypted MRI or CT scans to diagnose complex cases without exposing the raw imaging data.

Case Studies:

1. **Google and Healthcare Institutions:** Google collaborated with multiple institutions to enhance predictive models for sepsis and acute renal injury through FL. Each hospital must train the model on its local data and share updates with Google, which will aggregate these updates into a global model. This way, sensitive patient data remains on the local servers of each hospital.
2. **Owkin and COVID-19 Research**: Owkin, a French-American startup, used FL to study COVID-19 by collaborating with multiple hospitals. They developed models to predict patient outcomes and identify effective treatments, all while ensuring patient data remained private.

These examples demonstrate how FL has the potential to revolutionize the healthcare industry, inspiring a hopeful vision of the future of healthcare, by enabling security and collaboration in research and enhancing the accuracy of medical models [16].

15.3 DIFFERENTIAL PRIVACY TECHNIQUES

DP is a mathematical framework designed to ensure robust assurances of privacy regarding the analysis and dissemination of data. The general idea is to add random noise either to the data or results obtained from queries about the data such that the addition or removal of any single data point has limited effects on the outcome of the analysis; in particular, this makes it difficult to identify any specific individual in the dataset, hence protecting their privacy [17].

In the context of DP, privacy assurance is quantified by a parameter (ε), with lower values indicating stronger privacy protection. The two main mechanisms employed in DP are:

1. **The Laplace Mechanism:** This method injects noise sampled from the Laplace distribution into the numerical results of queries. Consider, for example, a situation where a hospital wants to publish the average age of patients with a particular disease. The Laplace mechanism would inject noise into the average age, rendering it impossible to identify any patient.
2. **Exponential Mechanism.** This approach is used to choose between a set of possible outputs. This technique gives different outputs a probability value based on a utility function and then injects noise into these probabilities to ensure privacy in the selection process. It is highly beneficial in areas such as finding the optimal model parameters in ML.

15.3.1 Applications of DP to the Analysis of Health Information

1. **Publishing Aggregate Statistics:** In the health domain, several applications publish aggregate statistics using DP. Consider an instance in which the hospital intends to publish a patient count for a specific diagnosis. In this regard, a DP mechanism adds noise to the count before printing to maintain the confidentiality of the patient co unt. This allows healthcare providers to discuss helpful insights and statistics without disclosing the identity of their patients.
2. **Genomic Data Analysis:** DP in genomic studies can enable the analysis of data in a way that prevents the disclosure of any participant's information as a consequence of a genetic study. For example, medical researchers conducting research on genetic markers of diseases can utilize DP techniques when analyzing genomic data. If the researchers add noise to their results, they can publish their findings without disclosing any personal information about the individuals they have studied.

3. **Health Surveillance with Personal Devices:** DP also finds application in health surveillance systems that utilize personal devices, including fitness trackers and smartwatches, which collect data. The devices generate an enormous amount of personal health information helpful to analyze for tracking public health trends. By applying DP, the data is anonymized to maintain the privacy of an individual while still providing meaningful analysis. These applications demonstrate the versatility and effectiveness of DP in enabling valuable data analysis in healthcare while preserving privacy.

15.4 HOMOMORPHIC ENCRYPTION

15.4.1 Overview of Homomorphic Encryption

Homomorphic encryption enables the execution of computations on encrypted data, eliminating the need for decryption while consistently preserving information privacy and confidentiality. This characteristic is particularly advantageous in scenarios where sensitive data must remain confidential while computational processes are needed, especially within healthcare and finance. Notably, the Paillier cryptosystem is one of the most prominent examples, as it supports additive homomorphic functionalities. Using the Paillier encryption scheme, the multiplication of two encrypted numbers yields the sum of their respective plaintexts when decrypted, thereby ensuring that confidentiality is maintained through computations. The Paillier cryptosystem is then tailored for application domains where privacy protection is crucial during analysis processes; examples include secure vote tallying and the processing of encrypted data in the cloud [18]. Figure 15.4 shows the process of secure federated learning for a multi-institutional scenario. Each institution holds a local dataset on which a regional model is trained. Subsequently, model parameters are aggregated securely to obtain the global model. In this way, institutions can collaboratively train a model while maintaining data privacy.

Paillier Cryptosystem

The probabilistic asymmetric algorithm, developed by Pascal Paillier in 1999, is used for public key cryptography. This is attributed to its additive homomorphic properties, which enable operations on encrypted data without requiring decryption. Hence, it is essential in applications where data privacy is fundamental, such as in healthcare.

The Paillier Cryptosystem applies to scenarios where only addition is permitted over sensitive health-related data. For instance, it can compute aggregate statistics across multiple hospitals, such as determining the average age of patients or the total number of cases, without compromising individual patient data. This cryptosystem can be implemented using Python libraries, such as PyCryptodome, or Java libraries, such as the Java Homomorphic Encryption Library (JHEL), which provide support for healthcare practitioners to perform secure and private computations on encrypted data. Equations 15.7 and 15.8 represent the general encryption of a homomorphic cryptosystem, including Paillier, which enables secure operations over encrypted values for both private computation and collaborative computation.

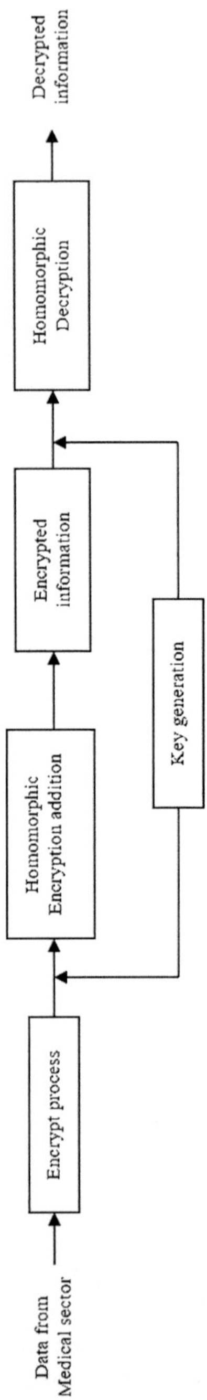

FIGURE 15.4 Homomorphic encryption process.

$$E(m) = g^m . r^m \bmod n^2 \tag{15.7}$$

where:

$g \text{ and } n: \text{public key}$

$r: \text{random number}$

The Homomorphic property is given by:

$$E(m_1). E(m_2) = E(m_1 + m_2) \tag{15.8}$$

where:

$m_1 \text{ and } m_2 \text{ are the plaintext messages being encrypted}$

The Brakerski-Fan-Vercauteren Scheme

The Brakerski-Fan-Vercauteren (BFV) is a homomorphic encryption technique that enables the arbitrary addition and multiplication of encrypted data, thereby achieving fully homomorphic encryption. Operations such as addition, as well as more complex operations like multiplication, can be performed on encrypted values without requiring decryption. The Microsoft Simple Encrypted Arithmetic Library (SEAL) is an efficient and optimized implementation of the BFV scheme for high-performance computations on encrypted data. Hence, SEAL is especially applicable in sensitive healthcare applications, as BFV was designed to support a variety of privacy-preserving computation scenarios, such as analyzing medical data where sensitive information must remain private but still be subject to mathematical operations on that data [19]. Equation 15.9 represents the encryption scheme, where a message. m can be encrypted into a ciphertext pair (a,b) For secure encoding, which allows operations over encrypted data, thereby supporting privacy-preserving computation.

$$E(m) = (a,b) = (a, b - a.s + m.q) \tag{15.9}$$

where:

$a,b: \text{ciphertext components}$

s : secret key

$q: \text{modulus}$

The following are different varieties of homomorphic encryption schemes.

1. **Partially Homomorphic Encryption (PHE):** Supports either addition or multiplication operations on encrypted data, but not both.
2. **Somewhat Homomorphic Encryption:** Allows a certain number of operations, both additions and multiplications.
3. **Fully Homomorphic Encryption (FHE):** Allows for an unlimited number of both addition and multiplication operations on encrypted data. It provides the most functionality but is computationally the most expensive.

15.4.2 Applications of HE in Medical Data Processing

1. **Securing Medical Data Analysis:** Homomorphic encryption can be applied to medical data analysis to secure sensitive patient information. For instance, a hospital encrypts its patient data and sends it to a third-party analytics service provider. The analytics service provider can perform computations on encrypted data and return the encrypted results to the hospital for decryption. This ensures the analytics service provider never gains access to the raw patient data.
2. **Multi-Institutional Collaboration Research:** Homomorphic encryption enables researchers involved in multi-institutional collaborative research to perform a collective analysis of the data while avoiding the actual sharing of raw data altogether. For example, different hospitals may share encrypted data and permit computation on their data jointly to determine disease patterns or treatment outcomes. The output derived post-decryption provides aggregated insights without revealing individual patient information.
3. **Cloud-based Healthcare Services:** Homomorphic encryption will enable secure cloud-based healthcare services. Healthcare providers can utilize the cloud to store encrypted patient data and process it without requiring decryption. It enables the safe storage and processing of data, ensuring that even if the cloud service provider is compromised, the patient's privacy remains intact.

These applications show the potential of homomorphic encryption in enhancing data privacy and security during the processing of medical data, thereby allowing safe and efficient healthcare services.

15.5 SECURE MULTI-PARTY COMPUTATION (SMPC)

15.5.1 Overview of SMPC Methodologies

SMPC is a cryptographic approach that enables multiple parties to collaboratively evaluate a function based on their inputs while ensuring the privacy of those inputs. Consequently, the data of each participant remains secure, preventing any party from obtaining information about the data inputs of others, except for what can be inferred from the resultant output.

The methodologies associated with SMPC encompass:

1. **Secret Sharing Schemes**: The data gets divided into multiple shares, which are then distributed among the participants. A minimum number of shares (threshold) is required to reconstruct the original information while preserving privacy. Ideal for sharing sensitive patient data between hospitals and healthcare organizations without exposing individual records. For example, hospitals can aggregate patient data securely for population health studies. Sharemind is an implementation of Shamir's Secret Sharing and other secret-sharing algorithms on a platform to aid multi-party computations in medical research collaborations.
2. **GMW Protocol (Goldreich-Micali-Wigderson)**: This protocol enables parties to jointly compute Boolean circuits through the secret sharing of individual bits and perform XOR and AND operations to evaluate functions securely. This protocol is particularly effective for privacy-preserving ML tasks in healthcare, such as secure logistic regression on distributed patient data across clinics, enabling collaborative analysis without compromising privacy. The Multi-Party – Somewhat Practical and Efficient Privacy-Preserving Distributed Computation framework provides an efficient implementation of the GMW protocol, enabling joint machine learning model projects across different healthcare organizations without compromising data confidentiality.
3. **Additive and Multiplicative Secret Sharing**: In the additive secret sharing setting, each party is given a random share of the data such that the sum of all shares equals the original value. On the other hand, multiplicative secret sharing gives random shares such that the product of all shares equals the original value. These techniques are widely applied in healthcare distributed networks for privacy-preserving data aggregation and cooperative model training among hospitals. For example, the additive secret sharing scheme is commonly used in a federated learning (FL) setting to securely aggregate model updates from different institutions. The frameworks TensorFlow Federated and PySyft provide support for additive secret sharing, hence preserving data privacy in collaborative healthcare research with secure model aggregation.
4. **Bulletproofs:** It is a zero-knowledge proof protocol that enables the verification of computations without revealing anything about the underlying data. It is non-interactive and does not need a trusted setup; hence, it becomes efficient in privacy-preserving applications. In healthcare, proving the correctness of computations over patient data while protecting the actual data would be most advantageously done using Bulletproof. They are also helpful in multi-institutional research, such as clinical trials, to prove the integrity of results across institutions securely. Cryptographic libraries, such as Libsnark, provide support for Bulletproofs, enabling healthcare institutions to perform verifiable computations with strong privacy assurances.

Two of the most significant techniques that SMPC has devised are Yao's Garbled Circuits and Shamir's Secret Sharing. Yao's protocol enables parties to perform computation on encrypted inputs without disclosing them. With this method, the inputs are encoded into garbled values such that each party can evaluate the circuit using only the encrypted data, without revealing any single individual's information. This could be useful in applications of genomic analysis in organizations where researchers need to collaborate on genomic-sensitive data to identify disease markers without sharing raw sequences. The Oblivious C library supports the design of garbled circuits, hence allowing complex computations to privatize sensitive health data. The Oblivious C framework enables health organizations to compute on encrypted datasets securely, thereby fostering advancements in genomic research while preserving personal data confidentiality. These methods enable multi-party computation with privacy for sensitive data [20]. The shares are generated using a polynomial of degree. $(t-1)$. Equation 15.10 represents a polynomial of degree, where $(t-1)$ It is a coefficient. These polynomials are commonly used in cryptographic protocols for encoding or evaluating secure computations; the structure required for privacy-preserving computations is maintained while allowing for complex transformations.

$$s(x) = a_0 + a_1 x + a_2 x^2 + \ldots + a_{t-1} x^{t-1} \tag{15.10}$$

where:

a_0: *is the secret*
t: *threshold number of shares needed for reconstruction*

15.5.2 Collaborative Healthcare Research Case Studies

1. **Genomic Research Collaboration:** Researchers from multiple institutions collaborated to analyze genomic data collectively. They achieved this by jointly using SMPC to uncover the genetic markers of diseases. Each party would keep its data private but would share encrypted inputs to the other parties. A party would execute the action based on these inputs, and the decrypted output gives generalized aggregate information. These features enable the collaboration of large-scale genomic studies without compromising the privacy of individual participants.
2. **Multi-Institutional Cancer Research:** A medical facility can encode its patient information and disseminate it in a secure format to other medical institutions for analytical purposes. Subsequently, this information can be decoded to evaluate the efficacy of cancer therapies. This methodology safeguards confidential patient data while simultaneously facilitating its contribution to joint cancer research among various establishments.

3. **FL for Predictive Modeling:** In the FL approach, hospitals employed SMPC to securely aggregate model updates across different institutions. Each hospital individually trains a local model on its patient data and encrypts model updates that it shares. The encrypted updates are summed up at the central server, which decrypts the final model to keep individual patient data private in the process

These case studies demonstrate the ability of SMPC to enable secure collaborative healthcare research, allowing institutions to leverage shared data insights without compromising privacy.

15.5.3 Emerging Technologies and Advanced Algorithms

1. **Integration of Differential Privacy (DP):** DP can be combined with SMPC to add a layer of privacy, ensuring that aggregated results are anonymized even in the event of a data breach. PySyft and TensorFlow Privacy are libraries that offer differential privacy mechanisms, which can be integrated with FL, thereby simplifying the application of DP in SMPC for healthcare applications.
2. **Post-Quantum Cryptography:** This approach encompasses lattice-based schemes that are being explored to enhance security in quantum computing. These algorithms are highly secure against quantum attacks and are promising for Homomorphic Encryption (HE) and SMPC in long-term healthcare applications. Microsoft SEAL and Google's OpenFHE provide support for lattice-based systems, laying the foundation for post-quantum security in the healthcare industry.
3. **Blockchain Technology for Secure Data Sharing:** Blockchain can provide decentralized trust and an immutable record for health data transactions in interoperability with HE and SMPC. It is helpful for sharing clinical trial results or patient records within multi-institutional networks in a secure way. Hyperledger and Ethereum are blockchain platforms that support smart contracts, enabling safe and transparent data sharing. This capability allows auditing and verification of data usage in the healthcare industry. Figure 15.5 utilizes blockchain technology to enable secure and immutable logging of model updates contributed by each participant, thereby enhancing trust and transparency within the FL framework. Additionally, the diagram includes a cloud server that securely aggregates locally trained model updates using blockchain to record each update, thereby allowing for transparency while preserving data privacy among participants.

Table 15.1 provides an overview of essential tools and technologies in HealthCare HE and SMPC.

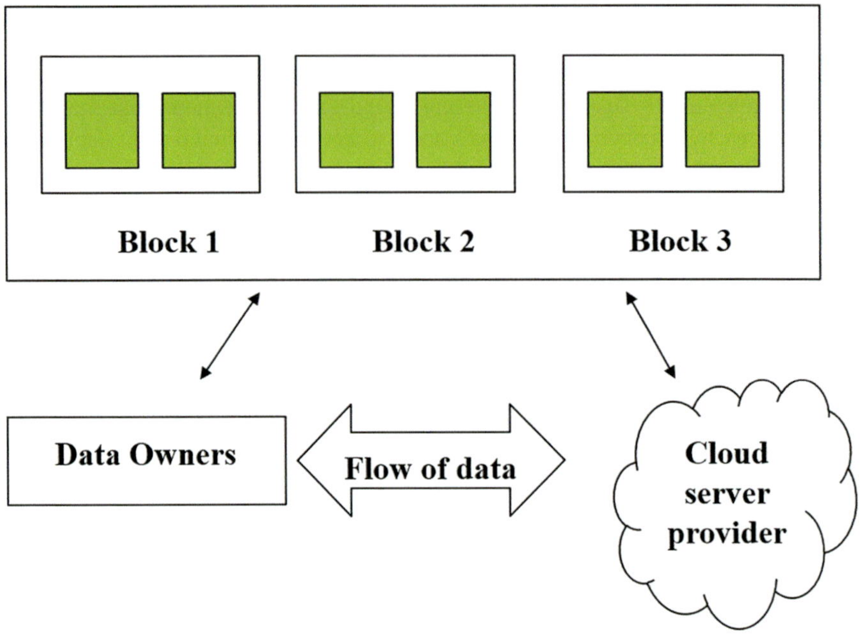

FIGURE 15.5 Blockchain-based integrity auditing for cloud data.

15.6 TECHNICAL CHALLENGES AND SOLUTIONS

15.6.1 Addressing Computational Efficiency and Scalability

1. **Computational Efficiency:** The high computational requirements of PPML methodologies, such as HE and SMPC, make their application very difficult. These techniques require significant processing power and time investments, making feasible implementations in large-scale healthcare settings very challenging. Therefore, it is a challenge for its possible implementation in extensive healthcare environments. Researchers and developers have considered improving algorithms and adopting hardware accelerators such as GPUs and TPUs. Additionally, the advanced HE reduces computational overhead, making it viable for real-time applications.
2. **Scalability:** Most healthcare data is usually high-dimensional, making it a challenge in terms of volume for many PPML techniques. The cloud-based solutions enable scalable infrastructure to dynamically allocate resources according to demand, ensuring that such PPML techniques can be scaled up for large datasets.

TABLE 15.1
Overview of Critical Tools and Technologies in Healthcare HE and SMPC

Algorithm/Protocol	Library/Tool	Healthcare Application
Paillier Cryptosystem	PyCryptodome, JHEL	Aggregate statistics across hospitals
BGV/BFV/CKKS Schemes	Microsoft SEAL, HElib	Genomic data analysis, secure patient records
Fully Homomorphic Encryption (FHE)	TFHE, OpenFHE	Deep learning over encrypted EHR data
Shamir's Secret Sharing	Sharemind	Sharing data in population health research
GMW Protocol	MP-SPDZ	Privacy-preserving ML
Secure Aggregation (FL)	TensorFlow Federated, PySyft	Federated learning for disease prediction
Bulletproofs	Libsnark	Clinical trial verification
Blockchain Technology	Hyperledger, Ethereum	Multi-institutional patient record sharing

15.6.2 Interoperability with Existing Healthcare Information Technology Systems

Interoperability Challenges

The incorporation of PPML methodologies into conventional healthcare IT infrastructures presents considerable challenges, primarily attributable to the prevailing absence of established standards concerning data formats and communication protocols. The interoperability among legacy systems remains notably constrained, resulting in inefficiencies such as redundant data entry and inconsistent patient information [21].

Solutions:

1. **Standard Protocols and APIs**: Standardized protocols and APIs can be developed to facilitate the integration of PPML techniques with legacy systems, ensuring that multiple systems share and communicate information effectively. Fast Healthcare Interoperability Resources (FHIR) is a popular standard employed in providing interoperability between modern and legacy healthcare systems.
2. **Hybrid Cloud Approaches**: Hybrid cloud solutions can be utilized for bridging legacy systems and state-of-the-art PPML techniques. Data is extracted from legacy systems and then made accessible on cloud-based platforms. Therefore, healthcare organizations can leverage state-of-the-art PPML techniques without overhauling their existing infrastructure.
3. **Middleware Solutions**: Web middleware serves as an intermediary layer that extends the communication of legacy systems with modern PPML

applications. Such solutions are likely to include conversions of data formats and protocols, thereby paving the way for compatibility and, consequently, successful integration.

Overcoming these technical challenges will enable healthcare organizations to implement PPML methodologies in practice, thereby increasing data protection, enhancing patient trust, and accelerating medical research, all while ensuring compliance with regulations concerning privacy.

15.7 BLOCKCHAIN TECHNOLOGY FOR DATA INTEGRITY

15.7.1 Improving Data Security and Integrity Using Blockchain

Blockchain technology inherently offers decentralization and immutability, which significantly enhance data security and integrity. Each block is connected to the previous block using a cryptographic hash and bears a timestamp, along with transaction information. It is henceforth evident that once the data gets recorded, it cannot be modified without affecting all subsequent blocks; therefore, the blockchain is considered tamper-proof [22].

Key Features:

1. **Cryptographic Hashing:** Transaction block hashes, wherein every modification to the data will result in a different hash, hence making it very easy to detect tampering.
2. **Decentralization:** Blockchain provides a highly distributed network, where a large number of nodes validate transactions occurring across the network, thereby reducing single-point failure and enhancing security.
3. **Public Key Infrastructure (PKI):** Blockchain secures the transactions with PKI. Each participant holds a pair of cryptographic keys, comprising a public and private key, through which the data will be accessed by authorized parties only.

Cumulatively, these features make blockchain a robust framework for ensuring the integrity and security of data, as well as being highly resistant to cyber-attacks and unauthorized access.

15.7.2 Applications of Blockchain in Healthcare

The significant applications of blockchain in healthcare are facilitating data security, transparency, and efficiency. Here are some key applications:

1. **Electronic Health Records (EHRs)**: Blockchain can provide an interoperable and secure framework for managing EHRs. The history of a patient can

be stored on a blockchain, where the data cannot be modified and remains accessible only to authorized parties. This enhances the integrity of data while reducing the likelihood of data breaches.

2. **Pharmaceutical Supply Chain**: With blockchain technology, it will be possible to track every stage that a pharmaceutical product goes through, from production to distribution. This ensures the authenticity of drugs and helps prevent counterfeit medications from entering the supply chain. For example, companies like Blockpharma use blockchain to verify the origin and authenticity of pharmaceutical products.
3. **Health Insurance:** Blockchain provides transparency in the health insurance system by maintaining tamper-proof records of all transactions. This system reduces fraudulent activities and enables faster, more efficient processing of claims. For example, firms like Guard Time rely on blockchain approaches to enhance the security of health insurance claims.
4. **Management of Patient Data:** Blockchain will empower patients with their health information. The blockchain enables the secure sharing of health information with providers when needed, ensuring the patient's privacy and data integrity. Platforms like Patientory enable patient data to be stored safely.

Each of these applications has demonstrated the power of blockchain technology in redefining healthcare processes, enhancing data security, promoting transparency, and improving operational efficiency.

15.7.3 Future Directions and Innovations

15.7.3.1 New Trends and Innovations in PPML

PPML is rapidly evolving, driven by a few emerging trends and innovations that enhance its effectiveness and applicability [22]:

1. **Advanced Cryptographic Techniques:** The latest cryptographic developments included in PPML are lattice-based and post-quantum cryptography. It will resist potential quantum computer attacks, providing long-term data protection.
2. **Hybrid Approaches:** FL can be integrated with DP, HE with secure multiparty computation, among other approaches. In these hybrid approaches, the strengths of each method are combined to achieve robust privacy while maintaining computational efficiency [23].
3. **Edge Computing:** The integration of PPML with edge computing enables data processing closer to the source of the data, which results in reduced latency and improved efficiency. This is particularly helpful in healthcare, for example, where real-time analysis of data is frequently required.

15.7.3.2 Challenges in Implementing PPML at Large Scale

Large-scale PPML deployment in healthcare faces significant challenges in four key areas: computational efficiency, scalability, interoperability, and regulatory compliance [24]. Addressing these challenges will enable healthcare organizations to implement PPML successfully, thereby enhancing data security, fostering patients' trust, and advancing medical research while ensuring compliance with regulatory provisions [25].

15.7.3.3 Legal Frameworks and Ethical Issues in Privacy-Preserving ML

The integration of legal structure and ethical considerations is crucial for ensuring that PPML complies with regulations such as the Health Insurance Portability and Accountability Act (HIPAA) and the General Data Protection Regulation (GDPR). These regulatory regimes demand stringent data protection protocols to safeguard patient privacy and ensure data integrity. In the United States, HIPAA establishes standards for protecting health information and mandates that healthcare providers implement administrative, physical, and technical safeguards. GDPR in Europe has stringent rules on data processing and grants individuals several rights over their data, including the rights of access, rectification, and erasure of their data [26]. PPML techniques, such as differential privacy or federated learning, comply with such regulations when the analysis is performed on sensitive data without exposing any information. For instance, differential privacy adds noise to data to prevent the identification of individuals, thereby adhering to the data minimization principle stipulated in the GDPR.

Ethical considerations, such as transparency, accountability, and informed consent regarding data processing, are crucial for establishing trust among patients. By confronting these moral and legal dimensions, healthcare organizations can provide assurances to patients that their data is utilized responsibly and securely.

15.7.4 Impact on the Healthcare Industry

The application of PPML holds significant implications in the healthcare sector [27]:

1. **Transformative Patient Care:** PPML enables secure and effective data analytics, facilitating personalized treatment plans and early interventions that improve patient outcomes.
2. **Operational Efficiency:** PPML enhances operational efficiency by facilitating secure data sharing and collaborative efforts among institutions, thereby minimizing redundancies and optimizing resource utilization.
3. **Improved Collaboration:** PPML facilitates secure collaboration among healthcare providers, researchers, and policymakers, leading to more comprehensive and effective healthcare outcomes.
4. **Innovation and Growth:** State-of-the-art PPML methodologies facilitate the development of new technologies and innovations in the healthcare sector, enhancing patient care and operational efficiency.

PPML in healthcare is the technological revolution that maximizes data usage while guaranteeing privacy and security. As these techniques advance, their effects on medical research and patient care, as well as the development of a safer and more efficient healthcare environment, will continue to grow.

15.7.5 Real-World Examples of Privacy-Preserving Techniques in Healthcare

Here are some more advanced, real-world applications of privacy-preserving techniques in healthcare:

1. **Blockchain in Secure Data Exchange:** The blockchain technology is being explored to create decentralized, immutable repositories of patient data that can be accessed only by authorized parties. For example, the MIT-developed MedRec utilizes blockchain to enable secure access to medical records for both healthcare providers and patients, thereby reducing the risk of unauthorized access and enhancing trust in data sharing among patients while protecting their confidentiality.
2. **Trusted Execution Environments (TEE) in Clinical Trials:** TEEs, such as Intel's SGX, provide a secure environment for the processing of sensitive data while reducing the risk of unauthorized exposure. Pharmaceutical companies and organizations involved in research use TEEs to manage data originating from clinical trials, ensuring that even sensitive data related to the efficacy of a drug is processed securely without violating patient confidentiality.
3. **Privacy-Aware Smart Wearables for Remote Monitoring:** Intelligent health devices, such as wearable cardiac monitors and glucose sensors, often employ privacy-preserving schemes to protect patients' data in real time. Companies like Apple and Fitbit are shifting toward privacy-sensitive data processing to ensure that personal health information collected from wearables is secure, while enabling healthcare providers to remotely monitor patients' health conditions.
4. **Privacy-Preserving COVID-19 Contact Tracing:** During the COVID-19 pandemic, privacy-preserving methodologies, such as decentralized data storage and narrow data collection practices, were employed by contact tracing applications from companies like Google and Apple. These apps, through the use of anonymous identifiers, warned users of potential exposure to the virus without disclosing personally identifiable information, thereby demonstrating privacy preservation in public health applications.
5. **Synthetic Data Generation for Research:** Healthcare organizations and research institutions are utilizing synthetic data, which is artificially generated to mimic factual patient information, to conduct research without compromising patient privacy. Tools like MDClone enable researchers to create realistic datasets for analysis and model training, allowing for robust health research while maintaining the confidentiality of actual patient data.
6. **PPML for Drug Discovery:** Pharmaceutical companies can adopt PPML techniques to collaborate on drug discovery. The MELLODDY platform (Machine Learning Ledger Orchestration for Drug Discovery), enables pharmaceutical companies to share models trained on sensitive data without revealing proprietary information. It is a much faster way of drug discovery, as it allows accessing broader datasets under the assurance of privacy and data security.

Computing and Informatics (IC3I), Gautam Buddha Nagar, India, pp. 2368-2372, 2023, doi: 10.1109/IC3I59117.2023.10397954.

[16] N. Chaudhary, V. Gupta, K. Sandhir, R. Gupta, S. Chhabra, and A. K. Singh, "Privacy-preserving ensemble learning classification model for mental healthcare," *2022 Seventh International Conference on Parallel, Distributed and Grid Computing (PDGC), Solan, Himachal Pradesh, India*, pp. 513-518, 2022, doi: 10.1109/PDGC56933.2022.10053268.

[17] V. K. Sheetal, V. S. SD, and P. K. Pareek, "Ensemble machine learning based blockchain model for privacy preserving of medical data in Fog computing," *2023 International Conference on Evolutionary Algorithms and Soft Computing Techniques (EASCT)*, IEEE, pp. 1-6, Oct. 2023.

[18] B. Kumar, P. Shukla, K. Mohan, A. Bharadwaj, Y. Shivam, and C. Kumar, "Medical dataset preparation and privacy preservation for improving the healthcare facilities using federated learning approach," *2023 International Conference on Electrical, Electronics, Communication and Computers (ELEXCOM), Roorkee, India*, pp. 1-6, 2023, doi: 10.1109/ELEXCOM58812.2023.10370601.

[19] K. Aggarwal, V. R. Vimal, U. Patil, S. C., A. Ingle, and T. S. Kumar, "Federated machine learning for cardiac disease detection using Internet of Medical Things," *2023 International Conference on Self Sustainable Artificial Intelligence Systems (ICSSAS), Erode, India*, pp. 1326-1331, 2023, doi: 10.1109/ICSSAS57918.2023.10331771.

[20] M. Gayathri Hegde, P. D. Shenoy, and K. R. Venugopal, "A comparative study of neural network and machine learning on privacy-preserving federated learning for healthcare applications," *2023 IEEE Technology & Engineering Management Conference - Asia Pacific (TEMSCON-ASPAC)*, Bengaluru, India, pp. 1-6, 2023, doi: 10.1109/TEMSCON-ASPAC59527.2023.10531360.

[21] B. Harini, M. P. Gouri, V. S. Balaji, K. Sangeetha, and A. Harshini, "Advanced sound detection and behavior examination for real-time intruder detection using deep learning: A comprehensive security framework," *2024 2nd International Conference on Artificial Intelligence and Machine Learning Applications Theme: Healthcare and Internet of Things (AIMLA)*, pp. 1-6, IEEE, Mar, 2024.

[22] M. Gupta, R. Kumar, S. Shekhar, B. Sharma, R. B. Patel, S. Jain, C. Iwendi, "Game theory-based authentication framework to secure internet of vehicles with blockchain," *Sensors*, vol. 22, no. 14, p. 5119, 2022.

[23] S. Mohammadi, A. Balador et al., "Balancing privacy and performance in federated learning: A systematic literature review on methods and metrics," *Journal of Parallel and Distributed Computing*, vol. 192, 2024.

[24] R. Kumari, D. K. Sah, S. Gupta, K. Cengiz, and N. Ivković, "Advancing medical recommendations with federated learning on decentralized data: A roadmap for implementation," *IEEE Transactions on Consumer Electronics*, vol. 70, no. 1, pp. 2666-2674, Feb. 2024, doi: 10.1109/TCE.2023.3334159.

[25] Regulatory Compliance Examples: 5 Illustrative Case Studies - Visualping. Available: Regulatory Compliance Examples: 5 Illustrative Case Studies - Visualping (accessed August 15, 2024).

[26] What Is an Example of a Regulatory Compliance Procedure? - OnPolicy. Available: What Is an Example of a Regulatory Compliance Procedure? -OnPolicy (accessed August 20, 2024).

[27] Sustainable compliance: Seven steps toward effectiveness and efficiency - McKinsey. Available: Sustainable compliance: Seven steps toward effectiveness and efficiency | McKinsey (accessed August 22, 2024).

[28] Regulatory Compliance Risk Management: Frameworks, Best Practices, & How to Do a Risk Assessment - Secureframe. Available: Regulatory Compliance Risk Management: Frameworks, Best Practices, & How to Do a Risk Assessment - Secureframe (accessed September 1, 2024).

[29] K. H. Krishnappa, and N. V. N. Gowda, "Dictionary-based PLS approach to pharmacokinetic mapping in DCE-MRI using Tofts model," *ICT Infrastructure and Computing. ICT4SD*, vol. 3, pp. 219-225, 2023, doi:10.1007/978-981-99-4932-8_21.

[30] R. Madhura, K. H. Krishnappa, R. Manasa, and K. P. Yashaswini, "Slack time analysis for APB timer using Genus Synthesis Tool," *ICT Infrastructure and Computing. ICT4SD*, vol. 3, pp. 207-217, 2023, doi:10.1007/978-981-99-4932-8_20. https://doi.org/10.1007/978-981-99-4932-8_20

[31] R. Shashidhar, P. Kadakol, D. Sreeniketh, P. Patil, K. H. Krishnappa, and R. Madhura, "EEG data analysis for stress detection using K-Nearest Neighbor," *2023 International Conference on Integrated Intelligence and Communication Systems (ICIICS), Kalaburagi, India*, pp. 1-7, 2023, doi: 10.1109/ICIICS59993.2023.10420898.

16 Soft Robotics in Healthcare

Pioneering a New Era in Medical Intervention and Rehabilitation

Prabhakar Gunasekaran, Meenakshi S, Shanthi J, and Revathy P

16.1 INTRODUCTION

The rapid advancements in soft robotics are driving a necessary revolution in the healthcare industry. Soft robots, in contrast to their rigid counterparts, are designed to be flexible, obedient, and adaptive, which makes them especially well-suited to interact with the human body in ways that were previously impossible. Soft robotics, utilizing advanced silicone materials, mimics the delicate movements of human sensitivity to tissues and incorporates bio-inspired designs, making them particularly useful in complex medical environments where accuracy and safety are crucial for rehabilitation and non-invasive surgery assistance [1]–[4]. The ability to intricately anatomize structures reduces the risk of injury and improves patient outcomes in various medical procedures, offering a promising future for healthcare.

The recent growth holds great potential in healthcare. It is safer, more efficient, and provides patient monitoring [5, 6] as well as assistive solutions [7]–[10]. This chapter concludes by outlining the principles underlying soft robotics, explores the design challenges specific to medical applications, and highlights the promise for the future in improving patient care, instilling a sense of optimism about the potential of soft robotics in healthcare.

The first study explores the challenges of Multiple Sclerosis. MS is a disorder that affects the central nervous system [11]. It is an autoimmune disease in which the body's immune system attacks the protective covering of nerve fibres, known as myelin [12], [13]. This disorder makes daily activities difficult. Assistive technologies, such as soft robotics, enhance the quality of life for individuals living with MS. Soft robotic systems aid with mobility. It addresses some of the mobility issues caused by the disease, enabling individuals to maintain greater independence. This stops communication between the brain and other parts of the body. It causes a wide range of physical, cognitive, and sensory impairments.

The disease is characterized by the development of scar tissue (sclerosis) along damaged nerves, which can result in muscle weakness, poor coordination and balance,

 DOI: 10.1201/9781003561309-16

fatigue, vision problems, and impaired mobility. The severity of the disease can vary widely among individuals. Some may have mild symptoms, while others may face significant disability. Relapses, or the sudden onset of symptoms, are common in MS, although they occur periodically.

This study investigates the potential of soft robotic devices in aiding patients with MS in managing their motor impairments. Soft robotics can potentially provide enhanced support for day-to-day activities and long-term rehabilitation. The versatile nature of soft robotics makes it an ideal candidate for designing and tailoring customized interventions for the specific needs of MS patients, thereby significantly improving their quality of life.

The second study addresses genetic diseases; Ankylosing Spondylitis is a hereditary disease [14, 15]. It is a chronic inflammatory disorder affecting the spine and sacroiliac joints. Finding effective interventions for Ankylosing Spondylitis is crucial in healthcare needs. A soft pneumatic spinal cord wearable assist for ankylosing spondylitis patients offers potential advancements in assistive technologies aimed at improving the quality of life for individuals affected by genetic diseases of the musculoskeletal system.

16.2 CASE STUDY: SOFT-ROBOTIC GLOVE FOR MULTIPLE SCLEROSIS (MS)

Animals and robots alike rely on their hands, or analogous structures, to grasp and manipulate objects in their environment. These actions are essential for interacting with the world, enabling a wide range of tasks that go beyond basic object handling. Grasping can be defined as the ability to pick up and hold an object securely, even in the presence of external forces or disturbances. Manipulation, on the other hand, refers to the ability to apply controlled forces to an object, causing it to rotate or move relative to the manipulator's reference frame. These two functions, grasping and manipulation, are foundational for both biological and robotic systems.

In addition to these core abilities, animals and robots can use their end effectors, which are the devices or tools at the end of a robotic arm or limb, for a variety of other tasks. For example, they may use these structures for movement, balancing, resting, or digging into surfaces. Other functions might include sorting objects, scratching, or performing fine motor tasks such as threading or picking delicate items. The versatility of end effectors enables a broad spectrum of actions that contribute to the system's adaptability in various environments.

Moreover, end effectors are not just mechanical tools for interaction; they can also serve as sensory devices. These structures can collect information about objects' physical properties, such as texture, temperature, shape, and weight. This sensory feedback is crucial for precise manipulation, helping the system adjust its actions based on the characteristics of the objects being handled. In both animals and robots, sensory-motor integration is crucial for performing complex tasks effectively.

Multiple sclerosis (MS) is a neurological autoimmune disease in which the body's immune system mistakenly attacks the central nervous system. This can disrupt the flow of information between the mind and body, resulting in impaired physical function and mobility. When it comes to young and middle-aged adults, it is the most frequent cause of neurologic disability. About 50% of MS patients will experience significant depression in their lives. To help individuals with multiple sclerosis improve and enhance their quality of life, a robotic exoskeleton has been developed. There was a presumption that multiple sclerosis was an irregular condition marked by areas of white matter myelin breakdown caused by inflammation. A decrease in quality of life in multiple sclerosis patients is associated with the frontal component of cognitive processes and involvement in behavioural memory.

16.2.1 Problem Statement and Proposed Methodology

Patients with multiple sclerosis suffer from various mental and physical health problems like depression, anxiety, headache, stress, and inability to regain their bodily movements. If they have an exoskeleton device with them, it means they will be able to recover their physical movements, but they still feel uncomfortable with that heavy device. Patients with multiple sclerosis can be helped to regain their physical mobility through smooth and high-force gripping gloves, which provide a more comfortable experience. They are lightweight and also user-friendly for patients with multiple sclerosis.

To develop a soft gripper robot with high gripping force, the gloves are designed using liquid silicone rubber gel. The gel is shaped using a specially designed mold. A pressure sensor is inserted at the centre of the glove. When pressure is exerted on the sensor, it causes the gripper to grasp the object. When the user wants to release the grasped object, the pressure in the gloves is released into the solenoid valve. With the help of this device, patients with multiple sclerosis can regain their mobility more easily. It also makes patients feel more comfortable compared to the exoskeletons that are available on the market for multiple sclerosis patients, which are heavy and bulky.

16.2.2 Overview of the Fabrication Process

This section provides detailed information on casting a PneuNets bending actuator. The PneuNets actuator consists of two parts: the main body, which contains compartments that swell when the actuator is inflated, and the bottom layer, which features a substance that relieves strain, such as paper. Each of the two components is independently moulded before being joined with cement. With the use of an oven to hasten the curing process, the actuator pieces can be cast and assembled in under an hour.

Figure 16.1 illustrates a **process overview** for the fabrication of a **soft pneumatic actuator**, which involves six key stages. Figure 16.2 portrays the 3D printing of the mould. Here's a step-by-step breakdown of each stage:

Stage 1: Pouring of Elastomer

- **Process**: In this step, the elastomer (a flexible material, likely silicone or Ecoflex™) is poured into a mould that shapes the top half of the actuator. The mould has ridges to create channels that will later be inflated.

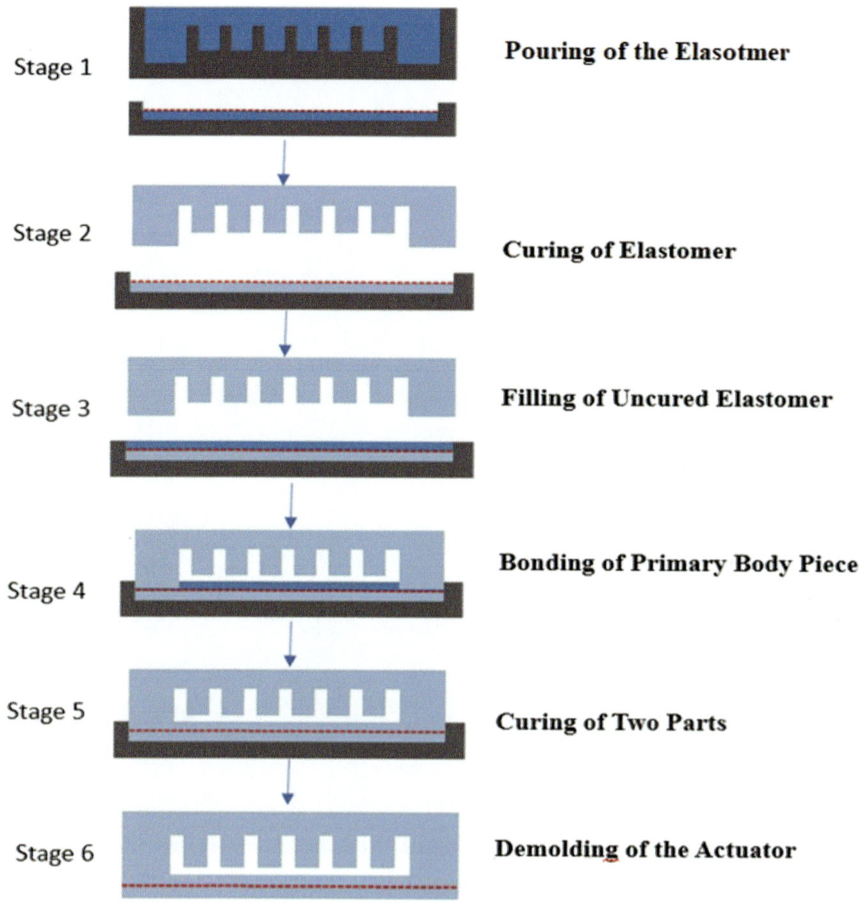

FIGURE 16.1 Overview of the fabrication process.

Stage 2: Curing of Elastomer

- **Process**: After the elastomer is poured, it is left to cure. This involves allowing the material to solidify, typically through a chemical process or by heating, depending on the type of elastomer used.

Stage 3: Filling of Uncured Elastomer

- **Process**: Once the first part has healed, the uncured elastomer is poured into the second mold, typically the bottom layer of the actuator.

Stage 4: Bonding of Primary Body Piece

- Process: The two required layers are kept together, aligned, and ensure they are adequately bonded to create the final actuator body.

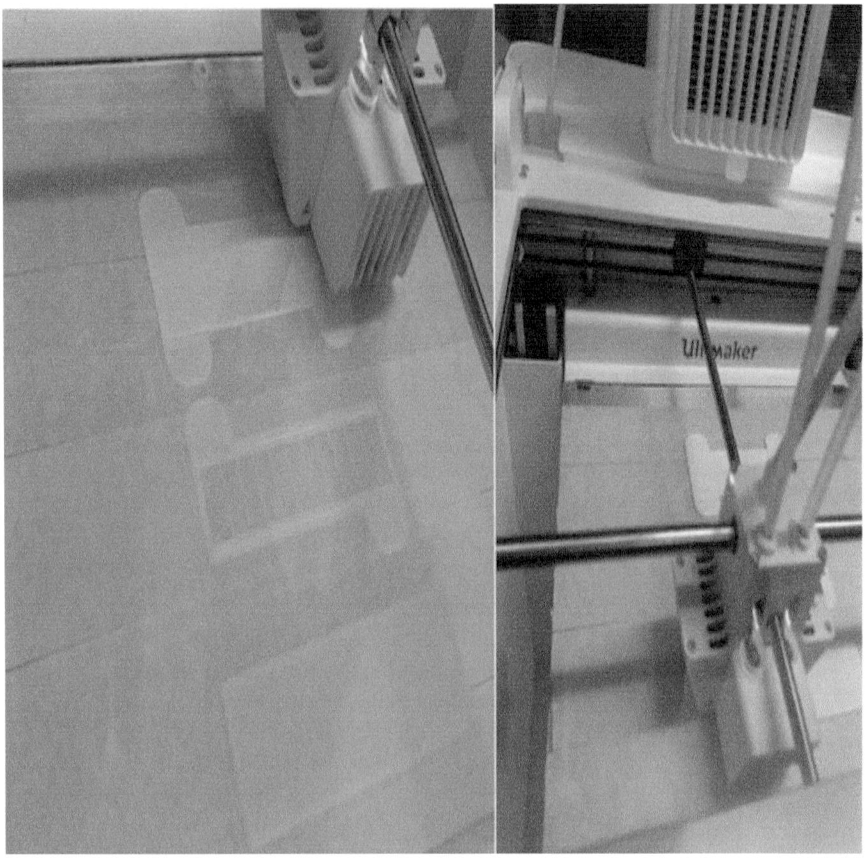

FIGURE 16.2 3D printing of the moulds.

Stage 5: Curing of Two Parts

- Process: The two parts are cured together, ensuring the elastomer parts adhere entirely, creating the soft actuator.

Stage 6: Testing of the Actuator

- Process: The final step involves testing its functionality.

This process is standard for soft pneumatic actuators [2], where the movement resulting from the application of high-pressure air is studied. By breaking down the process into six key stages—pouring, curing, filling, bonding, final curing, and testing—the fabrication ensures that the actuator is constructed with precision and durability. The careful bonding of the two main parts—the top compartmentalized body and the bottom strain-relieving layer—is essential for the actuator's successful operation. The use of elastomers, such as silicone or Eco flex™, and the proper curing methods are critical to achieving the desired flexibility and performance of the soft

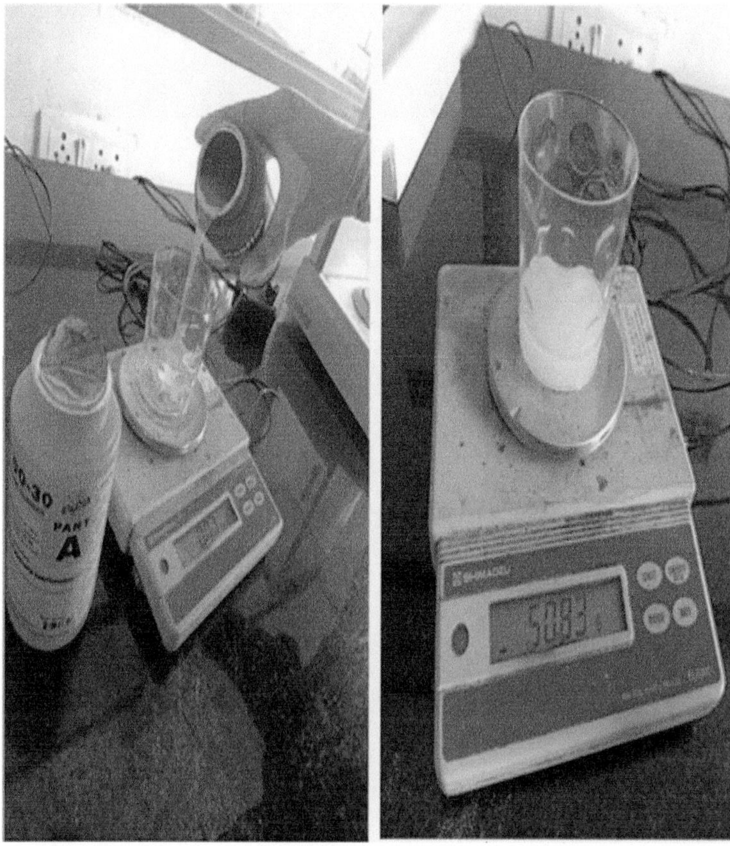

FIGURE 16.3 Measurements of the elastomer.

actuator. Additionally, testing the actuator's responsiveness under pressure ensures its reliability in applications that require soft robotic movements.

16.2.3 Real-Time Fabrication

Figure 16.3 illustrates mixing of Elastosil by combining **Part A** (red fluid) and **Part B** (white fluid) in a precise 1:9 weight ratio. For a total of **80g** of Elastosil, **8g** of Part A is carefully measured and poured into a cup, followed by **72g** of Part B. To maintain accuracy, any overshoot in Part A can be adjusted by adding more Part B, ensuring the correct proportion is maintained. If excess Part B is added, a spatula can be used to remove the extra material, guaranteeing a total of **80g** in the mixture.

The process begins by removing the cup holder/adapter from the mixer and balancing the mixer to the combined weight of the cup holder, cup, and elastomer assembly. After the mixing programme begins, the cup is added to the mixer. Upon completion, the cup is carefully removed, using a screwdriver if necessary to dislodge it. If visible streaks are present in the elastomer, the substance requires

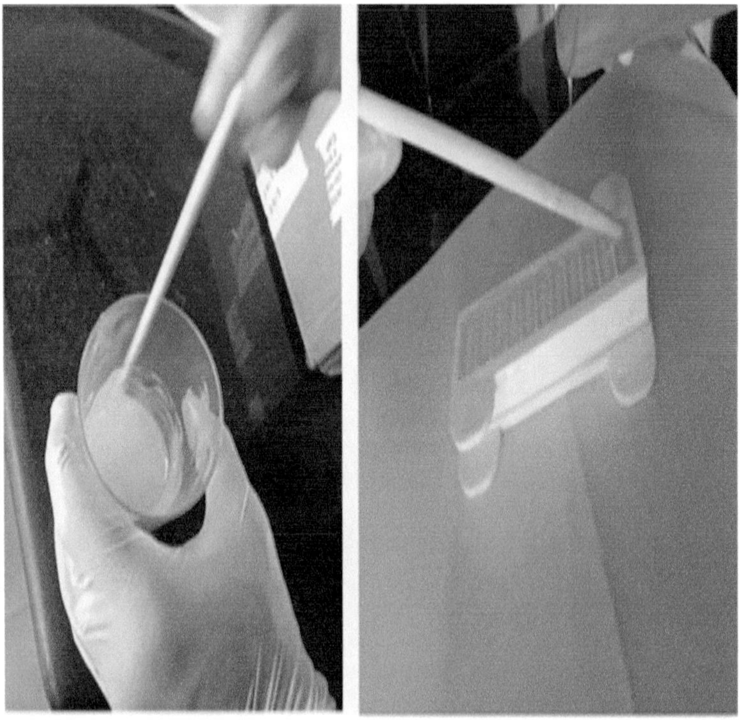

(a) (b)

FIGURE 16.4 Mixing of the elastomer b. Pouring of elastomer.

further mixing to ensure homogeneity (Figure 16.4). The mixture of elastomer, such as Elastosil, is carefully poured into the central chamber mould, filling one chamber at a time. The elastomer is poured into the base mould until it reaches halfway and is evenly spread by tilting the mould to ensure smooth distribution (Figure 16.5). To remove any air bubbles from the elastomer, the moulds are placed in a vacuum chamber. The vacuum pump is turned on, and the mixture is de-gassed for around 10 minutes, or until bubble production slows down. Care must be taken when reopening the valve to reintroduce air into the chamber slowly, as a sudden rush of air could knock over the molds.

Any surface bubbles that rise during the degassing process are gently popped using a spatula for aesthetic purposes, as unpopped bubbles may cause imperfections and affect the final product. The spatula should move gently over the surface without disturbing the material below. To ensure uniform chamber formation, any excess elastomer is removed using a straightedge or a trimmed piece of cardboard. This step ensures that the compartment dividers in the mould are still discernible, which

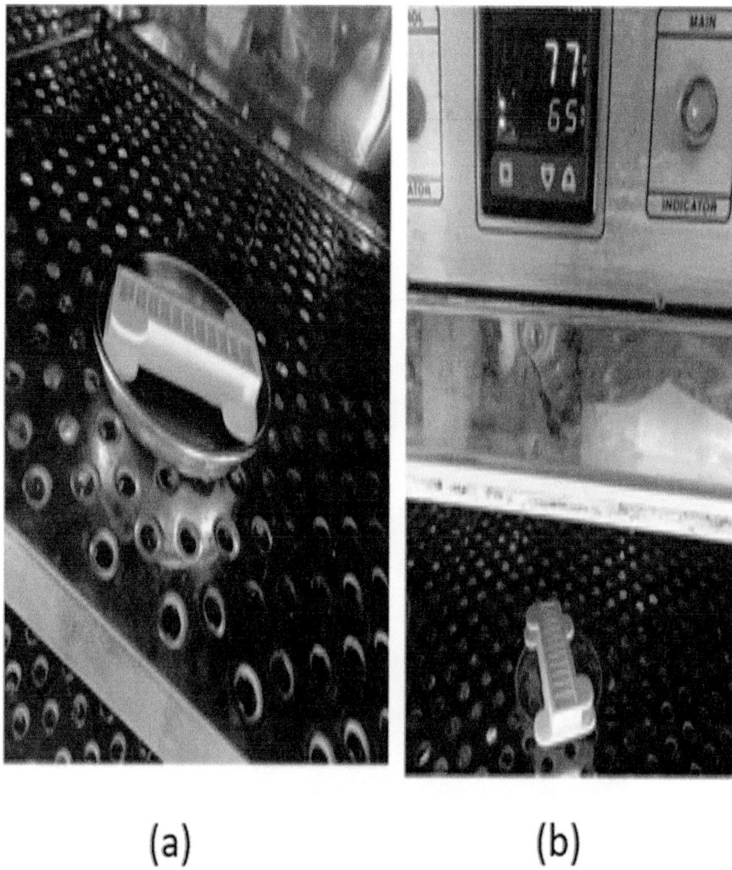

FIGURE 16.5 Curing of the elastomer.

is crucial for the proper formation of the actuator chambers. After popping any remaining air bubbles, a sheet of paper is placed on top of the elastomer in the base mould to ensure bonding. The sheet is lightly pressed down, ensuring it does not sink into the elastomer too much, which could affect the final structure. The moulds are then placed in an oven at 65°C for 10 minutes to cure the elastomer, solidifying the structure (Figure 16.5).

After curing, the main body of the actuator is removed from the moulds by gently prying them apart with a flathead screwdriver. Care must be taken not to pierce the actuator. The mould parts are separated using the tabs on the sides. If the mould deforms, it can be reheated and flattened for reuse (Figures 16.5a and 16.5b). A shallow groove along the actuator's axis allows for air to be supplied to the chambers. During assembly, care is taken not to block this groove, as doing so would prevent the actuator from functioning correctly. The two parts are bonded together

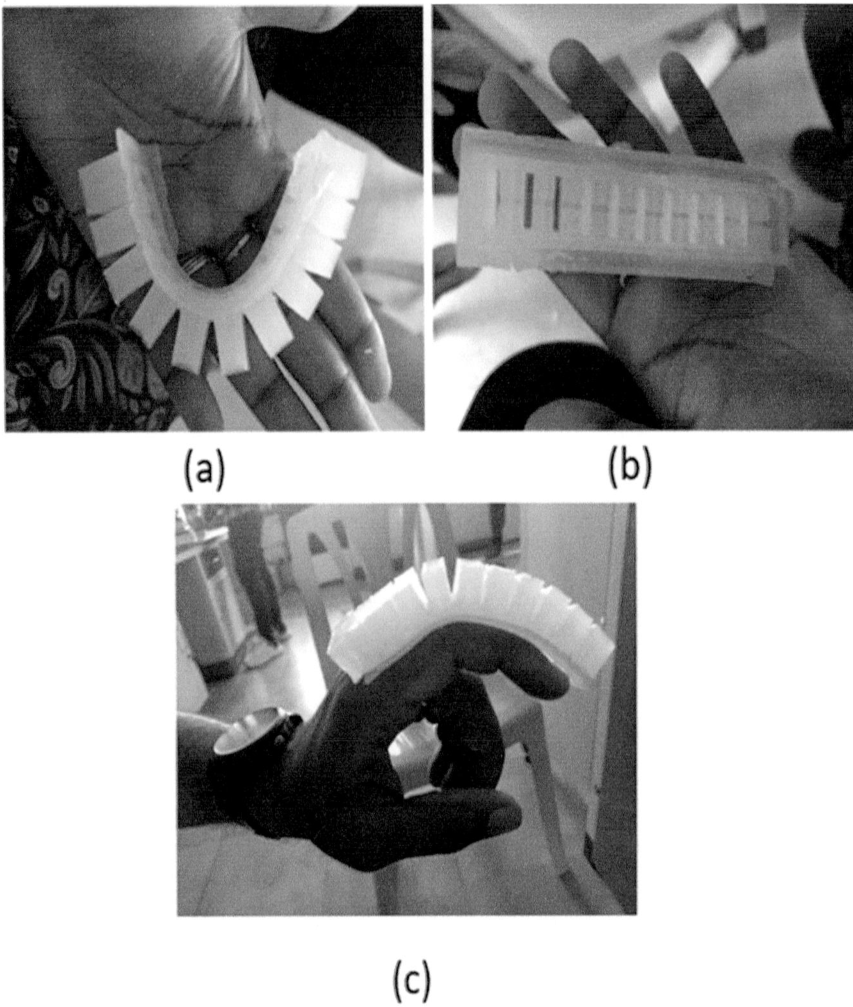

FIGURE 16.6 Removing the prototype from the mould and joining the main body and the base.

with uncured elastomer, ensuring a tight seal, and placed back in the oven for further curing (Figure 16.6).

Five fingers are fabricated using the previously described process and are then attached to the hand glove. To connect the air source, a small hole is made near the bottom of each actuator using a thin metal rod, ensuring the rod reaches the centre channel without damaging the actuator walls. Tubing is inserted through the hole, reinforced by a metal rod, and the rod is removed once the tube is securely

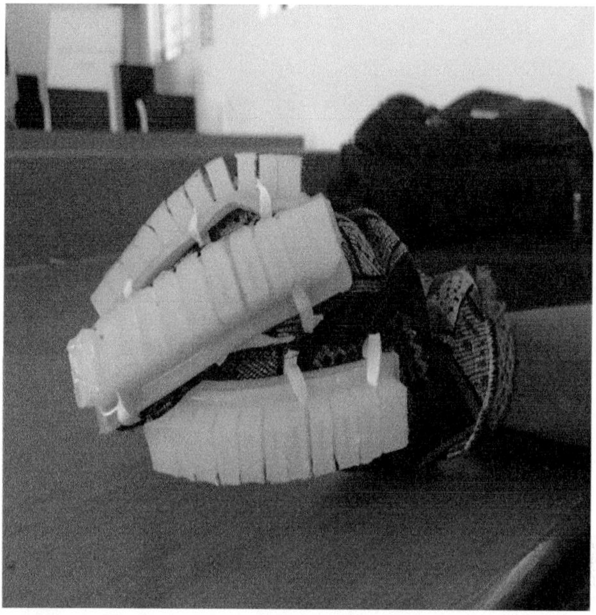

FIGURE 16.7 Fabrication and air source connection for actuated fingers.

in place. Finally, the actuators are inflated by connecting an air pump or another air source to the tubing, allowing the fingers to bend through pneumatic actuation. The fabrication and air source connection for actuated fingers is illustrated in Figure 16.7.

16.3 CASE STUDY: SOFT ACTUATOR FOR ANKYLOSING SPONDYLITIS

Ankylosing Spondylitis (AS), a form of arthritis primarily affecting the spine, presents significant challenges [16]–[18], including joint inflammation, spinal abnormalities, stiffness, and lower back discomfort, as illustrated in Figure 16.8. These symptoms contribute to reduced mobility and a diminished quality of life. Conventional treatments, such as medication and lifestyle modifications, offer limited relief and carry potential risks like dependency on painkillers.

16.3.1 Broader Implications of Spinal Issues

Beyond AS, spinal problems are prevalent among individuals such as IT professionals, engineers, and weightlifters, who often experience debilitating low back pain due to prolonged sitting. This trend highlights the increasing demand for innovative solutions to address spinal health challenges [19]–[21].

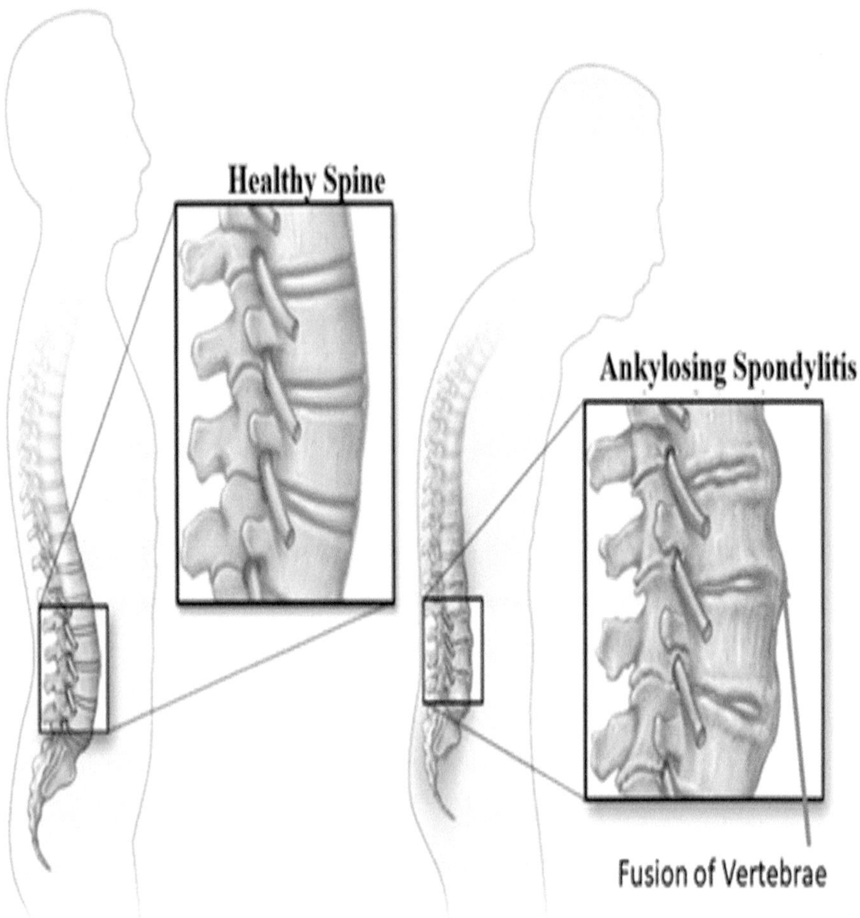

FIGURE 16.8 Ankylosing spondylitis. (www.mayoclinic.org/diseases-conditions/ankylosing-spondylitis/symptoms-causes/syc-20354808.)

16.3.2 Proposed Solution

The proposed solution is a **Soft Pneumatic Spinal Cord Wearable Assist**, explicitly designed for AS patients. This assistive device incorporates:

- **Soft Pneumatic Actuators** to support and correct spinal posture.
- **Acupressure therapy targets** specific pressure points in the lumbar area to alleviate pain and improve mobility.
- **Machine Learning-Based Control Models** to tailor support based on individual patient needs.

16.3.3 Challenges and Considerations

Developing a soft pneumatic spinal cord wearable assist requires addressing several critical challenges. A thorough understanding of the bending behavior of soft pneumatic actuators is essential to ensure their effectiveness in providing tailored support. Additionally, creating a robust control mechanism capable of personalized adaptability is vital for meeting the unique needs of individual patients. Furthermore, the diverse symptoms of AS, including inflammatory back pain, sacroiliitis grading, and active inflammation lesions revealed through MRI diagnostics, necessitate a comprehensive approach to design and functionality. These complexities underscore the importance of integrating advanced technologies and multidisciplinary insights to achieve practical solutions.

16.3.4 Innovative Features

The proposed wearable assist device incorporates advanced technologies and novel approaches to address the needs of patients with AS. Acupressure spikes are integrated to provide targeted therapeutic benefits, alleviating pain and promoting spinal alignment. Learning-based control models, utilizing deep learning techniques, ensure enhanced adaptability by tailoring the device's performance to individual needs. Additionally, the design and fabrication of soft pneumatic actuators are optimized to deliver superior performance in spinal posture correction, making the device both practical and user-friendly.

16.3.5 Research Objectives

1. Design, fabrication, and analysis of soft pneumatic actuators.
2. Development of a deep learning-based control model for enhanced adaptability.
3. Integration of acupressure therapy for pain relief and improved mobility.

16.3.6 Expected Outcomes

This research aims to alleviate pain and improve spinal posture for patients with AS, enhancing their overall quality of life. By addressing the challenges faced by individuals with musculoskeletal conditions, the study aims to provide effective and innovative solutions. Additionally, it offers valuable insights into the development of assistive technologies, particularly for aging populations, where the prevalence of such conditions is higher. Through these efforts, the research contributes to advancing healthcare interventions and improving patient outcomes.

16.3.7 Significance of the Research

The integration of soft robotics, acupressure therapy, and AI-driven control systems offers a transformative approach to addressing musculoskeletal challenges. This work holds promise for improving healthcare solutions for non-communicable diseases (NCDs), particularly in aging populations and those affected by occupational spinal issues.

16.4 CONCLUSION

Soft robotics plays a crucial role in medical rehabilitation and intervention. They are suitable for integration with the human body due to their versatility. Two case studies are presented regarding MS and AS, and a prominent solution is provided. The solution provided is based on soft robotics-assisted devices. This reduces risk and enhances a patient's lifestyle, incorporating AI to enable real-time and personalized care. To enhance the user experience, the system adapts by optimizing to provide a better experience.

16.5 FUTURE WORK

With the evolution of science and technology, and in response to current challenges, there is a growing need for more advanced bio-inspired materials. We can enhance the durability and functionality of soft robotics. By further advancing the scope of this research, an autonomous system could be achieved. This enables patients with severe mobility issues to perform more independently, without requiring human assistance, thereby boosting their confidence. Thus, this novel research work helps aid people with non-communicable diseases (NCD), such as ageing and older adults, by providing suitable assistive soft robots.

REFERENCES

[1] Joyee, E. B., & Pan, Y. (2019). A fully three-dimensional printed inchworm-inspired soft robot with magnetic actuation. *Soft Robotics*, *6*(3), 333–345. https://doi.org/10.1089/soro.2018.0082

[2] Leng, J., Sun, J., Guan, Q., & Liu, Y. (2020). Status of and trends in soft pneumatic robotics. *Science China Technological Sciences*, *50*, 897–934. https://doi.org/10.1007/s11431-020-1653-4

[3] Lei, J., Ge, Z., Fan, P., Zou, W., Jiang, T., & Dong, L. (2022). Design and manufacture of a flexible pneumatic soft gripper. *Applied Sciences*, *12*(13), 6306. https://doi.org/10.3390/app12136306

[4] Thalman, C., & Artemiadis, P. (2020). A review of soft wearable robots providing active assistance: Trends, common actuation methods, fabrication, and applications. *Wearable Technologies*, *1*, e3. https://doi.org/10.1017/wtc.2020.4

[5] Ding, L., Niu, L., Su, Y., Yang, H., Liu, G., Gao, H., & Deng, Z. (2022). Dynamic finite element modeling and simulation of soft robots. *Chinese Journal of Mechanical Engineering*, *35*, 24. https://doi.org/10.1186/s10033-022-00701-8

[6] Koenig, N., & Howard, A. (2004). Design and use paradigms for Gazebo, an open-source multi-robot simulator. In *Proceedings of the 2004 IEEE/RSJ International Conference on Intelligent Robots and Systems (IROS 2004)* (Vol. 3, pp. 2149–2154). IEEE.

[7] Robmann, J., Schluse, M., Rast, M., Kaigom, E., Cichon, T., & Schluse, M. (2015). Simulation technology for soft robotics applications. In A. Verl, A. Albu-Schäffer, O. Brock, & A. Raatz (Eds.), *Soft Robotics*. Springer. https://doi.org/10.1007/978-3-662-44506-8_10

[8] Elsayed, Y., Vincensi, A., Lekakou, C., Geng, T., Saaj, C. M., Ranzani, T., Cianchetti, M., & Menciassi, A. (2014). Finite element analysis and design optimization of a pneumatically actuating silicone module for robotic surgery applications. *Soft Robotics*, *1*(4), 255–262. https://doi.org/10.1089/soro.2014.0016

[9] Polygerinos, P., Wang, Z., Overvelde, J. T., Galloway, K. C., Wood, R. J., Bertoldi, K., & Walsh, C. J. (2015). Modeling of soft fiber-reinforced bending actuators. *IEEE Transactions on Robotics*, *31*(3), 778–789. https://doi.org/10.1109/TRO.2015.2428504

[10] Meenakshi, S., Prabhakar, G., Ayyanar, N., & Pugazhenthi, P. N. (2023). FEM-based design of a soft robotic gripper for seaweed farming. In *Proceedings of the 2023 International Conference on Energy, Materials, and Communication Engineering (ICEMCE)* (pp. 1–5). IEEE. https://doi.org/10.1109/ICEMCE57940.2023.10434066

[11] Walton, C., King, R., Rechtman, L., Kaye, W., Leray, E., Marrie, R. A., et al. (2020). Rising prevalence of multiple sclerosis worldwide: Insights from the Atlas of MS, third edition. *Multiple Sclerosis*, *26*(14), 1816–1821. https://doi.org/10.1177/1352458520970841

[12] Haki, M., Al-Biati, H. A., Al-Tameemi, Z. S., Ali, I. S., & Al-Hussaniy, H. A. (2024). Review of multiple sclerosis: Epidemiology, etiology, pathophysiology, and treatment. *Medicine (Baltimore)*, 103(8), e37297. https://doi.org/10.1097/MD.0000000000037297

[13] Tafti, D., Ehsan, M., & Xixis, K. L. (2024). Multiple sclerosis. In StatPearls [Internet]. StatPearls Publishing. www.ncbi.nlm.nih.gov/books/NBK499849/

[14] Sieper, J., Braun, J., Rudwaleit, M., Boonen, A., & Zink, A. (2002). Ankylosing spondylitis: An overview. *Annals of the Rheumatic Diseases*, *61*(suppl 3), iii8–iii18. https://doi.org/10.1136/ard.61.suppl_3.iii8

[15] Zhu, W., He, X., Cheng, K., Zhang, L., Chen, D., Wang, X., Qiu, G., Cao, X., & Weng, X. (2019). Ankylosing spondylitis: Etiology, pathogenesis, and treatments. *Bone Research*, *7*, 22. https://doi.org/10.1038/s41413-019-0057-8

[16] Akassou, A., & Bakri, Y. (2018). Does HLA-B27 status influence ankylosing spondylitis phenotype? Clinical Medicine Insights: *Arthritis and Musculoskeletal Disorders*, *11*, 1179544117751627. https://doi.org/10.1177/1179544117751627

[17] Sen, R., Goyal, A., & Hurley, J. A. (2022). Seronegative spondyloarthropathy. In John A. Hurley and Lawrence H. Brent (eds.), *StatPearls [Internet]*. StatPearls. www.ncbi.nlm.nih.gov/books/NBK459356/

[18] Shao, F., Liu, Q., Zhu, Y., Fan, Z., Chen, W., Liu, S., ... & Sun, Y. (2021). Targeting chondrocytes for arresting bony fusion in ankylosing spondylitis. *Nature Communications*, *12*, 6540. https://doi.org/10.1038/s41467-021-26750-6

[19] Muronosono, T., Nishiyama, T., Kawajiri, S., Imai, T., Arai, K., & Kobayashi, T. (2021). Research on rheumatoid arthritis detection support system. In *Proceedings of the 2021 IEEE 3rd Global Conference on Life Sciences and Technologies (LifeTech)* (pp. 122–123). IEEE. https://doi.org/10.1109/LifeTech52111.2021.9391830

[20] Park, J.-H., Stegall, P. R., Roye, D. P., & Agrawal, S. K. (2018). Robotic spine exoskeleton (RoSE): Characterizing the 3-D stiffness of the human torso in the treatment of spine deformity. *IEEE Transactions on Neural Systems and Rehabilitation Engineering*, 26(5), 1026–1035. https://doi.org/10.1109/TNSRE.2018.2821652

[21] Chua, M. C. H., Lim, J. H., & Yeow, R. C. H. (2019). Design and characterization of a soft robotic therapeutic glove for rheumatoid arthritis. *Assistive Technology*, *31*(1), 44–52. https://doi.org/10.1080/10400435.2017.1346000

Index